HANDBOOK OF SLEEP MEDICINE

Handbook of Sleep Medicine

JOHN M. SHNEERSON
MA, DM, FRCP, FCCP

Consultant Physician
Director of Respiratory Support and Sleep Centre
Papworth Hospital
Cambridge, CB3 8RE
UK

Blackwell
Science

DISTRIBUTORS

Marston Book Services Ltd
PO Box 269
Abingdon, Oxon OX14 4YN
(*Orders*: Tel: 01235 465500
          Fax: 01235 465555)

USA
Blackwell Science, Inc.
Commerce Place
350 Main Street
Malden, MA 02148–5018
(*Orders*: Tel: 800 759 6102
                 781 388 8250
          Fax: 781 388 8255)

Canada
Login Brothers Book Company
324 Saulteaux Crescent
Winnipeg, Manitoba R3J 3T2
(*Orders*: Tel: 204 837 2987)

Australia
Blackwell Science Pty Ltd
54 University Street
Carlton, Victoria 3053
(*Orders*: Tel: 3 9347 0300
          Fax: 3 9347 5001)

A catalogue record for this title
is available from the British Library
and the Library of Congress

ISBN 0-632-05135-3

For further information on
Blackwell Science, visit our website:
www.blackwell-science.com

Contents

Preface

Sleep disorders have been a neglected aspect of medicine, and all too often remain undetected. Sleep occupies approximately one-third of each person's life-time, but its impact on health and medical conditions remains largely unrecognized. The prevalence of sleep disorders is increasing in westernized societies where the potential for independence from natural influences on sleep, such as exposure to sunlight, is combined with social and economic pressures to shorten the time spent asleep. It is therefore surprising that so few books provide a readable but comprehensive account of sleep medicine. Many of these regard sleep disorders from a narrow viewpoint of a single specialty, whilst others are so large that they are daunting to the reader. The aim of this book is not to replace these texts, but to strike the balance with an up-to-date, broad-based account in which information is readily accessible.

The study of sleep and its disorders is advancing rapidly with new developments in their genetic, immunological and neurochemical basis and in the methods of investigation and treatment. Sleep medicine cuts across the conventional medical specialties so that it can be difficult to understand. The approach taken in this book is to integrate these various viewpoints within each section. I hope that those readers who see sleep disorders simply as a part of general internal medicine, as well as those who feel that it is a separate sub-specialty, will find that this approach brings them a wider outlook to sleep and its disorders.

The book is divided into three parts. The first contains chapters dealing with the fundamentals of sleep, how to assess sleep disorders and the important issue of how drugs interact with sleep medicine. The second part, which is the core of the book, consists of symptom-orientated chapters, each of which has a structured approach in order to guide the assessment and treatment of common sleep problems. Insomnia, excessive daytime sleepiness, experiences and awareness during sleep and behavioural abnormalities are all covered. The last part includes two chapters on the increasingly important respiratory consequences of upper airway dysfunction and changes in the control of breathing during sleep. The final chapter discusses the social aspects of sleep medicine.

I intend this book to appeal to all those who deal with sleep disorders. Sufficient detail has been included for the text to be of value to specialists in sleep medicine as well as neurologists, psychiatrists, respiratory physicians, those dealing with upper-airway disorders and general internal physicians. Most patients with a sleep disorder present to their primary care physician and this book should provide a ready guide to help with the recognition and treatment of the sleep problem and when to refer to a specialist. The links between the technical aspects, physiological processes and clinical problems should also be of interest to polysomnographic and other technicians who deal with sleep disorders. I hope that to all these groups it provides new perspectives, triggers the imagination and acts as a catalyst for the development of new ideas and interest in sleep medicine.

This book is based on my experience in the Respiratory Support and Sleep Centre at Papworth Hospital, Cambridge and could not have been written without the help and support of all the team who work in the Centre. I would also like to thank Margaret Flanigan for her most helpful comments and advice about the text, particularly the technical aspects of polysomnography. I am extremely grateful to Jill Dellar for skilfully and patiently typing the manuscript. Her speed in returning each draft has greatly eased its preparation. Lastly, my thanks go to Anne, my wife, who has constantly encouraged me throughout the 18 months that this book has taken to prepare and without whose support it could not have been written.

John M. Shneerson
Cambridge

1 Nature of Sleep and its Disorders

Sleep is recognizable by its contrast to wakefulness. It is a state of reduced awareness and responsiveness, both to internal and external stimuli. This reduced awareness is, however, selective [1]. It is an active process in which the significance of stimuli to the individual are interpreted and this determines whether arousal from sleep occurs. The crying of a child is, for instance, more likely to wake the parent than a different noise of the same intensity.

A second feature of sleep is motor inhibition (Table 1.1). The sleeping subject appears quiescent, but some movements occur, such as rapid eye movements. For each species there is a characteristic posture or type of movement that is adopted during sleep. Humans usually lie down, but many birds perch while asleep, horses may stand, vampire bats sleep upside down, dolphins and whales swim, and albatrosses can fly. In some of these animals, in contrast to humans, sleep is not accompanied by physical inactivity, but the repetitive locomotor movements are largely controlled by spinal and brain-stem reflexes. Humans usually sleep with the eyes closed, but some animals, such as cattle, sleep with their eyes open.

Sleep is a cyclical or episodic phase which alternates with wakefulness. There is a wide variation in the duration of sleep between species, but humans, moles and pigs sleep for about 8 out of each 24 h. An important characteristic of sleep which differentiates it from most other states of altered consciousness is that it is promptly reversible. This is usually recognized by the sleeper, but brief episodes of sleep or wakefulness (microsleeps and microarousals) may emerge from

Table 1.1 Characteristics of sleep.

Episodic
Promptly reversible
Reduced awareness
Reduced responsiveness
Motor inhibition

the background state without any subsequent recall of the events.

The margin between sleep and wakefulness is seldom sharp. The transition between wakefulness and sleep often lasts several minutes, and the moment of falling asleep may be impossible to determine. The point at which sleep is attained as judged by behavioural criteria may differ from, for instance, the moment of sleep onset defined by electrophysiological standards. A period of drowsiness or somnolence is often a transitional phase between wakefulness and sleep, but does not necessarily lead into sleep and may simply be a prolonged episode of subalertness followed by recovery of wakefulness. In a similar way the process of awakening can be sudden, particularly if there is a strong sensory stimulus; or gradual with a stage of partial recovery of wakefulness (confusional arousal). These represent phases when aspects of both sleep and wakefulness coexist. Similarly, awareness of the thoughts and images of dreams often persists into wakefulness after arousal from sleep.

Structure of sleep (sleep architecture)

External influences and some internal stimuli have less influence on the brain during sleep than during wakefulness. To an extent the brain becomes deafferentated, partially deprived of sensory stimulation. This has in the past led to the concept of sleep as a passive phase, contrasting with the active state of wakefulness. This concept has been discarded in the light of physiological findings over the last 50 years. Most parts of the brain are active in sleep, although their functions and interrelationships differ from wakefulness.

Until the 1950s it was assumed that sleep was a homogeneous or unitary phenomenon which was the opposite of wakefulness. Electrophysiological studies in the 1950s, however, clearly demonstrated that there were two main states of sleep, non-rapid eye movement (NREM) and rapid eye movement (REM)

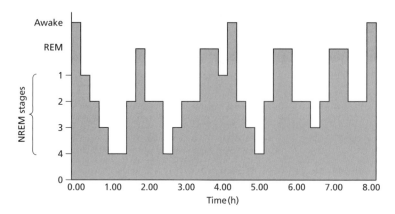

Fig. 1.1 Normal adult hypnogram.

sleep (Fig. 1.1). The fact that they usually occurred in sequence without an intervening episode of wakefulness probably delayed their recognition. Both NREM and REM sleep are themselves heterogeneous and at any one moment these two states and wakefulness may not be as distinct as has previously been thought. There is probably a continuous tendency to move in or out of one of these three states throughout the day and night. At any time, part of the brain may be predominantly in, for instance, REM sleep whereas another part may be tending towards NREM sleep. The current methods of categorizing sleep into one or other state by conventional electrophysiological criteria give a false sense of rigidity to the constantly changing functional processes within the brain.

The exact onset of sleep is often difficult to identify since precise criteria based on changes in subjective awareness, behavioural features or electrophysiological changes are hard to establish. The lighter stages of NREM sleep appear first, and often alternate with brief episodes of wakefulness before the deeper NREM sleep stages are entered. NREM sleep, and particularly its deeper stages, predominate early in the night, but REM sleep appears at around 90 minute intervals. There are usually 4–6 of these sleep cycles each night and as the night progresses the REM episodes become longer, and NREM sleep both shorter and lighter.

Brief arousals to wakefulness can be detected electrophysiologically and are a normal feature of sleep. They are usually brief, lasting up to 10–15 s and there is no awareness or recall of these events. A 40 s cycle of arousability (cyclic alternating pattern, CAP) related to changes in cortical activity has been identified and may underlie some of these arousals. They occur with increasing frequency in the lighter stages of NREM sleep with increasing age, and the threshold for arousal is highest in young children. Arousals may also occur because of external stimuli such as sounds, and internal stimuli from, for instance, gastro-oesophageal reflux, or upper airway obstruction during sleep.

Non-rapid eye movement sleep

Non-rapid eye movement sleep is present in all birds and mammals, but has not been clearly demonstrated in cold-blooded animals. This suggests that its evolutionary appearance may be related to the need to conserve energy at night when the ability to obtain food is greatly reduced. The motor inhibition and lower body temperature reduce the metabolic rate by 10–25% during NREM sleep early in the night, although to a lesser extent after 3.00–5.00 AM. Sleep would therefore have a survival value, but does increase the vulnerability of the subject to adverse environmental events unless rapid reversal to the wakened state in response to significant stimuli remained possible.

Non-rapid eye movement sleep also provides time for restorative processes to take place within the central nervous system (CNS) and other parts of the body. Cell division in many tissues is most rapid at this time. Protein synthesis is increased and other metabolic changes take place both in the glial tissue, particularly astrocytes, and the neurones. The reduction in physical and metabolic activity during NREM sleep switches the balance between catabolism and anabolism in favour of the latter and this is accentuated by the secretion of several anabolic hormones, such as growth hormone. Overall, NREM sleep appears to be a phase in which energy is conserved while food cannot be obtained, and both the central nervous and other systems are able to either recover from the activity of the previous episode of wakefulness or to prepare for the next episode (Table 1.2).

Four stages of NREM sleep are recognized on conventional electroencephalogram (EEG) criteria. These are categorized by the frequency and amplitude of the EEG, the presence of sleep spindles and K complexes, and electro-oculogram (EOG) and electromyogram (EMG) findings. Arousal from NREM sleep in response to external stimuli occurs most readily in its lighter stages and becomes progressively more difficult as the deeper stages are entered. The threshold for arousal is higher in children than in adults. Subjects woken during NREM sleep frequently report that they are aware of fragmented, thought-like processes, particularly in the lighter stages of NREM and later in the night. These contain less action than the dreams that occur during REM sleep. They may represent a process of reorganization of neural networks in an analogous, but different, manner to that which occurs in REM sleep.

The absence of most of the higher functions of the cerebral cortex during NREM sleep is paralleled by the loss of motor activity and depression of somatic and visceral reflexes. These become free of cortical control with the result, for instance, that tendon reflexes are reduced and 50% of subjects show an upgoing plantar (Babinski) reflex during NREM sleep. Autonomic reflexes are also altered in NREM sleep. There is a relative increase in parasympathetic activity which is amplified by the circadian rhythms compared to sympathetic activity. This is affected by the sleep–wake state, but not by circadian factors. This new balance remains fairly constant within each stage of NREM, but parasympathetic activity increases from stage 1 to stage 4.

Rapid eye movement sleep

Rapid eye movement sleep is present in all mammals and probably enables behaviour patterns and emotional responses to become established. The offspring of mammals are less mature and more vulnerable at birth than those of reptiles and birds which immediately lead an independent life. They have an urgent need to develop neural networks and programmes which can establish behaviour patterns that are essential for survival, such as maternal bonding. During REM sleep information obtained during wakefulness appears to be reprocessed and integrated into existing neural templates so that future responses can be modified or matured to reflect both the experience of the individual and the inherited potential [2]. This enhances memory and often gives images an emotional charge, helping, particularly through the limbic system, to bond new mental associations and to link them to established complex memory systems and other patterns.

The high proportion of the sleeping time occupied by REM in neonates and young children reflects the neurodevelopmental needs at these ages. The ability to form new neurones (neurogenesis) slows early in life and new behaviour patterns are mainly due to new functional interneuronal connections, rather than to brain growth. The contrary and older concept of REM sleep, and dreams in particular, as a mechanism of excretion of unwanted thoughts and associations, or of 'reversed learning' has found little support (see Table 1.2).

The characteristic electrophysiological features of REM sleep are the combination of a wide range of

Table 1.2 Comparison of NREM and REM sleep.

Characteristic	*NREM sleep*	*REM sleep*
Cerebral cortex	Prefrontal cortex inactive Frontal cortex partially active Limbic cortex inactive Deafferented	Prefrontal cortex inactive Parietal cortex partially active Limbic cortex active Active information processing Dreams
Somatic reflexes	Reduced	Intense inhibition
Movements	Constant for each stage (1–4) Reduced	Rapid eye movements
Autonomic function	Constant for each stage (1–4) Parasympathetic dominance	Fluctuates Overall parasympathetic dominance
Metabolic	Reduced metabolic rate Anabolic	Slightly reduced metabolic rate

Table 1.3 Nomenclature of sleep states and stages.

NREM	Quiet sleep (infants)
	Orthodox sleep
	Synchronized sleep
NREM stages 1 and 2	Light sleep
NREM stages 3 and 4	Deep sleep
	Slow-wave sleep
	Delta sleep
REM sleep	Active sleep (infants)
	Paradoxical sleep
	Desynchronized sleep

'desynchronized' EEG frequencies, loss of EMG activity and the presence of rapid eye movements (Table 1.3). The EEG reflects the intense cerebral cortical activity that distinguishes REM from NREM sleep, but its similarity to the EEG of wakefulness led to its old name of 'paradoxical' sleep. This is reflected in dreams which are characteristically full of activity, narrative, and incidents, especially those occurring later in the night. They differ from the more thought-like content of NREM sleep, and often, but not invariably, coincide with phases when rapid eye movements are present. The cortical processes responsible for dreams are not activated primarily by external and internal stimuli as in wakefulness, but by pontine centres.

Dreams vary in their vividness and in their extreme form can be so realistic that the subject is unaware whether the events in the dream have actually taken place or not. Some people can also apparently consciously alter the course of their dreams, a process known as 'lucid dreaming'. Recall of dreams declines rapidly during NREM sleep or wakefulness. This suggests that most subjects who claim not to dream probably have especially strong bonding between REM and NREM sleep so that their failure to wake at this transition stage renders them unaware of their dreams.

The content of dreams mainly reflects recent events and current issues, but those from the past may also feature frequently. This probably indicates that new experiences and ideas are being integrated into existing neural networks that represent these prominent issues [3]. There is, however, a limited number of main themes of dreams. These are connected to basic biological needs that are common to all individuals. Aggressive or hostile behaviour towards others or towards the dreamer, resulting in dominance or submission may be manifested in dreams by various actions and emotions. Dreams with a content of bonding to other people, a sexual content, or related to feeding are common. The prevalence of each of these dream themes varies with the subject's age, gender and stage of neural development, and probably reflects the current requirements and concerns. Dreams often have a strong emotional component and while a degree of anxiety may prepare the subject to respond to danger, it can become extreme and then represents a nightmare.

The sensory content of dreams varies, but around 75% of subjects dream in colour, and there is only a non-visual content if the individual becomes totally blind before the age of 5. There is an auditory component in around 75% of subjects. Sensations of falling, levitation or occasionally flying, are common and are probably due to inhibition of muscle spindle activity or occasionally to changes in vestibular function. Sensations of touch and taste occur in only around 1% of dreams and smell is even less frequent. Painful sensations during dreams are very unusual. These sensory differences reflect the ability of the brain-stem and thalamus to differentially gate the sensory pathways to the cerebral cortex. The varying tempo of dreams and their occasional discontinuities probably reflect variations in the speed and patterns of activity in the cortical association areas.

The cortical activity and desynchronized EEG are probably continuous ('tonic') throughout REM as is the loss of skeletal muscle tone. The intense motor inhibition of REM prevents dreams and other cortical processes from being enacted. It allows cortical activity to continue without any outward expression and it was probably the evolutionary step that allowed cortical activity during sleep to attain its important neuro-developmental role. Intermittent ('phasic') activity in some muscles does, however, persist during REM sleep. These include contraction of the middle ear muscles, but the most prominent are the rapid saccadic movements of the eyes. These occur particularly during dreams, but also at other times and are accompanied by bursts of small movements of the facial, limb and trunk muscles. Most of the respiratory muscles are inactive during REM sleep, except for the posterior crico-aryteroid muscles which abduct the vocal cords, the diaphragm, which has very few muscle spindles, and to a lesser extent the parasternal intercostal muscles.

In general, sympathetic activity is reduced and parasympathetic activity is increased, but their balance fluctuates rapidly, probably in synchrony with changes in cortical activity. The limbic cortex in particular is able to influence the hypothalamus which translates the changes in cortical activity into alterations in brain-stem autonomic and somatic function. Depression or loss of reflexes which are present during wakefulness is common. The tendon reflexes, for instance, may be lost. The reduction in sympathetic activity may be partly due to attenuation of sensory input at each relay in the brain-stem, as well as to active inhibition of sympathetic motor neurones as a result of the cortical activity.

Mixed sleep–wake states

Sleep and wakefulness are not totally distinct states. The constant flux in the activity of many parts of the brain may lead at any one time to either an overwhelming balance of activity in favour of one state or the other, or at other times to features of both appearing simultaneously. The fluctuations between NREM and REM sleep are also much more dynamic and complex than is usually appreciated. The instability of these states underlies the appearance of a range of mixed or incomplete states of wakefulness, NREM and REM sleep (Table 1.4).

The transitions between sleep and wakefulness may also be gradual, often lasting several minutes, rather than instantaneous. Consciousness and the awareness of activities for example, can become separated from the performance of movements. The spinal cord can coordinate repetitive flexion and extension movements, such as those seen in walking, without higher control and even complex activities can be organized by the basal ganglia and brainstem without the type of cerebral cortical involvement seen in wakefulness.

These mixed and transition states are very variable, but can be categorized according to the state from which they arise.

WAKEFULNESS
Intrusion of NREM sleep into wakefulness is manifested by automatic behaviour. This is the combination of often complex but inappropriate, behaviour patterns due to loss of the neurological movement control mechanisms which cause motor inhibition in sleep, combined with a lack of awareness of the environment and of activities. EEG recordings demonstrate 'microsleeps' with stages 1 and 2 NREM sleep lasting up to 15–30 s interrupting wakefulness.

Aspects of REM sleep can also intrude into wakefulness. The ability to recall dreams on awakening is a common example of this and the hallucinations associated with delirium, such as delirium tremens, probably represent partial REM intrusion into wakefulness. The loss of muscle tone with laughter (cataplexy) is an example of pathological REM intrusion into wakefulness. Sleep-onset sleep paralysis may also be regarded as intrusion of a fragment of REM sleep into wakefulness.

NREM SLEEP
Intrusion of REM into NREM sleep does not cause any symptoms since sleep is maintained, but intrusion of wakefulness is characteristic of 'disorders of arousal'. In these the transition from NREM sleep to wakefulness is incomplete or gradual and features of both states coexist temporarily. The commonest and mildest example is sleep inertia in which a nap is followed by drowsiness or at least a sensation of feeling unrefreshed and of being no more alert after the nap

Table 1.4 Mixed sleep–wake states.

Prior state	Effects of NREM sleep intrusion	Effects of REM sleep intrusion	Effects of wakefulness intrusion
Wakefulness: awareness, motor function	Unaware. Motor function retained (automatic behaviour)	Aware of dreaming. Loss of muscle tone (cataplexy and sleep paralysis)	—
NREM: unaware, no movements	—	—	Partially aware (sleep inertia and confusional arousal); motor function retained (automatic behaviour)
REM: unaware, REMs	—	—	Aware of lucid dreaming; motor function decreased (sleep paralysis) or increased (REM sleep behaviour disorder)

than beforehand, often combined with temporary disorientation. The EEG shows some features of wakefulness and of stages 1 and 2 NREM sleep. Sleep inertia may last for up to 2 h and is particularly prolonged if the overnight sleep phase is extended and awakening takes place out of NREM.

There is probably a spectrum of the degree of failure to arouse from NREM sleep which leads from sleep inertia through confusional arousals to activities such as sleep walking and sleep terrors. A confusional arousal (sleep drunkenness) is characterized by a similar combination of complex motor behaviour and lack of awareness as with automatic behaviour arising from wakefulness, except that it develops out of sleep.

REM SLEEP
Intrusion of wakefulness into REM sleep is responsible for sleep paralysis at the end of a period of sleep. Awareness of the environment coincides with the motor inhibition of REM sleep. Lucid dreaming, in which there is awareness of dreaming and the ability to direct its content, reflects the combination of the awareness which is characteristic of wakefulness, with continuing dream mentation. Retention of muscle 'tone' in the REM sleep behaviour disorder is dissociated from the continuing REM dream mentation with the result that cortical activities can be physically enacted, unlike normal sleep in which motor inhibition suppresses them.

Duration and timing of sleep

About 60% of the adult population obtain 7–8 h sleep per night, but around 8% sleep for less than 5 h and 2% for more than 10 h. The duration of sleep often differs considerably from what is needed. For most adults the optimal duration of sleep appears to be 8–9 h per night, but many people function almost as well on 6–8 h. Loss of NREM sleep, especially stages 3 and 4, probably causes more daytime sleepiness than loss of REM sleep. The sleep episode should be sufficient to lead to a feeling of being refreshed on waking and remaining alert throughout the day.

Oversleeping does not improve alertness, and during an extended sleep period the duration and depth of NREM sleep begins to increase since REM sleep takes the place of wakefulness in increasing the drive to enter NREM sleep. As a result sleep inertia becomes more prominent after prolonged sleep episodes and the subsequent night's sleep may become fragmented.

A regular time of going to bed, going to sleep, waking up and getting up in the morning is an important factor in stabilizing and synchronizing the circadian rhythms. The most important of these is the regularity of the waking time. The exact times that are adopted vary according to, for instance, age, social constraints such as work patterns, and the individual tendency to be a long or short sleeper (or a 'lark' or 'morning type' or an 'owl' or 'evening type'). Regular sleep patterns ensure that the homeostatic drive to sleep is strong since they allow a sufficient interval after the previous main sleep episode. In the elderly, restricting the nocturnal sleep phase to 6–7 h is usually preferable to sleeping for longer and often improves insomnia.

A common pattern of irregular sleep–wake schedules is that of restricting sleep during the working week, building up a sleep debt and then repaying this by sleeping longer at weekends. During these nights there is a high sleep efficiency, a short sleep latency and an increased duration of stages 3 and 4 NREM sleep. Waking later in the morning, however, causes a phase delay on the next day which is often followed by an early wake up time at the start of the working week. The duration of sleep is thereby considerably shortened and sleep deprivation begins again.

Daytime naps are normal in young children and common in the elderly. They are usually and most physiologically taken between 2.00 and 4.00 PM at a time when the circadian rhythms favour sleep. This is exemplified by the siesta that is taken in some societies. Naps should, where possible, be avoided in adults and minimized in the elderly unless excessive daytime sleepiness persists despite treatment of its cause and attention to other aspects of sleep and wake patterns. The structure of sleep in a nap depends mainly on the duration since the last sleep and on the position of the circadian rhythm. The later in the day the nap occurs the more likely it is that NREM, and particularly its deeper stages, will predominate unless the nap happens to coincide with the 90-minute REM sleep cycle which probably persists in a mild form throughout wakefulness as well as sleep.

Shift workers and others whose nocturnal sleep routines are unavoidably modified may require regular naps at other times of the day in order to achieve the necessary duration of sleep. Brief naps of 10–30 min usually increase alertness in narcolepsy and to a lesser extent in obstructive sleep apnoeas (OSAs), but longer naps are required in, for instance, idiopathic CNS hypersomnia and are often less refreshing. In addition to the sensation of tiredness and difficulty in concentrating (sleep inertia) motor performance may be impaired after a nap, particularly if it contains stages 3 and 4 NREM sleep, and there may be confusional arousals without recall of the events [4].

Sleep and age

The pattern of sleep varies considerably with age, partly because of intrinsic changes in the sleep–wake cycles and sleep structure (Figs 1.2 and 1.3), but also because of the presence of medical disorders and through the influence of external factors. These vary in type according to the subject's age and may induce psychological responses which affect the ability to sleep. The details of the individual conditions are discussed later, but in general the most important stages in the development of sleep patterns are as follows.

PRENATAL PHASE

A rhythmic cycling of motor activity is detectable at around 20 weeks gestation and at 28–32 weeks a regular sleep–wake cycle is detectable with alternating periods of body movements, rapid eye movements and irregular respiratory movements ('active sleep'), interrupted by brief episodes of inactivity ('quiet sleep'). By 24 weeks gestation the EEG recordings show intermittent high amplitude signals alternating with periods in which the EEG is 'flat', and which gradually become more prolonged. From 32 weeks onwards, active and quiet sleep become more easily distinguishable and resemble REM and NREM sleep respectively.

EARLY POSTNATAL PHASE

At birth the fetus moves from an environment of continuous darkness into one with intermittent light

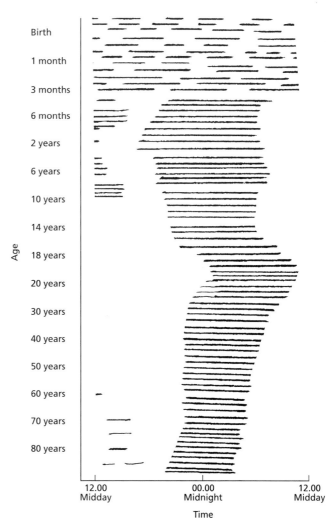

Fig. 1.2 Changes in sleep patterns with age. Horizontal lines indicate sleep episodes at different ages.

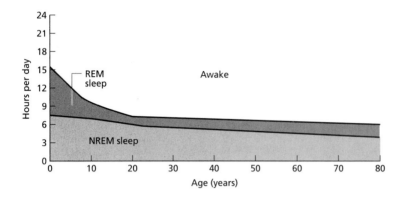

Fig. 1.3 Changes in duration of NREM and REM sleep with age. NREM, non-rapid eye movement; REM, rapid eye movement.

exposure, and the nature of other external stimuli such as feeding and social contact also changes vastly. Normal full-term infants show almost randomly timed phases of wakefulness, active sleep, and quiet sleep on behavioural criteria, although about 3% of their time is spent in an indeterminate state. Around 16 h per day is spent asleep, which is entered through REM sleep. Premature infants at 30 weeks appear to be in REM sleep for 80% of their sleeping time, at 36 weeks for 60% at 40 weeks for 50%, and unlike adults, sleep is entered through an initial phase of REM sleep.

3–12 MONTHS

At this age, as in the early postnatal phase, the interpretation of the electrophysiological tracings is difficult. Quiet sleep, thought to be equivalent to NREM, is first detectable at around 28–32 weeks in pregnancy, and predominates by around 3 months. Conversely, active sleep, thought to be equivalent to REM, occupies around 50% of the total sleep time in normal infants at birth and is responsible for only around 40% at 3 months and 30% at 6–12 months. The latency before entering REM sleep gradually increases during the first year.

By 3 months K-complexes and sleep spindles are detectable on the EEG and the latter increase in number by 6 months, although until the age of 2 years there is often interhemispheric asynchrony of spindles. High-voltage, low-frequency theta (4–8 Hz) or delta (0.5–4 Hz) waves are detectable, particularly over the occipital area from one month of age. By 6–12 months the 4 stages of NREM sleep are distinguishable electrophysiologically.

The sleep pattern until around 3 months is thought to be related to feeding which probably increases the tendency to sleep afterwards. Both sleeping and feeding occur at three- to four-hourly intervals, but by 3–6

months a circadian rhythm in the child's sleep patterns becomes detectable. This is initially free-running but gradually comes under the control of external stimuli, including light exposure. By 6 months it is common to sleep throughout the night and signs of a predominantly biphasic pattern with an afternoon sleep appear. Cycles of REM sleep develop by around 3 months. These are initially approximately of 45 min duration, but gradually lengthen to around 60 min by one year of age and 90 min by 5–10 years.

CHILDHOOD

By the age of one year children spend around 11 h asleep at night and up to 2½ h asleep during one or two naps in the daytime. Thirty per cent of their sleep is REM sleep. The morning nap is usually discontinued between the age of 2–3 years, but the afternoon nap is often retained until around 5 years.

During childhood the percentage of REM sleep and the total sleep time falls, but the 'best' quality of sleep is attained. The sleep latency is shorter than in later life at 5–10 min and 10 h consolidated sleep at night with few arousals are usually obtained by the age of 8. The sleep efficiency is around 95% and the percentage of stages 3 and 4 NREM sleep is greater than at any other age. There is a strong monophasic sleep cycle centred on the night time, possibly related to the high melatonin levels at this age, and there is little tendency to fall asleep in the afternoon. Excessive daytime sleepiness is a rare complaint.

Environmental factors often have a significant impact on sleep in childhood. Some physical disorders such as middle ear infections are more painful at night, but may not be recognized and nocturnal asthma or gastro-oesophageal reflux may also severely disrupt sleep. Bedtime fears and rituals may delay the initiation of sleep, and family situations can cause hyperarousal of the child shortly before the intended sleep time. Irregular sleeping times and peer group pressures may also lead to sleep problems.

PUBERTY
At this stage most children sleep for around 9 h, of which around 40% are stages 3 and 4 NREM sleep and 20–25% REM sleep. A biphasic sleep pattern begins to emerge with occasional complaints of daytime sleepiness, usually in the afternoon.

ADOLESCENCE
Most adolescents begin to go to sleep later and wake up later in the morning. The total sleep time increases slightly, perhaps related to the metabolic changes during the growth spurt. A mild delayed sleep phase syndrome is common, but whether this is due to an endogenous change in the circadian sleep rhythm or to social factors such as opportunities for late evening and night entertainment or work is uncertain. The sleep latency is usually longer than in childhood and 25% REM sleep is obtained.

Sleep restriction due to social pressures is common and irregular sleep–wake patterns often develop. Excessive caffeine or alcohol intake and recreational drugs may contribute to these patterns. Unrecognized depression and anxiety are also common.

YOUNG AND MIDDLE-AGED ADULTS
At the age of 20 years the sleep efficiency is still usually around 95%, but it then falls progressively. By 35 years the duration of stage 4 NREM sleep is only around 6% of the total sleep time which is only half of what it is at 20. Wakefulness at night is twice as prolonged and the duration of stage 1 NREM sleep is increased slightly at around 5% of total sleep time. The percentage of REM sleep remains constant at around 22–25% throughout early and middle adult life, but changes in the circadian rhythms prevent subjects over the age of around 45 from adapting as fast and as completely to changes in sleep patterns, e.g. shift work. Other environmental factors such as a reduction in exposure to light due to indoor employment, restriction of sleep time and medical and psychological disorders influence sleep patterns.

OLD AGE
The total sleep time during the night is reduced, but if daytime naps are frequent or prolonged, the total amount of sleep during each 24 h may be similar to younger subjects. The sleep efficiency falls to 70–80%

with an increase in the number of awakenings and a reduction in stages 3 and 4 NREM sleep [5]. This is around 18% at age 20 years, but may be only around 10% at the age of 60 and by 75 there may be no stage 4 NREM sleep. The amplitude of the delta waves falls by about 75% relative to childhood, probably as a result of loss of cortical synchronization due to degeneration of the sleep regulating processes and to cerebral atrophy which causes fewer cortical neurones to be sampled by the surface electroencephalogram (EEG). The duration of stages 1 and 2 NREM sleep is increased (up to 15% stage 1), sleep spindles become fewer, poorly formed, of small amplitude and their frequency may fall from 16 to 12–14 Hz.

The sleep pattern deteriorates in men at a younger age than in women, and men have more arousals from sleep than women between the ages 60 and 80. At these ages there is no detectable gender difference in the duration of REM sleep and its overall percentage remains almost constant at around 20% even into old age, although it may then fall slightly. REM sleep latency shortens to 70–80 min, but the first episode of REM sleep is often prolonged, possibly related to changes in the circadian rhythm. This results in REM sleep episodes of similar duration throughout the night rather than the pattern of lengthening REM cycles seen in younger subjects.

These changes in the sleep patterns of the elderly are influenced by the following factors.

Changes in circadian rhythms
There is no change in the endogenous length of the circadian cycle, which remains around 24.2 h, but the circadian rhythm reduces in amplitude and often alters its timing. The peak blood melatonin level, which is controlled by exposure to light, falls in the elderly and the amplitude of the temperature rhythm is attenuated. The sleep onset and time of wakening become almost 1 h earlier per decade after the age of 60 years. This is a form of the advanced sleep phase syndrome and is a continuation of the phase change from the delayed sleep phase syndrome of adolescence through the normal sleep phase of middle adult life. There may also be internal desynchronization of circadian rhythms, particularly of sleep, temperature and hormone secretion.

Reduction in homeostatic sleep drive
Disintegration of the sleep–wake controlling mechanisms increases the frequency of arousals which may be spontaneous, or due to a lower threshold for

arousal to, for instance, light and noise. The elderly wake closer to the peak of melatonin secretion and the temperature nadir than younger adults. The increased vulnerability of the elderly to these stimuli reduces the continuity of sleep and together with changes in the circadian rhythm leads to a polyphasic sleep pattern with frequent daytime naps. By the age of 70, 25% of men nap during the day and by 80 the figure rises to 45%.

Changes in environment

It is common for entraining factors of the circadian rhythms to be attenuated in old age. The exposure to light falls because the elderly remain indoors for longer, and often have cataracts and macular degeneration which reduce the amount of light stimulating the retina. Institutionalization in nursing homes, reduction in activity, either due to lack of opportunity or physical restrictions, social isolation and boredom all adversely affect the control of sleep. Conversely, some social habits such as regular meal times, bedtime and wake-up times tend to consolidate sleep–wake patterns. Exposure to bright light in the morning may exacerbate the advanced sleep phase syndrome. Light exposure at night, even if it is brief, may reduce melatonin secretion and worsen insomnia.

Co-morbidity

Other symptoms such as nocturia, heartburn and backache, as well as drugs may reduce the quality and duration of sleep. Sleep disorders such as OSAs and periodic limb movements in sleep are also more common in the elderly. Dementia, depression and anxiety are also frequent and the elderly develop drug reactions such as a hangover effect from hypnotics and caffeine intolerance more frequently than younger adults.

As a result of these factors, nocturnal insomnia is common with a difficulty in maintaining sleep and inappropriately early morning wakening. Insomnia may be multifactorial and due to medical, psychological, or social factors; or to pain, depression, reduction in physical activity, an increased number of naps during the day and intake of caffeine. Restlessness, agitation, confusion and brief arousals and more prolonged awakenings from sleep are frequent. Intolerance of irregular sleep habits, or time zone changes develops and daytime naps become more frequent.

Sleep and gender

There are only minor differences in sleep requirements between males and females. The duration of sleep appears to be slightly longer in females and their circadian rhythm may be a few minutes shorter. The changes in sleep structure seen in the elderly are delayed in women compared to men and the dreams of women are said to occur more often indoors than those of men, and to be less aggressive.

Sleep disturbances related to menstruation, pregnancy and the menopause are common, but have been poorly documented. Both insomnia and excessive daytime sleepiness may occur at each of these times (Chapters 5 and 6). Pregnancy is also associated with specific sleep disorders such as periodic limb movements and a worsening of OSAs. Obstructive sleep apnoeas are less common in premenopausal women than men, probably because of a difference in the bony structure surrounding the upper airway and because less fat is laid down in the necks of women than of men. These gender differences probably have a hormonal basis, but the cause of other gender differences such as the increased prevalence of insomnia in women is uncertain [6].

Sleep and the partner

Sleep disorders may affect the bed partner, family, friends, carers and even neighbours in addition to the patient. The partner may become concerned because of the implications of the sleep disorder, especially when the patient stops breathing, as in obstructive and central sleep apnoeas and Cheyne–Stokes respiration, appears to choke, make sudden vigorous movements as with epilepsy and REM sleep behaviour disorder and if there is a possibility of injury while sleep walking. Snoring and abnormal movements during sleep due to, for instance, the periodic limb movement syndrome (PLMS) may fragment the partner's sleep and cause a significant degree of excessive daytime sleepiness (EDS). Severe insomnia at night or sleep reversal can also put considerable strain on the family and carers, particularly if the patient also becomes confused at night and wanders from the bedroom.

These problems may lead to feelings of frustration, annoyance or anger which are often directed by the partner or family of the subject with the sleep disorder, who may come to feel guilty about causing the problem. Occasionally aggression or violence may be directed by the partner of the patient while the patient is asleep. Partners often taken hypnotics or alcohol, or both, in order to try to obtain adequate sleep. The patient and partner often decide to sleep in separate beds or separate bedrooms, at least for part of the night, or some nights, and the sleep disorder quite commonly is considered as a factor leading either to separation or divorce. The sleep disorder may also affect the partner less directly by imparing the daytime function of the patient. Excessive daytime sleepiness due to, for instance, OSAs or narcolepsy, restricts or even prevents family and social activities. Patients often fall asleep readily in the evenings and are unable to interact with other members of the household. The excessive sleepiness may cause difficulties at work with job insecurity, failure to be promoted and loss of earnings. Other symptoms such as cataplexy may prevent the patient from being left alone in the home or make it unsafe for the individual to care for children without another person being present. This can cause considerable difficulties and tensions.

The partner may also have to adjust to the treatment required for the sleep disorder. This may be intrusive as with nasal continuous positive air pressure systems for sleep apnoeas. Prescribed drugs may have side-effects which indirectly affect the partner's sleep.

The presence of a bed partner can also modify the patient's sleep and sleep complaints. The partner's snoring, movements during sleep or nocturia can cause frequent awakenings leading to sleep restriction. This may exacerbate the patient's underlying disorder, such as sleep walking, or worsen symptoms of conditions that lead to EDS such as sleep apnoeas or PLMS. Young children often wake their parents or carers during the night and the insomnia this causes can become a long-term problem. Similarly, pets in the home, such as cats and dogs, often prefer to sleep in the bedroom or in or on the bed and can disturb the individual's sleep. This may be due to movements,

purring or barking, but they may also lead to nocturnal asthma through an allergic mechanism, or by disturbing the dust in the bed and increasing its inhalation.

Effective treatment of the patient's sleep disorder has the advantage, compared with treatment of most other medical conditions, of often being directly of benefit to both the patient and the partner. Relief of OSAs, for instance, improves the patient's daytime sleepiness and reduces the disturbance to the partner's sleep. Treatment of REM sleep behaviour disorder not only reduces the risk of injury to the patient, but also of that to the partner. The partner's description of the changes in the patient's sleep disorder with treatment is often important in evaluating its effectiveness as it is in the initial assessment of the type and severity of the patient's sleep problem.

Control of sleep and wakefulness

The physiological control of sleep and wakefulness is complex and is discussed in detail in Chapter 2. The main components are described below.

Different types of sleep and wake drive

The homeostatic, ultradian, and adaptive drives interact with the influence of the circadian rhythms to determine whether sleep is entered or wakefulness occurs. These drives are modified by endogenous factors and environmental controls, especially light exposure (Fig. 1.4).

Circadian rhythms

These are generated by the internal clock in the suprachiasmatic nuclei (SCN) and control not only the sleep rhythms but also the temperature and endocrine cycles. The mechanisms by which the clock is entrained to environmental time are complex and involve the secretion of melatonin by the pineal gland.

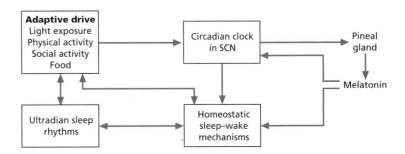

Fig. 1.4 Mechanisms of sleep–wake control. SCN, suprachiasmatic nuclei.

Neurophysiological and neuroanatomical mechanisms

The mechanisms responsible for generating NREM and REM sleep are different, but both converge on the thalamus which interacts reciprocally with the cerebral cortex to determine whether sleep or wakefulness occurs.

Neurochemical mechanisms

The classical neurotransmitters, such as noradrenaline and acetylcholine, interact with the large numbers of more recently recognized chemical mediators of neuronal activity to determine the sleep and wake drives. These are closely integrated with growth, repair and immune function and with the action of melatonin on sleep and circadian rhythms.

Pathophysiology of sleep disorders

The physiological mechanisms responsible for initiating and terminating sleep and establishing it in its various forms can all become disorganized, attenuated or exaggerated. These alterations are the basis of the sleep disorders which will be described in the later chapters of this book. The most important types of defects of sleep can be considered under the following headings, although many disorders fall into more than one category (Table 1.5).

Disorders of homeostatic sleep drive

Insomnia or excessive daytime sleepiness result from alteration of the homeostatic sleep drive, due, for instance, to organic lesions in the midbrain, hypo-thalamus or thalamus. An increase in this drive is probably responsible for habitual long sleepers, the prolonged deeper stages of NREM sleep in children, the long sleep times in idiopathic CNS hypersomnia and the excessive daytime sleepiness of hypothalamic disorders and some head injuries. If the sleep drive increases too rapidly during the day, it will lead to a need for naps which are not fully refreshing if the link between sleep and the inhibition of the homeostatic sleep drive is broken.

Disorders of the ultradian rapid eye movement sleep rhythm

The 90-minute REM sleep cycle is strongest during sleep but probably persists as a mild drive to enter REM sleep during wakefulness. It is rarely altered in length, but its intensity is enhanced in, for instance, narcolepsy. REM sleep or fragments of it intrude both into wakefulness and NREM sleep.

Disorders of adaptive drive

The level of arousal is increased in most subjects with insomnia, but may be lowered in some otherwise normal subjects and in narcolepsy which is often associated with subalertness. The level of stimulation by environmental factors influences the extent to which the variations in arousal level are expressed.

Circadian rhythm disorders

The circadian rhythms can be separated from environmental factors by, for instance, blindness, so that the sleep–wake and light–dark cycles become disconnected. Unusual environmental conditions such as

Table 1.5 Classification of important sleep disorders.

Disordered function	EDS	Insomnia	Behavioural abnormalities	Respiratory disorders
Homeostatic drive and NREM	ICNSH	Idiopathic insomnia	Disorders of arousal	—
Ultradian drive and REM	Narcolepsy	Narcolepsy	REM behaviour disorder	—
Adaptive drive	Poor sleep hygiene	Poor sleep hygiene	—	—
Circadian rhythms	DSPS, ASPS	Depression, DSPS, ASPS	—	—
Dissociation of sleep states	Sleep inertia	—	Confusional arousal	—
Arousals	OSA	Hyperarousal states	PLMS	—
Autonomic function	—	—	Sleep terrors	Asthma,
Behaviour in sleep	PLMS	PLMS	Epilepsy	OSA, CSA

ASPS, advanced sleep phase syndrome; COPD, chronic obstructive pulmonary disease; CSA, central sleep apnoea; DSPS, delayed sleep phase syndrome; EDS, excessive daytime sleepiness; ICNSH, idiopathic central nervous system hypersomnia; NREM, non-REM; OSA, obstructive sleep apnoeas; PLMS, periodic limb movements in sleep; REM, rapid eye movement.

residence at polar latitudes can have a similar effect on circadian rhythm matching with the environment. Imposed sleep–wake patterns such as shift work have the opposite effect. Instead of allowing the circadian rhythms to run free they impose a non-24 h pattern on them so that mismatch between the desired sleep–wake schedule and the circadian rhythms occurs regularly. Intrinsic abnormalities in the circadian control of sleep can cause it to be phase-advanced or delayed and the amplitude of the circadian rhythm falls with age.

Dissociation of sleep mechanisms

A range of these disorders including the separation of motor inhibition from sleep as in cataplexy and sleep paralysis are recognized. The intrusion of dream activity into wakefulness, which may make it hard to distinguish between the dream and reality, is a feature of narcolepsy.

Disorders associated with arousal from sleep

Physical disorders related to sleep such as the periodic limb movement syndrome and OSAs cause frequent arousals during sleep (sleep fragmentation). The conditions which lead to incomplete or an abnormal arousal from sleep should be distinguished from these. They include sleep walking and confusional arousals, in which often complex behaviour is carried out but with little relevance to environmental stimuli or subsequent recall of the event.

Disorders of autonomic and immunological function

The physiological changes in autonomic and immunological function in sleep can become accentuated, diminished or distorted. Examples include cluster headaches as a result of changes in vasomotor control, asthma due to alterations in bronchial smooth muscle function and inflammation within the airways, cardiac dysrhythmias caused by changes in parasympathetic innervation and paroxysmal nocturnal haemoglobinuria due to alterations in complement activation.

Disorders of motor control

Motor inhibition is characteristic of sleep, particularly REM sleep. This causes OSAs when the stabilizing effect of the dilator muscles of the upper airway is lost and central sleep apnoeas when there is insufficient respiratory muscle activity to generate airflow. Lack of motor inhibition leads to the REM sleep behaviour disorder, and repetitive transient failure of inhibition to PLMS. These should be distinguished from movements occurring at the time of arousal from sleep, for instance at the end of an OSA, and from movement disorders which are present during the day, but which are modified by sleep, e.g. Parkinsonism. Absence of movements during sleep may also be important, for instance in central sleep apnoeas.

Classification of sleep disorders

The pathophysiology and main symptoms of sleep disorders form the basis of the approach to these conditions in this book (see Table 1.5). The complaints of lack of sleep (insomnia) and excessive duration of sleep (excessive daytime sleepiness) are covered in Chapters 5–6 with the circadian rhythm disorders separately identified since they form a physiological entity. Abnormal experiences and events taking place during sleep are covered in Chapters 7 and 8; and the respiratory disorders of sleep, which are a subgroup of these, are discussed in Chapters 9 and 10. The links between the pathophysiology, clinical features and treatment of these sleep disorders are maintained throughout these chapters.

This scheme has many similarities to, but also some differences from, the widely used International Classification of Sleep Disorders (ICSD) produced by the American Sleep Disorders Association (ASDA) in association with other national and international sleep societies. The Third Revision (1997) [7] is summarized in Table 1.6. This groups insomnia and excessive daytime sleepiness as dyssomnias and distinguishes them from disorders occurring during sleep (parasomnias). It also has two other categories which are less satisfactory. Firstly, a group of medical and psychiatric disorders which includes epilepsy and mood disorders, all of which interact with the sleep mechanisms in a similar fashion to the disorders in the dyssomnia and parasomnia categories. The second group of 'proposed sleep disorders' is heterogeneous and emphasizes the descriptive aspects and includes partly developed concepts such as the 'sleep choking syndrome'.

In this book the disorders in these two groups have been integrated into the main categories of sleep disorders. The term 'parasomnia' has not been used because of the wide range and heterogeneous nature of the sleep conditions that this has come to represent. The important influence of drugs is recognized by a

Table 1.6 ASDA classification of sleep disorders 1997.

1 Dyssomnias

A Intrinsic sleep disorders
1 Psychophysiologic insomnia — 307.42–0
2 Sleep state misperception — 307.49–1
3 Idiopathic insomnia — 780.52–7
4 Narcolepsy — 347
5 Recurrent hypersomnia — 780.54–2
6 Idiopathic hypersomnia — 780.54–7
7 Post-traumatic hypersomnia — 780.54–8
8 Obstructive sleep apnoea syndrome — 780.53–0
9 Central sleep apnoea syndrome — 780.51–0
10 Central alveolar hypoventilation syndrome — 780.51–1
11 Periodic limb movement disorder — 780.52–4
12 Restless legs syndrome — 780.52–5
13 Intrinsic sleep disorder NOS — 780.52–9

B Extrinsic sleep disorders
1 Inadequate sleep hygiene — 307.41–1
2 Environmental sleep disorder — 780.52–6
3 Altitude insomnia — 289.0
4 Adjustment sleep disorder — 307.41–0
5 Insufficient sleep syndrome — 307.49–4
6 Limit-setting sleep disorder — 307.42–4
7 Sleep-onset association disorder — 307.42–5
8 Food allergy insomnia — 780.52–2
9 Nocturnal eating (drinking) syndrome — 780.52–8
10 Hypnotic-dependent sleep disorder — 780.52–0
11 Stimulant-dependent sleep disorder — 780.52–1
12 Alcohol-dependent sleep disorder — 780.52–3
13 Toxin-induced sleep disorder — 780.54–6
14 Extrinsic sleep disorder NOS — 780.52–9

C Circadian-rhythm sleep disorders
1 Time zone change (jet lag) syndrome — 307.45–0
2 Shift work sleep disorder — 307.45–1
3 Irregular sleep–wake pattern — 307.45–3
4 Delayed sleep–phase syndrome — 780.55–0
5 Advanced sleep–phase syndrome — 780.55–1
6 Non-24-hour sleep–wake disorder — 780.55–2
7 Circadian rhythm sleep disorder NOS — 780.55–9

2 Parasomnias

A Arousal disorders
1 Confusional arousals — 307.46–2
2 Sleepwalking — 307.46–0
3 Sleep terrors — 307.46–1

B Sleep–wake transition disorders
1 Rhythmic movement disorder — 307.3
2 Sleep starts — 307.47–2
3 Sleep talking — 307.47–3
4 Nocturnal leg cramps — 729.82

C Parasomnias usually associated with REM sleep
1 Nightmares — 307.47–0
2 Sleep paralysis — 780.56–2
3 Impaired sleep-related penile erections — 780.56–3
4 Sleep-related painful erections — 780.56–4
5 REM sleep-related sinus arrest — 780.56–8
6 REM sleep behavior disorder — 780.59–0

D Other parasomnias
1 Sleep bruxism — 306.8
2 Sleep enuresis — 788.36–0
3 Sleep–related abnormal swallowing syndrome — 780.56–6
4 Nocturnal paroxysmal dystonia — 780.59–1
5 Sudden unexplained nocturnal death syndrome — 780.59–3
6 Primary snoring — 786.09–1
7 Infant sleep apnea — 770.80
8 Congenital central hypoventilation syndrome — 770.81
9 Sudden infant death syndrome — 798.0
10 Benign neonatal sleep myoclonus — 780.59–5
11 Other parasomnia NOS — 780.59–9

3 Sleep disorders associated with mental, neurologic, or other medical disorders

A Associated with mental disorders — 290–319
1 Psychoses — 290–299
2 Mood disorders — 296–301, 311
3 Anxiety disorders — 300, 308, 309
4 Panic disorders — 300
5 Alcoholism — 303, 305

B Associated with neurologic disorders — 320–389
1 Cerebral degenerative disorders — 330–337
2 Dementia — 331
3 Parkinsonism — 332
4 Fatal familial insomnia — 337.9
5 Sleep–related epilepsy — 345
6 Electrical status epilepticus of sleep — 345.8
7 Sleep–related headaches — 346

C Associated with other medical disorders
1 Sleeping sickness — 086
2 Nocturnal cardiac ischemia — 411–414
3 Chronic obstructive pulmonary disease — 490–496
4 Sleep–related asthma — 493
5 Sleep–related gastroesophageal reflux — 530.81
6 Peptic ulcer disease — 531–534
7 Fibromyalgia — 729.1

4 Proposed sleep disorders

1 Short sleeper — 307.49–0
2 Long sleeper — 307.49–2
3 Subwakefulness syndrome — 307.47–1
4 Fragmentary myoclonus — 780.59–7
5 Sleep hyperhidrosis — 780.8
6 Menstrual–associated sleep disorder — 780.54–3
7 Pregnancy–associated sleep disorder — 780.59–6
8 Terrifying hypnagogic hallucinations — 307.47–4
9 Sleep–related neurogenic tachypnea — 780.53–2
10 Sleep–related laryngospasm — 780.59–4
11 Sleep choking syndrome — 307.42–1

separate chapter devoted to their effects, which are also referred to throughout the chapters dealing with the individual disorders.

References

1 Velluti RA. Interactions between sleep and sensory physiology. *J Sleep Res* 1997; 6: 61–77.

2 Jouvet M. Paradoxical sleep as a programming system. *J Sleep Res* 1998; 7: 1–5.

3 Cipolli C, Bolzani R, Tuozzi G. Story-like organization of dream experience in different periods of REM sleep. *J Sleep Res* 1998; 7: 13–19.

4 Jewett ME, Wyatt JK, De Cecco AR-De, Khalsa SB, Dijk D-J, Czeisler CA. Time course of sleep inertia dissipation in human performance and alertness. *J Sleep Res* 1999; 8: 1–8.

5 Hume KI, Van F, Watson A. A field study of age and gender differences in habitual adult sleep. *J Sleep Res* 1998; 7: 85–94.

6 Driver HS, Baker FC. Menstrual factors in sleep. *Sleep Med Rev* 1998; 2: 213–29.

7 International Classification of Sleep Disorders. (Revised). Diagnostic and Coding Manual. Rochester: American Sleep Disorders Association, 1997.

2 Physiological Basis of Sleep and Wakefulness

Control of sleep and wakefulness

Whether an individual is awake or asleep depends on the balance of forces promoting and inhibiting each of these two states [1]. At times the balance can be almost equal and the subject may begin to fall asleep if he or she had previously been awake, or to lighten from sleep if previously asleep. The mechanisms determining whether sleep or wakefulness predominates are poorly understood, but three processes interact with each other and with circadian rhythms.

Homeostatic (intrinsic) drive (process S)

This drive to enter sleep increases, possibly exponentially, with the duration since the end of the previous sleep episode. It declines once sleep has been initiated, again possibly exponentially. Although it is usually considered primarily a sleep drive, this process could equally well be regarded as a drive to wakefulness if looked at from the opposite view point. Whichever is the more appropriate, it reinforces the cyclical nature of sleep and wakefulness and equates sleep with other physiological needs such as hunger or thirst. The need to sleep increases with the length of time awake which is similar to the increase in hunger as the duration of abstinence from food increases.

This homeostatic sleep drive appears to control non-rapid eye movement (NREM) rather than rapid eye movement (REM) sleep. Sleep is normally entered through NREM rather than REM sleep in adults and an increase in the homeostatic drive will increase the duration and depth of NREM sleep at the expense of REM. On the first night after sleep deprivation NREM sleep rebound appears indicating, in sleep control terms, that the build up of the sleep drive is discharged by entering NREM rather than REM sleep. It is only once the NREM sleep debt has been repaid after one or two nights that an increase in REM sleep is seen.

Ultradian rapid eye movement sleep rhythm

The threshold for entering REM sleep is under the control of an ultradian rhythm with a 90-min cycle. This appears to continue through both wakefulness and sleep. In wakefulness it may be manifested only by a transient feeling of drowsiness or a tendency to daydream. This REM cycle is therefore not generated by sleep, but reflects an intrinsic process within the brain. This drive increases with REM sleep deprivation in a similar manner to the homeostatic drive for NREM sleep, but is distinct from this control system.

Rapid eye movement sleep is rarely entered directly from wakefulness which suggests that the expression of the tendency to REM sleep is somehow primed by the neurophysiological mechanisms of NREM sleep. Rapid eye movement sleep also occurs particularly during the second half of the night which coincides both with a waning homeostatic drive to NREM sleep and also with the onset of the rise of body temperature from its nadir which is usually between 3.00 and 5.00 AM. The significance of this is uncertain, particularly in view of the loss of homeostatic temperature control during REM sleep which results in the body temperature being influenced more by the ambient temperature.

Adaptive drive

This concept includes a variety of mechanisms that influence sleep but which are independent of the time spent awake and of circadian and ultradian rhythms. They modify the sleep–wake cycle according to changes in the environment which are significant for the individual. They are complex and ill-understood components of the sleep–wake control system, but have two main elements.

BEHAVIOURAL FACTORS
These include motivation, attention and other psychological responses to the environment. The voluntary choice of, for instance, deciding whether to take exercise or to move to a more stimulating situation influences the probability of remaining awake or falling asleep. Once asleep the comfort of the bed and the lighting, noise and temperature all influence whether

or not awakening will take place. The conscious or subconscious awareness of the significance of different sensory inputs is a further important factor which determines whether arousal from sleep occurs. Once aroused, the conscious brain is able to recognize the source of the stimulus and to respond accordingly. The conscious decision either to try to fall asleep or stay awake and knowledge of the clock time are factors which influence whether or not the individual stays awake or falls asleep.

Other important factors which prevent or promote sleep and which can be controlled are discussed below.

Psychological aspects
It is important to avoid mental stimulation in the hour before falling asleep and to use this time as a transition between the mental activities of the daytime and the moment of falling asleep. Worries and anxieties should be sorted out before going to sleep and it may be helpful to put some time aside regularly each evening to achieve this and to plan how to cope with any problems anticipated on the following day. Pre-sleep rituals, including washing and brushing the teeth, may also help if they become associated with successful initiation of sleep. Relaxation may be achieved by reading a monotonous book or newspaper or listening to background music. Television is usually stimulating because of its changing pictures, sounds and often exciting action. It can also induce sleep through boredom, immobility and the low ambient light levels.

The bedroom should become mentally associated with sleep and should be used only for this and sexual activity. It should not become a subsidiary office so that it becomes associated with alertness rather than sleep, or be used to watch television or videos. Most people also sleep better in a familiar environment than when they are, for instance, in a hotel or sleep laboratory. The 'first night effect' of this unfamiliarity reduces the sleep efficiency, and leads to less stages 3 and 4 NREM sleep and REM sleep, except in subjects with psychophysiological insomnia.

Bed comfort
A hard bed may help to reduce backache, but leads to more frequent changes of position during sleep. Many subjects sleep better with a partner, but this can disturb sleep, especially in the elderly or if the partner sleeps poorly, is restless or has a sleep disorder, particularly a behavioural disorder. Separate beds or sleeping in separate bedrooms may be helpful to one or both partners in these situations.

Social activity
This usually induces alertness but through its association with physical activity and exposure to light, may have complex effects on sleep. Sleep is more likely after social interactions, and the synchronization of sleep and wake patterns within a group or community may have a biological survival advantage.

REFLEX FACTORS
The general level or lack of sensory stimulation influences the sleep–wake state, but this is more specifically affected by the following factors.

Light exposure
Light exposure has complex and important effects on sleep and wakefulness [2]. The seasonal changes in the duration of daily light exposure lead to cyclical alterations in the duration of rest and activity. The duration of melatonin secretion and of sleep is longer in winter than in summer in non-tropical latitudes. At high latitudes with prolonged nights the nocturnal sleep phase in winter may break into two episodes with an intervening stage of quiet wakefulness. Seasonal changes in light duration also influence mood and behaviour, as exemplified by the seasonal affective disorder (SAD).

During sleep, around 10% of ambient light reaches the retina through closed eyelids. This has an alerting effect during NREM sleep, increasing the electro-encephalogram (EEG) frequency and often causing arousals from sleep with the result that after light exposure there may be a rebound increase in NREM sleep. The effects on REM sleep are less clear, but it can be promoted by brief episodes of darkness.

During wakefulness, light exposure increases the level of alertness. This effect is particularly marked at night and with bright light, which can lead to a significant increase in motor performance which is important for shift workers. A separate effect is the influence of light on the timing of the circadian rhythms. Exposure to light resets these each day so that they are coordinated with environmental time. An implication of this, however, is that exposure to artificial light in the evening may lead to a phase delay, making the initiation of sleep more difficult.

The effects of light on the circadian rhythms depend on the factors discussed below.

Intensity. The circadian rhythms can be altered by as little as 100 lux which is less than the light level in most domestic situations during the day.

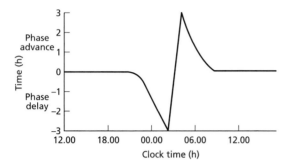

Fig. 2.1 Phase response curve to light. Bright light exposure in the early evening leads to a sleep phase delay, but after 3.00–5.00 AM advances the next sleep phase.

Duration. Brief light pulses can influence the circadian rhythms, but exposure for 10–20 min is required to have a significant impact.

Wavelength. The individual wavelengths of light probably influence the circadian rhythms differently. The most effective in resetting them appears to be around 480 nm.

Timing. The time within the circadian rhythm at which the subject is exposed to light has an important influence on the extent and type of response (phase response curve) (Fig. 2.1). The circadian rhythm is insensitive to light exposure during the day, but is affected by it at night, when there is usually little light and when melatonin is secreted. A rapid shift in the type of response to light occurs around the nadir of temperature and at the time of peak melatonin secretion, usually 3.00–5.00 AM. Light exposure before this phase-shift transition point delays the next sleep

phase, but afterwards leads to a phase advance. The magnitude of each of these effects is greatest close to the temperature nadir. There is no detectable phase delaying effect before around 9.00 PM or phase advance after around 10.00 AM. The sleep phases can be shifted by up to 1–2 h per day by light exposure, according to its timing and other factors affecting the circadian rhythms. These effects are mediated by the influence of light on the suprachiasmatic nuclei and melatonin secretion which parallels the changes in the sleep phase and which can also be temporarily suppressed by light (Fig. 2.2).

Noise

A quiet bedroom usually improves sleep but the threshold for arousal varies according to the age of the subject and the stage of sleep. Children sleep through more noise than adults and older subjects are readily aroused from sleep due to noise unless they are deaf. The threshold for arousal increases from stage 1 through to stage 4 NREM sleep. Arousal is therefore more likely later in the night after the initial episodes of stages 3 and 4 NREM sleep have been completed.

Arousal is also more likely if the noise is of significance to the sleeper. Adaptation to environmental noise occurs rapidly in many subjects, and people living, for instance, close to railways, motorways and even airports may sleep soundly. Measures to isolate sleepers from noise can be successful and include earplugs and double glazing.

Temperature

A constant environmental temperature of around 18°C (65°F) is ideal for inducing and maintaining sleep and for the optimal balance of NREM and REM

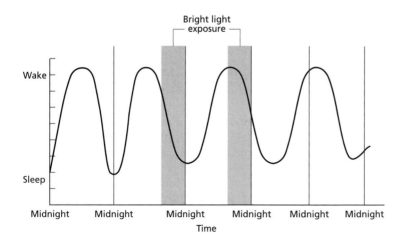

Fig. 2.2 Delay in sleep phase following exposure to bright light on the second and third evenings.

sleep. Rapid eye movement sleep is particularly sensitive to temperature changes and is promoted by a rising body temperature. Both high and low temperatures lead to fragmentation of sleep and a reduction of REM sleep is particularly a feature of the latter.

Physical exercise
In general, exercise promotes wakefulness not only at the time of the activity, but for around 2–3 h afterwards. Alertness is also more likely to be maintained if the subject stands or walks rather than lies down. This alerting effect is present both in normal subjects and also in, for instance, those with narcolepsy. Exercise within around 3 h of the desired time of sleep onset may delay this and cause the melatonin level to fall. Exercise early in the day may cause a phase advance, reducing the sleep latency on the next night. It increases the total sleep time and the duration of stages 3 and 4 NREM sleep, and may reduce the duration of REM sleep.

Food intake
Hunger is associated with wakefulness, but after eating, humans tend to relax and readily fall asleep. These patterns may have a survival advantage in that wakefulness is retained until sufficient food has been eaten.

Postprandial sleepiness may be partly mediated by reflexes. Dilatation of the jejunum by a balloon can induce sleep, but hormones such as cholecystokinin (CCK), which is secreted in the duodenum and jejunum, are also hypnogenic. Carbohydrates and milky drinks which contain tryptophan, a precursor of 5HT and melatonin, have a greater sleep-promoting effect than other foods presumably because of a specific chemical effect on the sleep control mechanisms. Conversely, high protein foods, which are rich in tyrosine may promote noradrenaline synthesis and lead to wakefulness.

Large meals taken before sleep can cause gastro-oesophageal reflux leading to heartburn and awakening. Large volumes of liquid should be avoided before sleep since they may lead to nocturia, especially if there is renal impairment or prostatic hypertrophy.

Very severe malnutrition, as occurred in prisoner of war camps, can induce excessive daytime sleepiness (EDS) and inactivity, but, in general, weight loss, whether it is due to anorexia nervosa, mania or thyrotoxicosis, leads to insomnia and hyperactivity. Weight loss in depression is associated with insomnia, but those who gain weight, as in SAD, often become excessively sleepy. There may a link in otherwise normal subjects between weight loss, hyperactivity and insomnia, and between weight gain, inactivity and EDS. The chemical basis of these associations is uncertain, but weight gain may also lead to EDS through a mechanical effect of increasing the quantity of fat around the upper airway and leading to obstructive sleep apnoeas (OSAs).

Sexual activity
Sexual intercourse usually promotes the onset of sleep, in contrast to other types of physical activity.

Circadian rhythms

Circadian rhythms have a periodicity of around a day which is longer than the ultradian rhythms of, for instance, REM sleep and shorter than infradian rhythms such as the menstrual cycle. All these endogenous rhythms are generated by an internal pacemaker, oscillator or biological clock, which can be modified by external factors (time givers, cues or zeitgebers). These entrain the internal clock and gear it to the external environment, but in certain situations the clock can become dissociated from the time givers, in which case it becomes 'free running' and desynchronized from the environment.

The suprachiasmatic nuclei (SCN) in the supraoptic region of the anterior hypothalamus contain cells responsible for the most important circadian rhythms. These two tiny bilateral nuclei about 3 cm behind the eyes each have a volume of only 0.1 ml and each contains around 10 000 neurones. Each SCN has a core of vaso-intestinal peptide (VIP) secreting neurones which respond particularly to light stimuli and which have melatonin receptors. There is a shell of vasopressin-releasing neurones which respond to non-photic stimuli. Gamma-aminobutyric acid (GABA)-secreting neurones occur in both the core and the shell.

Each of the cells in the SCN is capable of spontaneous depolarization. The coordination of these is the source of circadian rhythmicity, but within the SCN there are subpopulations of cells with different cycle times. These are usually entrained by diffuse chemical, rather than synaptic, mechanisms to a single rhythm but under certain circumstances they can become dissociated from each other. This may lead to desynchronization of the individual circadian rhythms of, for instance, sleep, temperature and hormone secretion. The SCN is active during the day, both in diurnal and nocturnal animals.

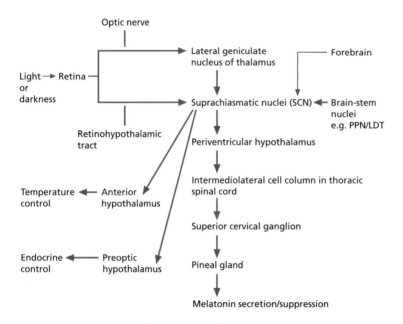

Fig. 2.3 Pathways linking retina, suprachiasmatic nuclei (SCN) and pineal gland. LDT, laterodorsal tegmental nuclei; PPN, pedunculopontine nuclei.

The characteristics of this rhythm generator or clock are largely genetically determined. Six genes have been identified on chromosome 5 which, through inhibiting protein transcription, form a complex negative feedback system which has the properties of an oscillator or clock. Its intrinsic rhythm is usually 24.2 h in humans, but there is considerable interindividual variation. This rhythm generator is not responsible for initiating sleep, but connects to the structures which control sleep onset and cessation.

Impulses reach the SCN from retinal receptors which lie particularly in the lower and nasal quadrant of the retina. The receptors have not yet been identified, but may be analogous to the horizontal cells in other species which produce opsins. They are distinct from the rods and cones which lead to the sensation of vision, and whose fibres run in the optic nerves, synapse in the lateral geniculate nuclei and connect to the primary visual sensory cortex in the occipital cortex. Impulses from the SCN-related receptors travel via retinal ganglion cells in the retinohypothalamic tract, which also runs within the optic nerves, but is independent of the visual pathways, and through the geniculohypothalamic tract which relays visual signals from the lateral geniculate nuclei of the thalamus. Light also activates nerve fibres reaching the pretectum and superior colliculus and these probably mediate the effects of light exposure on REM and NREM sleep respectively, but do not lead to any visual sensations.

The cholinergic pedunculopontine and laterodorsal tegmental (PPN/LDT) nuclei and basal forebrain neurones also project to the SCN, as do other areas of the brain-stem (Fig. 2.3). These probably mediate the effects of physical exercise on advancing or delaying the sleep phase. This is also influenced by melatonin which inhibits the activity of the SCN and forms part of a negative feedback loop which promotes sleep.

Fibres leave the SCN to reach the ventrolateral preoptic area of the anterior hypothalamus which is closely involved in sleep–wake control, temperature regulation and hormone secretion. Fibres also travel multisynaptically to the pineal gland. These take a tortuous course descending through the periventricular hypothalamus into the intermediolateral cell column of the thoracic spinal cord from which preganglionic sympathetic neurones project to the superior cervical ganglion and then postganglionic sympathetic fibres travel along the internal carotid artery to reach the pineal gland.

The pineal gland contains a circadian pacemaker in some vertebrates, such as perching birds (passerines), but in humans this function is taken over by the SCN in the anterior hypothalamus and this controls the cycle of pineal melatonin secretion. The human pineal gland contains glial cells and pinealocytes which have similarities to the photoreceptors of amphibia, but in humans are only indirectly, not directly, light sensitive. The pinealocytes secrete several hormones and related chemicals such as GABA and 5HT, but their most important hormone is melatonin.

The clock in the SCN has a circadian influence through its neurological connections, not only on sleep, but on other functions, especially temperature control and hormone secretion. Removal of the SCN causes a loss of most of these rhythms, but does not prevent sleep from taking place or temperature from being controlled. In normal circumstances these functions have a constant relationship, but they can become desynchronized. This may occur even if the SCN is working normally, perhaps due to independent action of subpopulations of cells within the SCN with different timings, or to different connections outside the SCN. Dissociation of these rhythms is seen particularly in unusual environmental situations which can disturb their coordination. The potential for this internal desynchronization varies between the various circadian rhythms.

The most important SCN-related circadian rhythms are as follows.

Sleep rhythms

The diurnal cycling of sleep–wake rhythms maintains sleep and wakefulness in line with environmental time, but by itself is insufficient to initiate sleep. In effect, it alters the threshold of the other sleep drives for initiating sleep or wakefulness. It does not selectively promote either NREM or REM sleep. The circadian sleep rhythm usually promotes wakefulness during the day, except between 2.00 and 4.00 PM, and particularly in the evenings shortly before the usual time of sleep onset which is when the homeostatic drive to sleep is greatest. The circadian rhythm opposes this and leads to the 'forbidden zone' when it is often difficult to fall asleep just prior to the usual time of sleep. The end point of this zone occurs when the homeostatic drive, together with an input from the adaptive drive, overcomes this circadian influence. The circadian drive to wakefulness is at its least at the habitual wake-up time of the subject in the morning. This helps to consolidate sleep at the end of the night when the homeostatic drive to sleep is waning.

Temperature cycle

The sleep and temperature cycles are usually closely coupled, although in free-running experiments the sleep cycle usually becomes around 1 h longer than the temperature cycle. The temperature of the blood is sensed in the anterior hypothalamus which reacts to its rise by increasing heat loss through cutaneous vasodilatation and sweating. If the temperature falls, the posterior hypothalamus causes heat conservation by cutaneous vasoconstriction and increased heat production through skeletal muscle activity, including shivering, and pilo-erection.

The amplitude of the circadian temperature cycle is 0.5–0.75°C with a nadir at 3.00–5.00 AM. The temperature rises to a peak of 37°C at 3.00–5.00 PM and only falls slowly until around 9.00 PM. The drop in core temperature which frequently precedes sleep is associated with an elevation of skin temperature, presumably due to cutaneous vasodilatation. The temperature continues to fall after sleep onset, due to a reduction in physical activity and metabolic rate, and to vasodilatation during NREM sleep. The assumption of the supine position also tends to lower the temperature through a postural reflex. Secretion of melatonin lowers the core body temperature and the peak melatonin serum level coincides with the temperature nadir at around 3.00–5.00 AM (Fig. 2.4). The subsequent temperature rise is linked to the increase in duration and density of REM sleep, although thermoregulation is much less precisely controlled in REM sleep than in NREM sleep or wakefulness.

Endocrine cycles

There is an important circadian pattern to the secretion of hormones, many of which are controlled by the hypothalamus [3]. Those needed to adapt the individual to respond to external influences during wakefulness, such as adrenaline and cortisol, are secreted especially during the day. Cortisol secretion in response to adrenocorticotrophic hormone (ACTH) is closely related to the circadian rhythm. It rises towards the end of the nocturnal sleep episode and peaks around the time of wakening. The secretion of ACTH is slow to change and it may be several weeks before it alters in response even to gross changes in sleep routines. It is hardly affected by sleep itself, but can modify sleep, particularly by increasing the duration of time awake, in the lighter stages of NREM sleep and reducing the duration of stages 3 and 4 NREM sleep. The secretion of thyroid stimulating hormone (TSH), which is highest just before sleep, is controlled partly by the circadian rhythm but is also inhibited by sleep itself.

Other hormones which have a primary anabolic function have a different pattern of secretion. Growth hormone is secreted in pulses during stages 3 and 4 NREM sleep. Two-thirds of it is released in the first NREM episode during sleep and prolactin is also secreted in pulses during stages 3 and 4 NREM sleep. Aldosterone levels rise during REM sleep, whereas

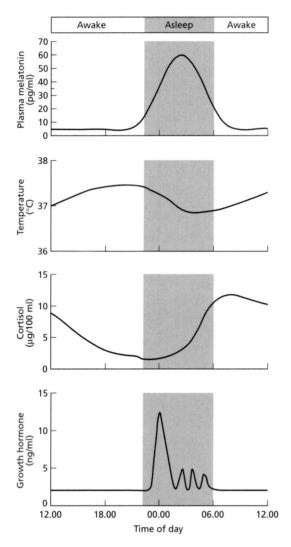

Fig. 2.4 Diurnal changes in melatonin, temperature, cortisol and growth hormone.

renin is secreted mostly in stages 1 and 2 NREM sleep. Luteinizing hormone (LH) and follicle-stimulating hormone (FSH) are secreted in pulses during the night and testosterone blood levels are highest in REM sleep.

Neurophysiology and anatomy of sleep and wakefulness

The activity of the cerebral cortex is critical in determining whether sleep or wakefulness occurs, but it does not generate the drive to enter sleep or wakefulness. Cortical activity is largely determined by interactions between the thalamus and the cortex itself,

and differs between NREM and REM sleep. In both of these states, however, the prefrontal cortex which is involved particularly in temporal organization of behaviour, short-term memory and motor attention, is inactive. The limbic cortex which gives representation for autonomic function such as cardiovascular and gastro-intestinal control and is involved in behaviour related to emotion, is inactive in NREM but active in REM sleep. The parietal cortex is less active in REM than in wakefulness, and the same has been observed of the frontal cortex in NREM sleep.

The thalamus is the final common path for most of the information reaching the cortex from receptors, apart from olfaction, and from the brainstem. The thalamus modifies these inputs, in effect acting as a gate determining which of the stimuli reach the cortex and in what form, although thalamic activity is itself regulated by the cerebral cortex.

The thalamic reticular nucleus is especially important in interacting with the cerebral cortex and determining the state of arousal. It has groups of excitatory neurones which release glutamate and inhibitory neurones which release GABA at their synapses. Intrathalamic relay neurones modify thalmic activity whereas other neurones form the thalamocortical projection fibres. Thalamic excitation is followed by inhibition by corticothalamic impulses. Their timing determines the frequency of the bursts of thalamic stimulation of the cortex which varies from 0.6 to 1 Hz [4]. GABA-secreting neurones also inhibit brainstem centres that are capable of leading to arousal.

The extent of convergence of the many inputs to the thalamus determines the extent to which they influence its activity and synchronize its output so that it can become, in effect, a cortical pacemaker. The divergence of the projection fibres within the cerebral cortex and their radiation to subcortical centres regulates the extent of this influence. The thalamic pacemaker protects the cortex from other incoming electrical impulses so that it is deafferentated or sensorily deprived, unless stimuli can break through the imposed thalamic rhythm. This only occurs if the stimuli are particularly intense or of particular significance to the individual. The limbic cortex suppresses brainstem transmission of sensory information to the thalamus during REM sleep, helping to maintain the thalamic control of the cortex. The effectiveness of this varies with the strength of the drive to remain asleep or to arouse to wakefulness. As the drive to sleep wanes, the ability of the reticular activating system, and in particular the reticular

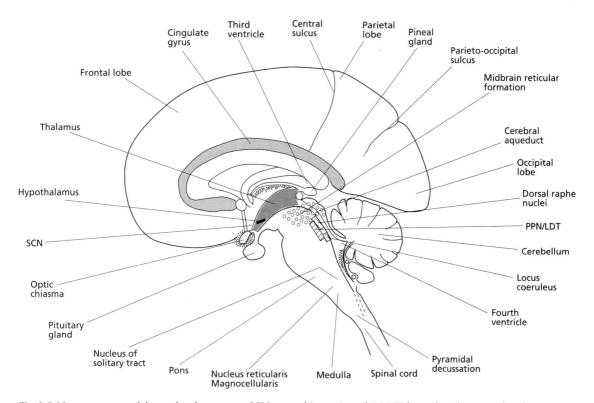

Fig. 2.5 Neuro-anatomy of sleep-related structures. SCN, suprachiasmatic nuclei; LDT, laterodorsal tegmental nuclei; PPN, pedunculopontine nuclei.

nucleus of the thalamus, to block transmission to the cortex weakens and arousal may occur.

The thalamus is driven by impulses from various sites within the brain so that it promotes wakefulness, NREM or REM sleep (Fig. 2.5). Wakefulness and NREM sleep are mainly controlled by homeostatic and adaptive drives, REM sleep by the ultradian drive, and the circadian rhythms act on each of these states.

Wakefulness-related mechanisms

The reticular activating system (RAS) is a physiological entity which promotes wakefulness when it is active and allows sleep when it is inhibited or inactive (Fig. 2.6). It was originally thought to be a homogeneous system, but the complexity of its structure and function is now being realized. It governs the homeostatic drive, many of the reflex factors of the adaptive sleep drive, and is closely connected to the circadian sleep rhythms.

The RAS is largely contained in the brain-stem reticular formation (RF) which is a loosely connected structure with small groups of cells and nuclei, large numbers of short interneurones and complex ascend-

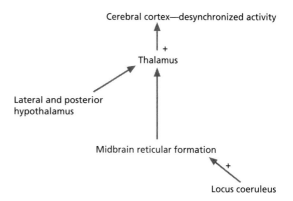

Fig. 2.6 Main mechanisms involved in wakefulness.

ing and descending interconnecting tracts. Most of the RF lies in the central core or tegmentum of the pons and midbrain, but it also extends into the medulla, hypothalamus and thalamus. It has a complex microstructure and GABA is secreted at most of its synapses. It has an extensive influence over the sensory input to the brain-stem, motor function of the cranial nerve nuclei and spinal cord, and the state of sleep or wakefulness. It also has close links, through the hypothalamus, with endocrine control.

The locus (nucleus) coeruleus in the lateral floor of the fourth ventricle in the pons activates the ascending RAS, particularly in the midbrain. The RF in the lateral and posterior hypothalamus and particularly in the tubero-mammillary region also promotes wakefulness. These areas, together with connections from the ascending RAS in the midbrain, project to various nuclei within the thalamus especially the reticular nucleus. This is part of the RAS and influences other thalamic nuclei and the cerebral cortex in a way that promotes wakefulness.

NREM sleep-related mechanisms
The regulation of NREM sleep is poorly understood in anatomical terms, probably because the mechanisms responsible for it change according to the activity of other sleep–wake controlling pathways and the fluctuating balance of neurotransmitters and cotransmitters (Fig. 2.7). In general, however, NREM sleep appears when the activity of the RAS dwindles. The RAS can be inhibited by centres in the medulla, such as the nucleus of the solitary tract and the ventral reticular nucleus. The dorsal raphe nuclei (DRN), which lie near the midline in the ventral part of the periaqueductal grey matter from the level of the rostral pons to the caudal midbrain, also inhibit the RAS and promote NREM.

The ventrolateral preoptic area inhibits the tubero-mammillary region and promotes NREM sleep; the medial preoptic area of the anterior hypothalamus also promotes NREM sleep. 5HT and adenosine are secreted at some of the latter's synapses. This area has complex connections with many other parts of the brain, including the RF in the midbrain, the PPN and LDT nuclei, thalamic nuclei and the cerebral cortex including the limbic cortex and the magnocellular area of the basal forebrain. It is close to the centres for temperature regulation which have an important influence on sleep, and to the SCN which regulates the circadian rhythms, including sleep rhythms. It also influences the autonomic nervous system, increasing parasympathetic activity and leading to slowing of the heart rate, lowering of the blood pressure and pupillary constriction.

The combination of RAS inhibition by medullary centres, the DRN, the medial preoptic area of the anterior hypothalamus and its connections, particularly the PPN/LDT nuclei and basal forebrain, can reduce the arousal drive from the RAS sufficiently for impulses reaching the thalamus and basal forebrain to switch the cortical activity to that of NREM sleep.

REM sleep-related mechanisms
The PPN/LDT nuclei are located dorsolaterally at the pontine midbrain junction adjacent to the locus coeruleus (Fig. 2.8). The PPN/LDT nuclei contain magnocellular areas and while many of the PPN neurones are cholinergic, those in adjacent areas secrete other neurotransmitters such as histamine, glutamate and in the locus coeruleus, noradrenaline and in the DRN, 5HT [5].

The drive to enter REM sleep appears to originate in this area, probably as a result of changes in the balance between cholinergic and other neurotransmitter agents in these various nuclei. Cessation of activity in, for instance, the DRN which secrete 5HT with nitric oxide as a cotransmitter, and in the locus coeruleus shifts the balance towards cholinergic dominance. 5HT, nitric oxide, GABA, opiates and adenosine all cause hyperpolarization of the PPN/LDT neurones and inhibition of REM sleep and wakefulness.

The tendency towards cholinergic dominance promotes REM sleep through projections from the PPN/LDT nuclei to the ascending RAS, particularly in the pons and midbrain, the hypothalamus, thalamus and limbic system, including the basal forebrain. It is pro-

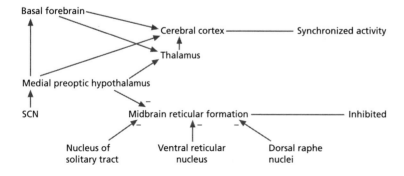

Fig. 2.7 Main mechanisms involved in non-rapid eye movement (NREM) sleep. SCN, suprachiasmatic nuclei.

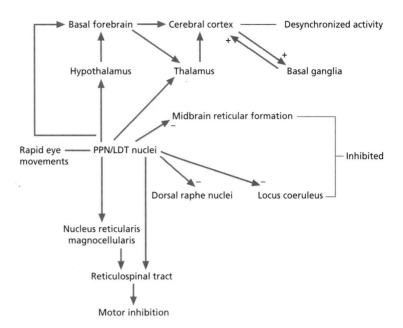

Fig. 2.8 Main mechanisms involved in rapid eye movement (REM) sleep. LDT, laterodorsal tegmental nuclei; PPN, pedunculopontine nuclei.

bably also responsible for the ponto-geniculo-occipital (PGO) waves which arise just before and during REM sleep and which can be recorded over the pons, lateral geniculate nuclei of the thalamus and occipital cortex. These waves are more prominent in animals such as cats than in humans and are rarely detectable with conventional scalp surface electrodes in humans. The activity of the PPN/LDT is probably the source of the high-frequency thalamocortical bursts which result in the desynchronized EEG characteristic of REM sleep.

The PPN/LDT nuclei influence sleep-related eye movements, which are controlled by the oculomotor nuclei, particularly the rapid movements characteristic of REM sleep. They are also responsible for initiating the loss of muscle tone that is characteristic of REM sleep. They have a direct output to the reticulospinal tract and an indirect one through projections to the nucleus reticularis magnocellularis in the medial medulla. They cause supraspinal inhibition of both alpha and gamma motor neurones in the ventral horns of each spinal cord segment. This reduces reflex responsiveness and muscle tone, particularly in the postural muscles. The diaphragm, which has very few gamma fibres, shows little change in activity in REM sleep and is the main chest wall respiratory muscle that remains active in REM sleep.

The loss of muscle tone is more marked in REM than in NREM sleep, despite the continuous activity of the cerebral cortex and its formation of complex

behaviour patterns and movements which are transmitted to the basal ganglia (Fig. 2.9). These remain active in REM sleep, in contrast to NREM sleep in which the cortex does not generate the type of behaviour patterns seen in REM sleep. The basal ganglia, in which dopamine is the main transmitter, interact with the limbic system and corticospinal pathways to coordinate and control skeletal muscle movement. These pathways are intensely inhibited during REM sleep so that the cortical and basal ganglia behaviour patterns experienced as dreams are not physically enacted.

Neurochemistry of sleep and wakefulness

The theory that sleep and wakefulness are determined by the balance of activity in various nuclei and tracts within the brain only partially explains the way in which these states are controlled. There is a continual flux in the relative importance of the various areas concerned in sleep–wake control as well as in the activity within each of these areas. This instability is largely controlled by chemical influences. The long-standing theory of a neurotransmitter as a single compound liberated by the presynaptic membrane passing across the synaptic cleft and inducing depolarization of the postsynaptic membrane has required modification. Some neurones produce two or more chemicals which influence the depolarization of the postsynaptic

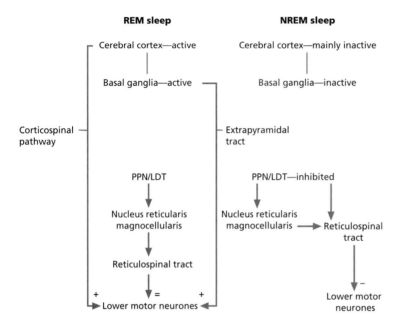

Fig. 2.9 Control of movements in non-rapid eye movement (NREM) and rapid eye movement (REM) sleep. In rapid eye movement (REM) sleep, reticulospinal tract inhibition of lower motor neurones overcomes stimulation arising from cerebral cortex and basal ganglia. In NREM sleep the cerebral cortex and basal ganglia are largely inactive and there is little movement, although inhibition via the reticulospinal tract is less intense. LDT, laterodorsal tegmental nuclei; PPN, pedunculopontine nuclei.

membrane. One of these (a cotransmitter) may also alter the responsiveness of the membrane to the other transmitter by, for instance, modifying the sensitivity of the receptors. The cotransmitter may also control the synthesis or release of the main transmitter (neuromodulation). Many of these chemicals are amines, amino acids or peptides, and have other important, but often less clearly defined, effects. They may act as growth factors, altering the pattern of formation of dendrites, remodelling synapses and influencing neurological development. Many of these chemicals secreted in the brain also play a role in the immune system, whose control is closely linked to the control of sleep and wakefulness, (pages 29, 177). Growth, tissue repair and immune function are closely related and all three are facilitated by the metabolic and endocrine changes during sleep that promote anabolic processes.

The awareness of the functions of locally released chemicals overlaps with the concept of sleep factors (hypnotoxins, somnogens, sleep regulatory substances) which are chemicals found in the brain and cerebrospinal fluid which promote sleep and which increase in concentration during wakefulness. Some of these sleep factors are probably cotransmitters which have been released into synapses, but others may be secreted either by neurones or glia to act as local neurohormones and which influence the threshold for depolarization of the postsynaptic membranes. Some

systemically released classical hormones probably also cross the blood–brain barrier and have similar effects on the control of sleep and wakefulness. These chemicals all interact with the recognized nuclei and pathways which influence sleep and wakefulness, and are capable of altering widespread patterns of neuronal activity and sensitizing to or protecting neurones from other influences. Some are released in response to synaptic activity and then induce new synapses through their growth factor action, modify the ways in which information is processed and change the activity in neuronal networks. These coordinated effects may form a major component of the homeostatic drives to sleep and wake, and the activity of the RAS.

The details of these neurochemical influences on sleep are poorly understood, but the chemicals can be grouped into the following categories.

Amines

Most of the classical neurotransmitters are amines (Table 2.1), but melatonin is an important additional regulator of sleep–wake control.

NORADRENALINE (NOREPINEPHRINE)

This is thought to promote wakefulness and to inhibit REM sleep through its alpha, but not beta, adrenergic actions. There is a dense noradrenergic innervation in the medulla of nuclei which control the autonomic nervous system and cranial nerve nuclei, e.g. solitary

Table 2.1 Comparison of neurotransmitter amines.

Effect	Noradrenaline	Acetylcholine	5HT	Dopamine	Histamine	Melatonin
Promotes	Wakefulness	Wakefulness, REM	NREM	—	Wakefulness	NREM
Inhibits	REM	—	REM	—	REM	—
Other actions	Influences mood and behaviour	Motor inhibition in REM	Influences mood, behaviour and motor control	Influences thoughts, emotions, behaviour and motor control	—	Regulates circadian rhythms and immune function

NREM, non-rapid eye movement; REM, rapid eye movement.

tract nucleus. Neurones in and close to the locus coeruleus release noradrenaline. They inhibit REM sleep through their action on the PPN/LDT nuclei and promote wakefulness through effects on the posterior hypothalamus, thalamus and cerebral cortex. They also reach the limbic system and may influence mood and behaviour.

Acetylcholine

Cholinergic neurones are concentrated in the reticular formation, particularly in cells arising from the PPN/LDT nuclei which promote REM sleep and wakefulness through their ability to induce thalamocortical desynchronization. These neurones also lead to the loss of muscle activity in REM sleep and connect to the hypothalamus, thalamus and basal forebrain. Acetylcholine is involved in movement control in the basal ganglia where its action appears to be opposite to dopamine. Its effects on wakefulness are antagonized by adenosine.

5-Hydroxytryptamine (5HT, serotonin)

This is synthesized through L-tryptophan to 5-hydroxytryptophan and then to 5-hydroxytryptamine (5HT). 5HT 1 receptors are particularly important, but there are also 5HT 2 and 3 receptors. In general, 5HT reduces REM sleep and increases NREM sleep. Cells in the DRN release 5HT with nitric oxide as a cotransmitter and interact with the PPN/LDT nuclei to inhibit REM sleep. 5HT releasing neurones also control mood and behaviour, motor control, feeding, thermoregulation and may be involved in hallucinatory states generated from the brain-stem and with cataplexy seen in narcolepsy. 5HT secreting axons descend from the brainstem to the medulla and spinal cord.

Dopamine

This is synthesized by phenylalanine being converted to L-tyrosine and then to L-dopa which is converted to dopamine which can then be metabolized to noradrenaline and then to adrenaline. Dopamine acts on D1 and D2 receptors within the central nervous system (CNS), but there are also D3 receptors which are located in the mesolimbic pathways associated with cognitive and emotional function.

Dopamine is not thought to have any direct effect on sleep or wakefulness. It is mainly located in the basal ganglia which regulate movements of the skeletal muscles and which link to the cerebral cortex including the limbic cortex, and influence cognitive, emotional and reward behaviour. Dopaminergic fibres are involved in endocrine control within the hypothalamus and pituitary and in the response of the carotid body to increase ventilation in response to hypoxia.

Histamine

There are H1, H2 and H3 receptors within the CNS. Histamine appears to inhibit REM sleep generation by the PPN/LDT nuclei and to promote wakefulness and arousal. Histamine is released from neurones in the tubero-mammillary nucleus of the posterior hypothalamus which project widely to the thalamus and cerebral cortex.

Melatonin

Melatonin (N-5-methoxytryptamine) is synthesized from trytophan after it has been converted to 5HT [6]. Its synthesis can be increased by oral tryptophan or vitamin B6, a coenzyme in tryptophan metabolism. Little melatonin is stored in the pineal gland, but it is synthesized and secreted in pulses in response to noradrenaline release at synapses within the pineal. Its release is increased by selective serotonin re-uptake inhibitor (SSRI) antidepressants and antipsychotic drugs, but is inhibited by caffeine, beta blockers, benzodiazepines and non-steroidal anti-inflammatory drugs. It is also produced in the retina and gastro-intestinal tract.

Without any exposure to light the endogenous rhythm of the SCN leads to a circadian rhythm of melatonin secretion of around 24.2 h by the pineal gland. Melatonin is a marker of the circadian clock function, but it also acts as a hormone of darkness to reinforce the synchronization of sleep with the light–dark cycle of the environment. The pineal gland in effect acts as a transducer, converting a photo-period signal into a chemical signal.

Melatonin secretion starts shortly before darkness, usually after around 9.00 PM, but its rhythm can be modified by the following.

LIGHT EXPOSURE
Light exposure can phase advance or delay melatonin secretion. Light exposure in the evening delays melatonin secretion and darkness in the morning prolongs it and helps maintain sleep. This mechanism underlies the phase response curve of the circadian sleep rhythm to light. Regular light–dark cycles probably entrain melatonin secretion by altering the duration for which it is synthesized each night.

A brief light stimulus at night also inhibits melatonin secretion temporarily. Complete suppression requires more than 1000 lux for more than 2 h, but as little as 100 lux may halve melatonin secretion.

AGE
Under the age of 3 months little melatonin is secreted and there is no variation with light exposure. A nocturnal secretion pattern then emerges and the peak nocturnal concentration rises to around 1400 pmol/l at around the age of 3 years. This then declines, especially during puberty, to a level which is then maintained until around 40 years of age before it falls further. The peak nocturnal level in adults is reached between 2.00 and 4.00 AM and is 250–500 pmol/l. A total of 30 μg is usually secreted in each circadian cycle, but melatonin is often undetectable (less than 40 pmol/l) during the day. The peak melatonin level is reached 1 h before the transition point of the phase response curve to light (3.00–5.00 AM). Exposure to light early in the morning induces an earlier onset of melatonin secretion the next evening, but exposure to bright light in the evening delays the onset of melatonin secretion.

Melatonin is lipid soluble and is released both into the cerebrospinal fluid and blood so that it becomes widely distributed within the brain and the rest of the body, to which it acts as an indirect chemical messenger of the SCN. The concentration in the periventricular areas of the brain, which are exposed to the cerebrospinal fluid, may be very much higher than the blood levels. It has a half-life of 30–45 min in the blood and is mainly inactivated in the liver by conversion to 6-hydroxymelatonin and then conjugated with sulphuric or glucuronic acid. These metabolites are excreted in the urine, particularly 6-sulphatoxymelatonin whose concentration runs in parallel, but with a delay of around 2 h, with the serum melatonin concentration.

The effects of melatonin have not been fully clarified (Fig. 2.10). The cells in the core of the SCN contain mel1a receptors. Mel1b receptors are located in the retina and brain, especially the pars tuberalis of the pituitary gland suggesting that it may have a role in hormone control. Melatonin binds to calmodulin within the cells, but the details of its biochemical actions are unclear.

Melatonin appears to have two effects on the SCN which are mediated either by a direct effect on the

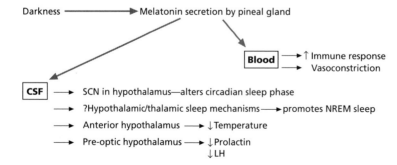

Fig. 2.10 Effects of melatonin secretion. CSF, cerebrospinal fluid; LH, luteinizing hormone; NREM, non-rapid eye movement; SCN, suprachiasmatic nuclei.

Table 2.2 Effects of amino acid and other neurotransmitters on sleep.

	Wake promotion	NREM sleep promotion	REM sleep inhibition
	PGE2	GABA	GABA
		PGD2	
		Adenosine	
		?Nitric oxide	

GABA, gamma-aminobutyric acid; NREM, non-rapid eye movement; PGD2, prostaglandin D2; PGE2, prostaglandin E2; REM, rapid eye movement.

circadian rhythm generating cells or by activation of GABA-ergic neurones within the SCN which inhibit its activity. Firstly, it modifies the timing of its circadian rhythms and reduces the body temperature, predisposing towards NREM rather than REM sleep and influencing the timing of sleep. This action is greatest in the evening when the circadian drive to wakefulness is strongest. It causes a phase advance of the sleep pattern with opening of the 'gate' for sleep through loss of the normal 'forbidden zone' for sleep shortly before the usual sleep time which is due to the strong wakefulness drive. Secondly, melatonin may synchronize other circadian rhythms, such as temperature and cortisol secretion, either through an action on the SCN or directly on the centres controlling these rhythms. The sleep and temperature rhythms, for instance, can be dissociated either because of incoordination of subpopulations of cells in the SCN which control the two rhythms or through divergences in the mechanisms controlling them outside the SCN.

Melatonin also has a soporific effect which is independent of its actions on the SCN and which is greatest during the day. This may be through a direct action on the sleep mechanisms, perhaps in the thalamus or hypothalamus. Its effect is probably mediated by activation of inhibitory GABA-ergic neurones, possibly through the action of cytokines. It does not appear to alter the proportions of NREM and REM sleep, but if given during the day usually leads to stages 1 and 2 NREM sleep.

Melatonin is a vasoconstrictor, has a mild anticonvulsant action and modifies reproductive function, including reducing prolactin and LH levels and delaying puberty. The fall in its serum concentration at puberty may enable sexual development to take place. The steadily changing seasonal duration of exposure to light alters the duration for which melatonin is secreted each night. This may influence reproductive

activity although humans are less sensitive to this photoperiod signal than many animals which have well defined seasonal reproductive cycles.

Melatonin has an important influence on immune function which is shown by the immunosuppression and changes in the thymus that follow resection of the pineal gland which secretes melatonin. Its influences are:

1 augmentation of natural killer (NK) cell activity in killing tumour and virus infected cells;
2 binding to T-lymphocytes, especially CD4+, and augmenting T-helper cell activity increasing their production of interferon gamma and interleukin-1 (IL-1), and release of IL-2;
3 increasing antibody responses, probably by augmenting T-helper cell function;
4 preventing apoptosis of T-lymphocytes; and
5 antagonizing corticosteroid-induced immunosuppression, probably through its effects on cytokine availability.

Amino acids

The importance of these chemicals as neurotransmitters has probably been underestimated (Table 2.2). They fall into two groups.

EXCITATORY

Glutamate

Glutamate is the main excitatory neurotransmitter in the CNS. It is located particularly in the brain-stem where it interacts with the PPN/LDT nuclei. It is also the transmitter of the thalamocortical projection fibres which are responsible for synchronizing cortical activity during NREM sleep.

Aspartate

The role of this excitatory neurotransmitter in sleep–wake control is uncertain.

NREM promotion	NREM inhibition	REM promotion	REM inhibition
GHRH	Nil known	Somatostatin	Opioids
DSIP		VIP	IL-1
CCK		Prolactin	TNF-α
Insulin			
IL-1			
TNF-α			
IFN			

Table 2.3 Effects of peptide neurotransmitters on sleep.

CCK, cholecystokinin; DSIP, delta sleep inducing peptide; GHRH, growth hormone releasing hormone; IFN, interferons; IL-1, interleukin-1; TNF-α, tumour necrosis factor alpha.

INHIBITORY

Gamma aminobutyric acid
This is synthesized from glutamate, and both $GABA_A$ and $GABA_B$ receptors are present, particularly in the brain-stem reticular formation, basal ganglia, hypothalamus and thalamus. It is the most important neurotransmitter in the reticular formation and is present in over 30% of synapses within the CNS. It is secreted by SCN neurones and in the thalamus it influences sensory transmission and appears to have an opposite action to glutamate. In general, GABA promotes NREM sleep, possibly by inhibiting the locus coeruleus, and inhibits REM possibly through its action on the PPN/LDT nuclei.

Glycine
This is located mainly in the brain-stem and spinal cord, but its role in sleep–wake control is uncertain.

Taurine
This is one of the most widely distributed amino acids in the brain and its postsynaptic inhibitory action is blocked by strychnine, a CNS stimulant.

Peptides
This important group of chemicals includes most of the sleep factors and cytokines which, like melatonin, also have an important influence on the immune response (Table 2.3).

GROWTH HORMONE AND RELATED COMPOUNDS
Growth hormone releasing hormone (GHRH) is a peptide produced in the hypothalamus which increases growth hormone synthesis. Somatostatin regulates the timing of its release. Growth hormone releasing hormone promotes NREM sleep and growth hormone is produced mainly in the first cycle of stages 3 and 4 NREM sleep, although its secretion may precede sleep. The effects of GHRH may be mediated by its release at synapses in the basal forebrain from neurones projecting to the median eminence. Somatostatin can promote REM sleep. Corticotrophin-releasing factor (CRF), adrenocorticotropin hormone (ACTH), glucocorticoids and alpha melanocyte stimulating hormone (α MSH) all inhibit sleep.

VASOACTIVE INTESTINAL PEPTIDE AND PROLACTIN
Vaso-active intestinal peptide-containing neurones are present in the core of the SCN and elsewhere in the hypothalamus, where they project to the median eminence where VIP acts as a releasing factor for prolactin. Prolactin secretion increases slightly in the first sleep cycle, although larger pulses are secreted in the second half of the night. Vaso-active intestinal peptide increases REM sleep and prolactin has a similar effect.

DELTA SLEEP INDUCING PEPTIDE
Delta sleep inducing peptide (DSIP) increases NREM sleep and may inhibit secretion of ACTH.

CHOLECYSTOKININ AND INSULIN
Cholecystokinin is secreted as a 33-amino acid peptide (CCK33) from the duodenum and jejunum. It stimulates pancreatic enzyme secretion and gall bladder contraction. It is also present in the CNS as an 8-amino acid peptide (CCK8) fragment of CCK33 and both these types of CCK induce NREM sleep, reduce motor activity and mediate satiety after food

intake. The drowsiness that often follows eating is partially due to CCK, but also to the release of insulin as the blood glucose level rises. Insulin promotes NREM sleep but does not affect REM. Non-rapid eye movement sleep is often reduced in duration in diabetes mellitus.

Cholecystokinin-8 is present in the reticular formation, for instance, in the DRN and in the hypothalamus. It is an excitatory neurotransmitter, usually acting as a cotransmitter either with 5HT, as in the DRN, or elsewhere with dopamine.

OPIOID PEPTIDES
These interact with endorphins, enkephalins and dynorphins, which are located particularly in the medulla, hypothalamus, thalamus, basal ganglia and limbic system. They tend to inhibit REM sleep partly through their action on the PPN/LDT nuclei.

SUBSTANCE P
This peptide is released at 40% of the synapses with PPN/LDT neurones. Its role in sleep is unknown but may be related to control of sensory transmission through the brain-stem.

CYTOKINES
These are peptides which are chemically similar to peptide hormones such as growth hormone, but are produced by helper T-lymphocytes and other cells including microglia in the brain in response to a specific stimulus. They modify the immune response and within the brain act on nearby cells. Several of the cytokines are recognized to act as sleep factors.

Interleukin-1
This is produced in the hypothalamus and other areas of the brain in response to endotoxin, tumour necrosis factor alpha (TNF-α) and muramyl peptides derived from peptidoglycans in bacterial cell walls. Their production is inhibited by prostaglandin E2 (PGE2) and glucocorticoids, both of which inhibit sleep. Interleukin-1 increases the duration of NREM sleep through an action on the anterior hypothalamus and slightly inhibits REM sleep. These actions may be mediated by IL-1's augmentation of GABA receptor function and its ability to increase GHRH secretion. They are inhibited by corticotrophin releasing factor (CRF) and alpha melanocyte stimulating hormone (MSH). Interleukin-1 is also a neuronal growth factor, acts as a pyrogen to raise the body temperature,

controls CRF release, has immunological effects, and blocks the metabolism of anandamide, the receptor for tetradihydrocannabinol.

Other interleukins such as IL-2 and IL-6 have little or no effect on sleep.

Tumour necrosis factor alpha
This cytokine, which is produced by macrophages is released mainly at night, increases stages 3 and 4 NREM sleep and reduces REM sleep.

Interferons
Interferons (IFN) such as IFN alpha 2 are produced by leucocytes in response particularly to viral infections and enable phagocytes to kill infected cells. The peak gamma interferon level is seen at around 10.00 PM with the minimum at 6.00 AM. Interferons increase NREM sleep.

Neurotrophin-2
This cytokine acts as a sleep and growth factor, enhancing the development and activity of GABA-releasing neurones. Its production and release are increased by acetylcholine and glutamate.

HYPOCRETINS
Hypocretins (orexins) are peptides which are widely distributed in the CNS especially in the hypothalamus and its projections to, for instance, the cerebral cortex, thalamus and reticular activating system. A prehypocretin protein is split to form two related peptides, hypocretin 1 and 2 (orexin A and B) which are located in the synaptic vesicles. These are excitatory neurotransmitters with specific receptors and which appear to interact with noradrenaline, dopamine and acetylcholine. Hypocretins may limit the duration of REM sleep and genetically determined abnormalities in hypocretins or their receptors may contribute to the development of narcolepsy.

Other neurotransmitters

PROSTAGLANDINS
Prostaglandins are polyunsaturated fatty acids with a 5-carbon ring structure. Prostaglandin D2 (PGD2) acts in or near the ventrolateral preoptic area of the hypothalamus to induce sleep and reduce body temperature, whereas PGE2 acts in or near the posterior hypothalamus to promote wakefulness and raise body temperature. The prostaglandins are fatty acids and PGE2 inhibits IL-1 production.

ADENOSINE

This is a nucleoside which is produced from adenosine triphosphate (ATP) and adenosine diphosphate (ADP) and is converted into inosine and then to hypoxanthine. It promotes NREM sleep, especially stages 3 and 4, and its action is antagonized at A1 receptors by xanthines. It is present in the basal forebrain where its concentration rises during wakefulness and falls during NREM sleep. It appears to inhibit the ventrolateral preoptic nuclei as well as the locus coeruleus and these effects may be important factors in determining the homeostatic sleep drive.

NITRIC OXIDE

This is a cotransmitter with 5HT in the dorsal raphe nuclei, and is unusual in that it spreads from the point of its release to influence and coordinate neuronal function over a wide region. It is able to alter the intrinsic rhythm of the SCN. It is also a vasodilator and probably integrates local cerebral blood flow with the neuronal activity.

References

1 Johns M. Rethinking the assessment of sleepiness. *Sleep Med Rev* 1998; 2: 3–15.
2 Cajochen C, Krauchi K, Danilenko KV, Wirz-Justice A. Evening administration of melatonin and bright light: interactions on the EEG during sleep and wakefulness. *J Sleep Res* 1998; 7: 145–57.
3 Gronfier C, Brandenberger G. Ultradian rhythms in pituitary and adrenal hormones: their relations to sleep. *Sleep Med Rev* 1998; 2: 17–29.
4 Huguenard JR. Anatomical and physiological considerations in thalamic rhythm generation. *J Sleep Res* 1998; 7 (Suppl. 1): 24–9.
5 Rye DB. Contributions of the pedunculopontine region to normal and altered REM sleep. *Sleep* 1997; 20: 757–88.
6 Brzezinski A. Melatonin in humans. *N Engl J Med* 1997; 336: 186–95.

3 Drugs and Sleep

Introduction

The main indications for pharmacotherapy in sleep disorders are as follows.

1 To modify circadian rhythms.

2 To promote alertness and wakefulness (central nervous system (CNS) stimulants). The most frequent use is in excessive daytime sleepiness (EDS).

3 To promote and improve the quality of sleep (hypnotics). The most frequent use is in insomnia.

4 To treat the large group of sleep disorders which lead to abnormal awareness, autonomic and immunological activity and behaviour during sleep, usually by modifying the nature or duration of individual sleep stages.

Two other groups of drugs also have important effects on sleep although these are usually not the primary indication for their prescription.

1 Drugs used to treat psychiatric or neurological disorders. These are used to influence, for instance, mood or thought processes and behaviour (psychotropic drugs), but can have a profound effect on the state of wakefulness and sleep.

2 Drugs used for non-psychiatric or non-neurological disorders. Most of these agents affect sleep and wakefulness by altering neurotransmitter function within the brain.

In this chapter these major groups of drugs will be considered. No distinction is made between drugs that have a licence for medical disorders, 'over the counter' preparations, drugs in commonly used foods and drinks, socially used drugs such as alcohol and nicotine, or illicit (recreational) drugs such as lysergic acid diethylamide (LSD). The aims are to:

1 describe the principles of action of each class of drug;

2 give examples of important individual drugs;

3 highlight the advantages and disadvantages of each drug; and

4 provide a brief indication of the use of the drugs in sleep disorders.

Details are given in the later chapters regarding the use and effectiveness of the drugs in individual sleep disorders. It is important to emphasize that drug treatment should only be used after the sleep disorder has been assessed and a working diagnosis made, and as part of the total management plan. Insomnia, for instance, may respond to analgesics or antidepressants to relieve pain or depression rather than to a hypnotic to promote sleep.

Circadian rhythm modifiers

Introduction

The range of drugs which can modify circadian rhythms is very limited. Melatonin is the only one that has a significant effect that is sustained. The lack of available drugs is unfortunate since disorders of circadian rhythms are frequent, especially those due to shift work, and effective treatment could have widespread application.

Antidepressants and hypnotics

Lithium and some monoamineoxidase inhibitors (MAOIs) delay the sleep phase. Short-acting benzodiazepines can entrain the circadian rhythm, but usually only for a few days. These drugs are rarely prescribed for the primary purpose of altering circadian rhythms.

Melatonin

Melatonin is produced in the pineal gland and its effects are described in Chapter 2. This section is restricted to the administration of exogenous melatonin.

PHARMACOLOGY

Melatonin is rapidly absorbed from the gastrointestinal tract and the peak plasma concentration is reached within around 60 min. It has a half life of 30–45 min. It is lipid soluble and therefore enters most tissues, including the brain. It is inactivated in the liver.

EFFECTS ON SLEEP

Melatonin has two effects on sleep.

Sleep-phase alteration

Endogenous melatonin is secreted in the absence of light exposure and influences the timing of the suprachiasmatic nuclei (SCN). Exogenous melatonin has an identical action and acts on the circadian sleep rhythm like an episode of darkness. It advances the next phase of sleep and of endogenous melatonin secretion. This effect is greatest late in the evening. It causes a delay of the next sleep phase if it is taken late in the night or in the early morning since the exogenous melatonin is superimposed on the endogenous secretion. Exogenous melatonin taken in the middle of the day retains its soporific effect, but has little influence over circadian rhythms or the total sleep time.

Hypnotic effect

It is a mild hypnotic when given in the day at the time when endogenous melatonin levels are low. This effect is detectable within 1 h of administration, lasts for 1–2 h and is dose related. Melatonin also causes a fall in body temperature. This is usually associated with sleep onset, but its soporific effect is present before any change in body temperature, suggesting that this has a different mechanism.

OTHER ACTIONS AND SIDE-EFFECTS

Melatonin is a vasoconstrictor, has a slight hypotensive effect, and inhibits reproduction. Daytime sedation is not a problem with melatonin administered in the evening.

PROBLEMS WITH USE

Preparations of melatonin

The availability of melatonin varies between countries. It is taken regularly by several million people in the USA where it is classed as a nutritive or dietary supplement. This does not require review of the quality of the preparations by the Food and Drug Administration (FDA) and one study showed that one third of the brands contained no melatonin and in 75% there was significantly less than advertised. Most melatonin is synthesized, but some is prepared from bovine pineal glands.

Uncertainty about dose

The recommended dose of melatonin ranges from 0.1 mg to 5 or 10 mg daily [1]. Doses up to 0.5 mg give plasma levels similar to those generated by endogenous secretion and 1–5 mg give blood levels around 10–100 times the physiological values. Only 0.03 mg is normally secreted every 24 h, but these high doses may be needed to elevate cerebrospinal fluid and brain tissue concentrations to physiological levels. A dose of around 0.5 mg appears to be sufficient to entrain the circadian rhythm when taken on a regular basis, but 5 mg is probably more effective in making acute changes to the sleep phase. This dose may also increase the total sleep time slightly.

Lack of data

There is little data regarding the safety or efficacy either in the short-term or with long-term use of melatonin, probably because of its variable status as a drug in different countries.

Drug interactions

There are no known drug interactions with exogenous melatonin, but its effect also depends on the endogenous secretion which can be increased by selective serotonin re-uptake inhibitor (SSRI) antidepressants and antipsychotic drugs and reduced by beta blockers, benzodiazepines and nonsteroidal anti-inflammatory drugs.

Effects on reproduction

Melatonin is recognized to affect reproduction, inhibiting ovarian function and reducing prolactin and luteinizing hormone (LH) levels. The importance of these effects is uncertain, but because of them it should be avoided in children, women wishing to conceive and whilst breastfeeding.

Effects on inflammation

Melatonin enhances the immune response and although there is little data regarding this it should be avoided in autoimmune diseases which may deteriorate during melatonin treatment.

INDICATIONS IN SLEEP DISORDERS

Some of the claims for the efficacy of melatonin have been exaggerated and there have been few controlled studies, particularly of its long-term use. Different doses and timing of administration of melatonin have been used in these reports, and some of the results are conflicting.

It has two main indications as described below.

Chronobiological (chronobiotic) agent

This relies on its ability to reset the sleep phase. Its efficacy depends more on the timing than the size of the dose, although 5 mg is usually recommended initially. A fast release preparation is required to advance the sleep phase and is given 1–2 h before the time of the previous night's onset of sleep. It can be used in the short and long term.

Short-term. It accelerates the adaptations of the circadian rhythms to time zone changes causing jet lag. It should be taken in the evening before and after the flight on eastward travel in order to cause a phase advance, and in the morning with westward flights to delay sleep onset. Similar principles underly its use in shift workers and it may also be useful in re-establishing sleep patterns after withdrawal from drugs, such as alcohol and cocaine.

Long-term. Melatonin can promote more regular sleep–wake cycles in those who are blind and experience insomnia or EDS due to the failure to entrain their circadian rhythms to environmental light exposure. It can also be used to advance the sleep phase when it is taken in the evening in the delayed sleep-phase syndrome and retard sleep when it is taken in the morning in the advanced sleep-phase syndrome. Disorders of the pineal gland, such as pineal tumours, are usually associated with low endogenous melatonin secretion, and melatonin administration may be of benefit, acting as a hormone replacement or supplement treatment.

Hypnotic
Melatonin is a weak hypnotic, but can cause sleepiness during the day. It may have a use in treating the early morning wakening (EMW) pattern of insomnia when there is a deficient secretion of endogenous melatonin. Sustained release preparations may be effective in the elderly, in whom melatonin levels are often low, and has been proposed for treating EMW in depression.

Melatonin agonists
Several melatonin agonists are being developed, but are not yet available for clinical use. They have the potential advantages over melatonin of higher standards of preparation and of confidence in their purity, that they will have undergone superior safety and efficacy studies, and that their dose ranges would have been better established. Their potential physiological advantages over melatonin may be a longer half-life, increased bio-availability and lack of a vasoconstrictor effect.

Central nervous system stimulants
Introduction
The most commonly taken CNS stimulants to combat EDS are caffeine and nicotine which are usually self administered. Of the prescribed drugs, amphetamines, which have been available since around 1930, have been the most widely used. The ideal drug would have a completely selective action on the CNS so that it only increased alertness and reduced sleep. None of the stimulants are this specific. They all influence other aspects of neurological function, particularly the older drugs such as strychnine and ephedrine which are now hardly ever prescribed for EDS. Caffeine, the amphetamines and related drugs also have several unwanted effects due to generalized CNS stimulation, but modafinil is more specific in promoting wakefulness.

The use of CNS stimulants is also limited by the risk of drug dependency, withdrawal symptoms, tolerance, side-effects, drug interactions and the dangers of overdose. The risks of each of these unwanted effects varies between the different drugs. The issues that determine the choice of stimulant are discussed in detail in Chapter 6.

Caffeine and other xanthines
PHARMACOLOGY
Xanthines are alkaloids and while caffeine (1, 3, 7-trimethylxanthine) is a trimethylxanthine, theophylline and theobromine are dimethylxanthines. They are all well absorbed from the gastrointestinal tract. The peak blood level of caffeine is reached 30–60 min after ingestion. It has a plasma half-life of 3–4 h although there is considerable interindividual variability. It is prolonged in pregnancy and with the oral contraceptive pill. It crosses the placenta, enters breast milk and readily crosses the blood–brain barrier to reach the CNS. It is metabolized in the liver by microsomal enzymes and its metabolites are excreted in the urine. One of these, paraxanthine, can be detected in the serum and can be used as marker of caffeine intake.

DOSE
The usual dose of caffeine in tablet form is 50–200 mg. Caffeine is a constituent of a wide range of food and drinks, such as tea, coffee, cola and other soft drinks, drinking chocolate and cocoa, and is also present in many analgesic preparations, appetite suppressants and tonics. The quantity of caffeine in some of these preparations is shown in Table 3.1.

Table 3.1 Doses of caffeine in food and drinks.

Food and drink	Quantity	Caffeine (mg)
Tea	1 cup (150 ml)	25–50
Instant coffee	1 cup (150 ml)	60–80
Brewed or percolated coffee	1 cup (150 ml)	100–150
Decaffeinated coffee	1 cup (150 ml)	3
Cocoa	1 cup (150 ml)	15
Cola drink	330 ml	40–60
Plain chocolate	100 g	40
Milk chocolate	100 g	15
White chocolate	100 g	0

MECHANISMS OF ACTION

Xanthines competitively inhibit phosphodiesterase which degrades cyclic 3–5 AMP (adenosine mono-phosphate) and thereby increases its intracellular concentration. They act as antagonists at adenosine receptors within the CNS, and thereby stimulate it at all levels, especially the higher centres. In high doses xanthines also stimulate the medullary vagal, vaso-motor, and respiratory centres.

Caffeine has a greater effect on the CNS and skeletal muscle than other xanthines, but other drugs in this group such as aminophylline, theophylline and theobromine (which is present in cocoa) have greater effects on other systems.

EFFECTS ON SLEEP

Caffeine and other xanthines reduce the total sleep time, increase the sleep latency, reduce the duration of stages 3 and 4 non-rapid eye movement (NREM) sleep and of rapid eye movement (REM) sleep [2]. They cause insomnia, particularly if they are taken in the evening, by the elderly, or if the total daily dose is greater than 500 mg. This may worsen daytime sleepiness so that more caffeine is taken which worsens the insomnia.

EFFECTS ON WAKEFULNESS

They increase mental activity, improve attention and vigilance and performance of complex logical mental tasks, especially if the subject is fatigued. They do not improve mental function requiring originality, but increase psychomotor coordination, except in high doses, or if they have caused sleep deprivation or anxiety.

OTHER ACTIONS AND SIDE-EFFECTS

1 Respiratory effects. Theophylline is a respiratory stimulant and bronchodilator.
2 Diuresis. This is due to an increase in the renal blood flow and glomerular filtration rate.
3 Tachycardia, cardiac dysrhythmias and hypertension.
4 Nausea, vomiting, abdominal pain and gastro-oesophageal reflux.
5 Tremor and muscle twitching.

PROBLEMS WITH USE

1 Tolerance to CNS effects.
2 Withdrawal symptoms. Withdrawal may cause headaches, irritability, anxiety and dizziness.
3 Drug interactions. Smoking and drugs that induce microsomal enzymes in the liver, such as phenytoin, increase the clearance of caffeine and reduce its half-life.
4 Insomnia.

INDICATIONS IN SLEEP DISORDERS

Excessive daytime sleepiness

Caffeine is a moderately effective CNS stimulant which is widely available and is frequently used to relieve EDS due to sleep deprivation, irregular sleep–wake patterns, shift work, jet lag and to prevent and relieve sleepiness during driving. The alerting effect of 500 mg caffeine is approximately equivalent to 5 mg dexamphetamine. It is usually ineffective in EDS due to primary neurological disorders, such as narcolepsy and idiopathic central nervous system hypersomnia (ICNSH).

Central sleep apnoeas and Cheyne–Stokes respiration

Aminophylline 225–450 mg bd is the most effective of the xanthines for these conditions.

Nocturnal asthma

Theophylline or aminophylline, which is metabolized to theophylline, are effective bronchodilators. Sleep fragmentation due to nocturnal asthma is reduced, but the stimulant effect of these drugs may cause insomnia.

Nicotine

PHARMACOLOGY

Nicotine is a pyridine alkaloid which is rapidly absorbed when inhaled or chewed. Approximately 1 mg is absorbed from smoking each cigarette. It has a half-life of 1–2 h.

MECHANISMS OF ACTION

Nicotine acts on nicotinic cholinergic receptors in autonomic ganglia, at the neuromuscular junction and within the CNS. In low doses it is excitatory at nicotinic synapses but in higher doses it inhibits these receptors.

EFFECTS ON SLEEP

There has been surprisingly little research into the effects of nicotine on sleep, but it reduces the total sleep-time, increases sleep latency, reduces sleep efficiency and the duration of REM sleep.

EFFECTS ON WAKEFULNESS

Nicotine in a low dose leads to mental relaxation, is a mild sedative and promotes sleep, but in higher doses it increases arousal and may cause agitation. It can improve motor performance, but commonly causes muscle tremors and in overdose leads to dizziness, fits and delirium.

OTHER ACTIONS AND SIDE-EFFECTS

1 Loss of appetite and nausea.
2 Tachycardia.

PROBLEMS WITH USE

1 Tolerance.
2 Withdrawal symptoms. Nicotine is addictive and its withdrawal may cause irritability and insomnia.

INDICATIONS IN SLEEP DISORDERS

Nicotine can promote sleep but smokers commonly have fragmented sleep possibly due to the stimulant effect of nicotine, or to regular nicotine withdrawal effects each night. Nicotine reduces the total sleep time and is a mild stimulant in higher doses. Nicotine is rarely prescribed for EDS, but is usually taken in tobacco or occasionally as a gum or skin patches.

Glucocorticoids

These increase alertness and motor activity in the day and reduce the total sleep time, increase the number of awakenings from sleep, especially NREM, and may slightly reduce the duration of REM sleep and increase the duration of stage 2 NREM sleep. These effects are probably mediated through interactions with cytokines.

Glucocorticoids are rarely specifically prescribed as CNS stimulants and occasionally cause depression or a steroid psychosis which, when it occurs, is dose related. The insomnia that they cause is usually well tolerated because of the increased alertness and hyperactivity that compensates for it.

Strychnine

Strychnine is an alkaloid extracted from the seeds of *Strychnos nux-vomica*. It was the most commonly prescribed drug in the UK until the early 1920s and was used as a 'tonic' to improve alertness, sensory acuity and wakefulness. It has fallen out of use and is almost never prescribed. It abolishes CNS inhibitory postsynaptic potentials due to the release of taurine as a neurotransmitter and thereby reduces inhibition of reflexes. In overdose it causes muscle spasms, fits and death, although these actions can be antagonized by barbiturates. It has a poor toxic to therapeutic ratio and is usually fatal in a dose of 60–90 mg.

Sympathomimetics

These include adrenaline (epinephrine) and ephedrine. They reduce the duration of sleep and improve alertness, but also cause tachycardia, hypertension, anxiety and tremor. Ephedrine in a dose of 30–60 mg orally, 2–4 hourly was used to treat narcolepsy before amphetamines became available, but it is now rarely prescribed because of its side-effects.

Pemoline

This stimulant is structurally unrelated to amphetamines. It has a long half-life of 9–14 h and its clinical effects last for 8–10 h. Sixty per cent of pemoline is metabolized in the liver and 40% excreted unchanged in the urine. The usual dose is 40–120 mg. It increases mental alertness, has a mild euphoric action and increases motor activity, possibly through its action as a dopamine agonist. It causes relatively little peripheral nervous system stimulation, but can lead to insomnia and is an effective appetite suppressant. A rise in the liver enzymes is common and acute liver necrosis, which may be fatal, occasionally occurs. This has led to its virtual withdrawal from the UK market, although it is effective in treating mild and moderate daytime sleepiness.

Mazindol

This is an imidazole derivative which differs chemically from the amphetamines. It is readily absorbed, has an onset of action within 30–60 min and its peak effect is at around 2 h. It is excreted in the urine. The usual dose is 2–12 mg daily given either as one or two doses. Two milligrams are equivalent in effectiveness to around 10 mg dexamphetamine.

Its mechanism of action is uncertain, but it may inhibit noradrenaline and dopamine re-uptake, particularly in the limbic system. It has little effect on total sleep time, but reduces REM sleep. It increases alertness and may cause insomnia, but not euphoria. Loss of appetite, nausea, abdominal pain, constipation, hypertension, tremor and urinary retention may occur. Tolerance and abuse are also recognized.

Mazindol is an effective stimulant but its side-effects and lack of availability have limited its use.

Selegiline

This is a selective, irreversible inhibitor of monoamine oxidase type B which is responsible for dopamine catabolism. It therefore increases dopamine levels, particularly in the thalamus and brainstem, but its stimulant action is probably mainly due to its metabolism to levo-amphetamine and levo-metamphetamine. It does not have an antidepressant effect because of its lack of type A action. It has been used as a stimulant in narcolepsy in a dose of 10 mg daily, but may provoke vivid dreams and hallucinations. It should not be used in conjunction with an SSRI antidepressant.

Amphetamines and related drugs

PHARMACOLOGY

Amphetamines are well absorbed through the gastrointestinal tract. Approximately 50% is hydroxylated in the liver and oxidized to benzoic acid, and 50% excreted in the urine as glucuroxide or glycine conjugates.

MECHANISMS OF ACTION

All the amphetamines enhance activity at dopamine, noradrenaline and 5HT synapses. They cause pre-synaptic release of preformed transmitters, and also inhibit the re-uptake of dopamine and noradrenaline. These actions are most prominent in the brain-stem reticular activating system and the cerebral cortex. Amphetamines also cause release of noradrenaline from peripheral nerve terminals which leads directly to enhanced sympathetic activity. The alerting effects of amphetamines are probably due either to noradrenaline or 5HT release or to both of these. Their effects on motor function are probably mainly due to potentiation of dopamine activity in the basal ganglia and limbic cortex, but their action in relieving cataplexy may be due to the enhancement of 5HT (Table 3.2).

INDIVIDUAL DRUGS

Amphetamines are listed under Schedule 2 of the Misuse of Drugs Act 1971, and prescriptions have to comply with controlled drug requirements. The most important individual drugs are as follows.

Amphetamine

This was the first amphetamine to be used clinically. It is a racemic mixture of dextro- and levo-amphetamines. It has relatively more central than peripheral action than ephedrine, but fewer central and more peripheral action than dexamphetamine. Dose 5–60 mg daily.

Dexamphetamine

This is the dextro- or d-isomer of amphetamine and is three to four times more potent than levo-

Table 3.2 Effects of CNS stimulants on neurotransmitters.

Drug	Noradrenaline	Acetylcholine	5HT	Dopamine	GABA	Adenosine	Cytokines	Taurine
Caffeine	–	–	–	–	–	†	–	–
Nicotine	–	*low dose	–	–	–	–	–	–
	–	†high dose						
Glucocorticoids	–	–	–	–	–	–	†	–
Strychnine	–	–	–	–	–	–	–	†
Sympathomimetics	*	–	–	–	–	–	–	–
Pemoline	–	–	–	*	–	–	–	–
Mazindol	*	–	–	*	–	–	–	–
Selegiline	*	–	*	*	–	–	–	–
Amphetamines and related drugs	*	–	*	*	–	–	–	–
Modafinil	–	–	–	–	†	–	–	–

* promotes action of neurotransmitter; † inhibits action of neurotransmitter; 5HT, 5-hydroxytryptamine; GABA, gamma-aminobutyric acid.

amphetamine. The peak blood level is reached around 2 h after ingestion. It has a half-life of 8–12 h and a duration of action of 6–10 h. Dose 5–60 mg daily usually taken in two to three divided doses.

Levo-amphetamine
This has no clinical advantage over dexamphetamine. Dose 20–60 mg daily.

Metamphetamine
This is the most rapidly absorbed amphetamine. Its peak blood level is reached 1 h after ingestion and it has a half-life of 12 h. It has more peripheral actions than dexamphetamine and is rarely used clinically. It is subject to drug abuse and known as methedrine and speed. Dose 5–15 mg daily.

Methylphenidate
This is a piperidine derivative which is structurally similar to amphetamine. It is rapidly absorbed and is de-esterified to an inactive metabolite, ritalinic acid, in the liver and is then excreted in the urine. Its peak blood level is reached within 1–2 h. It has a half-life of 2–4 h and a clinical effect for 3–6 h. Dose 10–60 mg daily in three to four divided doses. It acts particularly on the thalamus and cerebral cortex, but causes more sympathetic side-effects than amphetamines.

Phenmetrazine
This drug is now rarely used, but can cause euphoria and psychosis. Dose 25–75 mg in one to three divided doses.

Cocaine
This is very similar structurally to methylphenidate. It potentiates the effects of noradrenaline and adrena-

line. It increases alertness, relieves fatigue, has a euphoric action and increases motor activity. It reduces the total sleep time, increases sleep latency and reduces both stages 3 and 4 NREM and REM sleep. In overdose it may lead to fits and delirium and chronic use causes sleep deprivation. Abrupt withdrawal leads to depression and prolonged sleep with REM sleep rebound, especially if it has been used in high dose for a prolonged time. Tolerance frequently develops and chronic use is associated with death from cardiac dysrhythmias, myocardial infarction and strokes.

Ecstasy
This is chemically related to metamphetamine. It is a stimulant, mood altering and hallucinogenic drug, which occasionally causes hyperpyrexia. It leads to a reduction in REM sleep and its use may be followed by depression.

EFFECTS ON SLEEP
Amphetamines reduce total sleep-time, increase sleep latency, slightly reduce the duration of stages 3 and 4 NREM sleep, increase REM latency and reduce the duration of REM sleep, often to as little as 10%. They cause sleep fragmentation and if taken late in the day cause difficulty in initiating sleep (DIS) (Table 3.3).

EFFECTS ON WAKEFULNESS
Amphetamines prolong wakefulness, increase the level of alertness, reduce the sense of fatigue, increase confidence, concentration and loquacity, increase the capacity for physical and mental activity, lead to euphoria and a sense of excitability. They improve psychomotor and mental performance for simple, but not complex tasks, particularly when fatigue is

Table 3.3 Effects of CNS stimulants on sleep.

Drug	TST	SL	Awakenings	1 and 2 NREM sleep	3 and 4 NREM sleep	REM sleep latency	REM sleep	Dreams
Caffeine	↓	↑	–	–	↓	–	↓	–
Nicotine	↓	↑	–	–	–	–	↓	↑
Glucocorticoids	↓	–	↑	↑	↓	–	Slightly ↓	–
Mazindol	0	–	–	–	–	–	↓	–
Amphetamines and related drugs	↓	↑	↑	–	Slightly ↓	↑	↓	–
Modafinil	↓	–	–	–	–	–	–	–

NREM, non-rapid eye movement; REM, rapid eye movement; SL, sleep latency; TST, total sleep time.

present. They can lead to agitation, aggression and occasionally to a paranoid psychosis, with auditory hallucinations, which is indistinguishable from schizophrenia. Depression and fatigue often follow the phase of psychic stimulation. The need to sleep usually returns suddenly as the amphetamine blood level is falling and this 'crash' is more profound with high doses of amphetamines.

OTHER ACTIONS AND SIDE-EFFECTS
1 Appetite suppression.
2 Respiratory stimulant.
3 Peripheral sympathetic and motor effects, including a rise in body temperature, tachycardia, palpitations, mild hypertension, nausea, vomiting, abdominal cramps, dry mouth, headaches and tremor. Hypertension may be severe, particularly during exertion, and lead to intracranial haemorrhage. Amphetamines should be avoided in those with hypertension, ischaemic heart disease and cardiac dysrhythmias, but have been used in these situations with betablockers to minimize the risks of sympathetic side-effects.
4 Growth retardation with prolonged treatment in children.

PROBLEMS WITH USE

Short duration of action
Amphetamines give quick relief from sleepiness, but the offset of their action is equally quick and patients frequently find this 'crash' and return of their symptoms unpleasant.

Tolerance
Around 30% of narcoleptics become tolerant to amphetamines, especially when doses above 60 mg daily of dexamphetamine are used. 'Drug holidays' which are spells of a few days off amphetamine treatment have been used to try to minimize tolerance to these drugs. There is little evidence that they help, and they may cause recurrent episodes of withdrawal symptoms.

Dependency
The euphoria of amphetamines has led to their widespread use and abuse. Withdrawal causes fatigue, depression, hypersomnia, an increase in appetite and occasionally paranoia and agitation. The total sleep time increases, and REM sleep rebound may be present for up to two months after cessation of amphetamines.

Table 3.4 Precautions with amphetamines.

Patient problems	Drug effects
Addictive personality	Tolerance
Psychiatric disorders	Dependency
Ischaemic heart disease	Overdose
Hypertension	Drug interactions
Children	Psychosis

Drug interactions
Amphetamines are metabolized by hepatic microsomal enzymes and any drug that influences these will alter the rate of their metabolism. Tricyclic and MAOI antidepressants inhibit their metabolism, potentiate their effects and require the amphetamine dose to be reduced by around one third. Beta blocking agents, such as propranolol, and lithium may antagonize the effects of amphetamines.

Overdose
This causes intense sympathetic nervous system stimulation with hypertension, tachycardia, hyperthermia and a toxic psychosis, often with paranoid delusions and violence accompanied by epileptic fits, and occasionally a stroke due to hypertension, particularly during exercise. Amphetamines cross the placenta, reach the fetus and also enter breast milk. They should be discontinued during pregnancy and while breast feeding.

INDICATIONS IN SLEEP DISORDERS
Amphetamines are effective stimulants, but their use is limited by their side-effects, abuse, potential tolerance and withdrawal symptoms (Table 3.4).

Excessive daytime sleepiness
Amphetamines have been used to relieve EDS due to unavoidable sleep restriction for social reasons, to increase performance at work and in competitive sport, both in humans and in animals (such as horses and greyhounds), but their medical indications are in treating the following.

Excessive daytime sleepiness due to central nervous system disorders. These include narcolepsy and ICNSH. Amphetamines are effective, but their short action leads to a rapid return of sleepiness. Little benefit is obtained by increasing the dose above 60 mg dexamphetamine daily, and tolerance to amphetamines occurs in around one third of subjects with narcolepsy. Their use is limited by side-effects, including psychoses and insomnia. There has been less experience of use of amphetamines in neurological disorders other than narcolepsy, but they are probably as effective as in ICNSH.

Excessive daytime sleepiness due to opiate treatment. Amphetamines may be of value through increasing wakefulness during treatment with opiates without antagonizing their analgesic action.

Cataplexy. Amphetamines have a mild anticataplectic action, possibly due to their effects on 5HT release, which is often useful in treating narcolepsy.

Modafinil

PHARMACOLOGY
Modafinil is well absorbed from the gastro-intestinal tract. The peak blood level is reached at 2–3 h, although this can be delayed by food. Its half-life is 10–12 h. It is metabolized in the liver to modafinil acid and sulphone, both of which are inactive. Ninety per cent of the drug is excreted through the kidneys in these forms and 10% as unchanged modafinil.

DOSE
The initial dose is 200 mg daily, often increasing to 400–600 mg daily. It is usually given twice daily with the larger dose on waking and a smaller dose in the middle of the day. The dose should be reduced in the elderly and in the presence of renal and hepatic impairment.

MECHANISMS OF ACTION
The mechanism of action is uncertain, but may be related to a selective reduction of the release of gamma-aminobuyric acid (GABA) in regions of the CNS that promote wakefulness. Modafinil increases the activity of histaminergic neurones in the tubero-mammillary nuclei of the posterior hypothalamus, which promotes wakefulness. This may be partly through inhibition of the ventro-lateral preoptic area of the anterior hypothalamus. It has no effect on dopaminergic synapses or melatonin secretion, but increases activity in hypocretin (orexin) containing neurones in the lateral hypothalamus and through this action may limit the duration of REM sleep.

EFFECTS ON SLEEP
Modafinil has little effect on sleep if it is taken in the morning [3], but taken later in the day it can cause insomnia. It has no effect on circadian rhythms or secretion of melatonin, cortisol or growth hormone [4].

EFFECTS ON WAKEFULNESS
Modafinil promotes alertness and wakefulness, but, unlike amphetamines, it does not increase motor activity or have any effects on the sympathetic nervous system. It does not increase anxiety or lead to a sleep debt with sleep rebound as occurs with amphetamines. It does not cause euphoria or any other mood change and is not hallucinogenic.

OTHER ACTIONS AND SIDE-EFFECTS
1 Headaches and a dry mouth may occur early in treatment, but are usually transient.
2 Mental hyperactivity may occur with high doses.

PROBLEMS WITH USE

Tolerance
This has not been well documented, but may develop in some narcoleptics.

Dependency
Modafinil has little potential for drug dependency since it does not cause any euphoria. Cessation of treatment does not lead to any withdrawal symptoms or REM sleep rebound.

Drug interactions
Modafinil does not interact with amphetamines, but since it is metabolized in the liver it may cause oral contraceptives to be less effective. Products containing at least 50 μg of oestrogen, such as ethinyl-oestradiol should be used, or alternative methods of contraception employed. On theoretical grounds care should be taken if modafinil is administered with anticonvulsants. It may increase the blood level of tricyclic antidepressants such as clomipramine.

INDICATIONS IN SLEEP DISORDERS
Modafinil is a selective wakefulness promoting drug which has been recently introduced for treating EDS (Table 3.5). It is indicated when this persists after treatment of the cause and if there has not been any response to first-line stimulant treatments such as caffeine. It is preferable to amphetamines and related

	Amphetamines	*Modafinil*
Efficacy	+	+
Duration of action	Short	Long
Specificity of action	Low	High
Dependency	Moderate risk	Low risk
Withdrawal symptoms	Common	Absent
Tolerance	30% narcoleptics	Unknown
Side-effects	Multiple, often serious	Few, mild
Contraindications	Multiple	Few
Drug interactions	Occasional	Rare
Effects of overdose	May be fatal	Insomnia

Table 3.5 Comparison of amphetamines and modafinil.

drugs, because although they are equally effective and modafinil has a slower onset of action, it has the advantages of a more specific effect on sleep–wake control, fewer side-effects, low potential for dependency, no withdrawal symptoms, few drug interactions and is safer in overdose. Its main indications are as follows.

1 Excessive daytime sleepiness due to neurological disorders. It has been most widely used in narcolepsy, but it is probably equally effective in ICNSH, and EDS due to other conditions such as myotonic dystrophy. It does not improve cataplexy, which therefore may worsen if patients with narcolepsy are transferred from dexamphetamine to modafinil.

2 Exessive daytime sleepiness that persists despite optimal treatment of the cause. It may remain a problem despite conventional treatment in, for instance, Parkinsonism, multiple sclerosis and even occasionally in periodic limb movements in sleep (PLMS) and obstructive sleep apnoeas (OSAs). Modafinil may improve EDS without the risk of the side-effects of amphetamine treatment, but there are little data regarding its precise indications.

3 Severe and unavoidable sleep deprivation.

Hypnotics

Introduction

Synthetic hypnotic drugs were developed in the nineteenth century. Bromides became available in 1857, chloral has been used since 1869 and barbiturates were introduced in 1903. These were largely superseded by the benzodiazepines in around 1960 and, despite doubts about their effectiveness and advisability for long-term use, they have continued to be used in increasing quantities. World-wide sales of hypnotics are increasing by around 8% per year, particularly in the USA and many European countries. Within Europe the sales are least in the UK, Holland and Belgium, and greatest in France, Germany and Italy.

The main use of hypnotics is in the treatment of insomnia [5]. The aim of treatment should not be simply to increase the quality and duration of sleep, but also to improve alertness during wakefulness. The balance between these two effects is difficult to achieve with the currently available hypnotics. The ideal drug would promote sleep but not result in any residual sleepiness during the next day, or cause any other features of CNS depression. None of the available drugs have this combination of actions. Most have other effects such as respiratory depression or a muscle relaxant effect and they usually interact with other hypnotics. The issues that determine the choice of a hypnotic are described in detail in Chapter 5. The main groups of drugs are described below.

Benzodiazepines

PHARMACOLOGY
The benzodiazepines contain a benzene ring linked to a seven-member diazepine ring. They are rapidly absorbed from the gastro-intestinal tract, although this is slowed by food and particularly by antacids. Most of the benzodiazepines are lipophilic, cross the blood–brain barrier readily and have a wide distribution within the body. A clinical effect is apparent with most of these drugs within 1 h and the peak plasma level is usually reached between 1 and 3 h after ingestion.

All the benzodiazepines are metabolized by hepatic microsomal enzymes and are conjugated with

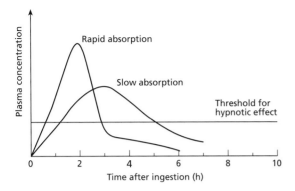

Fig. 3.1 Effects of rate of absorption on hypnotic action.

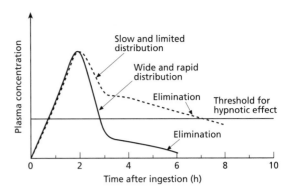

Fig. 3.2 Effects of distribution on hypnotic action.

glucuronic acid to form water-soluble metabolites which are excreted in the urine. Some benzodiazepines such as triazolam and midazolam have few active metabolites, but diazepam, for instance, is metabolized to desmethyldiazepam which is active and has a half-life of 50–100 h. This metabolite is not produced by lorazepam, oxazepam or temazepam. The metabolism of benzodiazepines is slower in the elderly, in whom there is also a greater neurological sensitivity because of the ageing processes within the brain.

Despite these similarities, there are quantitative differences between the individual benzodiazepines which have important implications for the timing and extent of their effects. They only have a hypnotic action if their level in the brain and cerebrospinal fluid is above a threshold which differs for each drug. This threshold may vary according to the balance of the sleep–wake drives, circadian rhythm and if tolerance to the drugs develops, but it is mainly affected by pharmacokinetic issues. The most important factors are as follows.

Rate of absorption
Rapidly absorbed drugs exceed the hypnotic threshold level quickly and have an early onset of action. Triazolam and diazepam are the most rapidly absorbed and have a quick effect, but oxazepam, which is the most slowly absorbed, has a slower onset of hypnotic effect (Fig. 3.1).

Distribution
The volume of distribution of the benzodiazepines varies considerably. Lipophilic drugs, such as diazepam, cross the blood–brain barrier readily and the brain and plasma concentrations quickly equilibrate. Lipophobic drugs such as oxazepam, lorazepam and

clonazepam have a smaller volume of distribution. The rate and volume of distribution is important in determining the effects of a single dose. Drugs that cross the blood–brain barrier have a quick onset of action, but if they also have a large volume of distribution they are removed from the receptors in the brain rapidly and the brain and blood levels soon fall below the threshold for the hypnotic effect so that the duration of action is short (Fig. 3.2).

Elimination
This comprises both metabolism and excretion of the drug. Drugs that are rapidly eliminated reach a low blood level before the next dose is administered, and this prevents them accumulating. A steady state blood level is reached after 4–5 times the half-life of the drug and if this is sufficiently long for the drug to fail to be eliminated before the next dose is given there will be a gradual increase in the blood level with a risk of sedation during the daytime (Fig. 3.3).

MECHANISMS OF ACTION
The benzodiazepines do not have any direct action on neurological function, but enhance the effects of GABA. Gamma-aminobutyric acid is a widely distributed inhibitory amino acid transmitter which is secreted particularly by interneurones. Benzodiazepines interact with $GABA_A$ rather than $GABA_B$ receptors (Fig. 3.4). These consist of a GABA binding site on the cell membrane close to the chloride channels which are opened by GABA so that the postsynaptic membrane becomes hyperpolarized. This inhibits the activity of the neurone and reduces its firing frequency.

Benzodiazepines bind to this macromolecular GABA-receptor complex close to the GABA binding

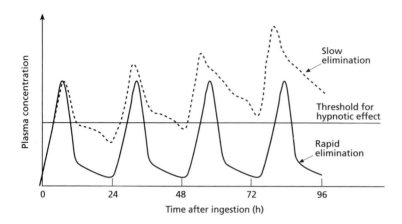

Fig. 3.3 Effects of rate of elimination on hypnotic action.

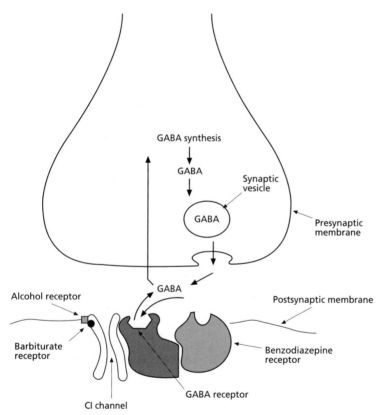

Fig. 3.4 GABA$_A$ receptor and hypnotics. Cl, chloride; GABA, gamma-aminobutyric acid.

site and the chloride channels, and at a location close to, but distinct from, the binding site for barbiturates and alcohol. Subtypes of the benzodiazepine receptors (e.g. BZ1, omega-1; BZ2, omega-2) have been identified but their significance is uncertain. BZ1 receptors may mediate sedation and BZ2 cognition, memory and psychomotor function. Benzodiazepines cause a change in the conformation of the GABA-receptor, increasing its affinity for, and enhancing the effects of,

GABA. They also increase the affinity of the barbiturate and alcohol receptors for these compounds and potentiate the effects of these drugs.

The action of benzodiazepines on the GABA-receptor complex is most marked in the hypothalamus, thalamus and limbic system, and the inhibition of these regions underlies the sedative and hypnotic effects of the benzodiazepines as well as their anxiolytic, muscle relaxant, and antiepileptic effects.

Table 3.6 Individual benzodiazepines.

Drug	Dose	Effect of single dose on sleep	Effect of regular dose in daytime	Uses
Triazolam	0.125–25 mg	Short acting	Nil	Brief daytime and nocturnal sleep, DIS
Midazolam	7.5–15 mg	Short acting	Nil	DIS
Flunitrazepam	0.5–1 mg	Short acting	Mild sedation	DIS
Diazepam	2.5–10 mg	Short acting	Sedation	Transient DIS, DMS and EMW with anxiety
Temazepam	10–20 mg	Intermediate	Mild sedation	DIS, DMS
Lormetazepam	0.5–1 mg	Intermediate	Nil	DIS, DMS
Oxazepam	15–30 mg	Intermediate	Nil	DMS, EMW with anxiety
Flurazepam	15 mg	Moderately long	Mild sedation	DMS, EMW
Nitrazepam	2.5–5 mg	Moderately long	Sedation	DMS, EMW with anxiety
Clorazepate	7.5–15 mg	Long acting	Sedation	DMS, EMW with anxiety
Clonazepam	0.5–1 mg	Long acting	Sedation	DMS, EMW with anxiety

DIS, difficulty in initiating sleep; DMS, difficulty in maintaining sleep; EMW, early morning awakening.

Table 3.7 Effects of hypnotics on sleep.

	TST	Sleep latency	1 and 2 NREM sleep	3 and 4 NREM sleep	REM sleep latency	REM sleep
Most GABA receptor-acting drugs	↑	↓	↑	↓	↑	↓
5HT agonists	↑	↓	? ↑	↑	Little effect	Little effect
Melatonin	No effect	↓	↑ during day	No effect	No effect	No effect

NREM, non-rapid eye movement; REM, rapid eye movement; TST, total sleep time.

INDIVIDUAL DRUGS

Details of the individual benzodiazepines are given in Table 3.6. The drugs are distinguished particularly by their speed of onset, potency, extent of distribution in the body, elimination half-life and ability to accumulate in the body, particularly in the brain. The availability of benzodiazepines varies considerably between different countries. Triazolam, for instance, was withdrawn from use in 1991 in the UK because of its pronounced rebound insomnia and anterograde amnesia, but is still available in the USA. Flunitrazepam has been removed from the list of prescribable drugs under the National Health Service (NHS) in the UK, but is available in other countries.

EFFECTS ON SLEEP

Benzodiazepines in low dose have a sedative effect and in higher dose induce sleep, and may even lead to coma. They reduce the spontaneous activity and response to afferent stimuli of the reticular activating system (RAS) and block the electroencephalogram (EEG) responses that are evoked by RAS stimulation. The EEG during wakefulness shows a reduction and slowing of the alpha-rhythm with an increase in the beta-rhythm, particularly in the frontal cortex.

Benzodiazepines increase total sleep time, shorten sleep latency, reduce the number of awakenings and provide a sense of a deep and refreshing sleep. Rapid eye movement sleep latency is prolonged, the duration of REM sleep is reduced, there are fewer eye movements and less dreaming during REM sleep except with short-acting drugs, such as triazolam, which cause a rebound in REM sleep late in the night. Sleep is consolidated in that there are fewer sleep-stage transitions, but the duration of stages 3 and 4 NREM sleep is reduced in parallel with that of REM sleep. The duration of stage 2 NREM sleep increases. The clinical significance of these changes in sleep architecture is uncertain (Table 3.7).

Withdrawal of benzodiazepines leads to REM sleep rebound, which may be associated with vivid dreams and nightmares for several weeks.

EFFECTS ON WAKEFULNESS

Daytime sedation is most pronounced with benzodiazepines with a long duration of action, such as flurazepam, particularly if the drugs are given for prolonged periods and in high dose. A steady-state blood level is reached at four to five times the half-life, which implies that if the drug has a 72 h half-life it may take up to 15 days before a steady state is reached. Elimination of the drugs is slowed in the elderly, who are also more predisposed to sedation. The degree of sedation during the day also depends on the balance between the improvement in sleep quality and the 'hangover' effect of persisting sedation. Tolerance to the sedative effect often develops, but it is accentuated if other sedatives, particularly alcohol, are taken.

The sedative effect of benzodiazepines impairs motor skills, attention, memory and judgement, and if severe may lead to confusion and incoordination. The risk of accidents, including road traffic accidents, is increased, particularly in those who take alcohol as well. Accidents, such as falls, may also occur during the night if the subject becomes confused and leaves the bed.

OTHER ACTIONS AND SIDE-EFFECTS

The benzodiazepines have little effect on the autonomic nervous system, but can cause the following.

1 Anxiolysis. This is seen with lower doses than are required to induce sedation or sleep and is common with long-acting hypnotics taken at night. Their anxiolytic effect probably has a similar underlying mechanism to the hypnotic effect. Oxazepam has relatively more anxiolytic and less hypnotic effect than other benzodiazepines.

2 Muscle relaxation.

3 Amnesia. Transient global anterograde amnesia is independent of the level of sedation and is probably mediated by a different mechanism from the hypnotic action of these drugs. It is particularly marked with short-acting drugs such as triazolam and flunitrazepam.

4 Anticonvulsant effect.

5 Depression. Depression is common but occasionally disinhibition occurs.

6 Respiratory failure and OSAs may be precipitated in susceptible patients, particularly with a high dose of benzodiazepines. This complication can be reversed by the specific benzodiazepine antagonist, flumazenil.

PROBLEMS WITH USE

Tolerance

This is common and often develops within a few weeks, but occurs to a lesser extent than with barbiturates. The loss of efficacy may require an increase in the dose.

Withdrawal symptoms

Cessation of benzodiazepines may lead to a recurrence of the original symptoms, or even to a transient worsening, or rebound of these. A specific withdrawal syndrome may also appear and is characterized by disturbed sleep, vivid dreams and nightmares, associated with an increase in REM sleep and in stages 3 and 4 NREM sleep. Autonomic symptoms such as excessive sweating, a psychosis, delirium and fits may occasionally be induced as well as a tachycardia and hypertension.

These problems are most common if the benzodiazepine has been used in high dose, is of high potency and has been used for a long duration. They are often sufficiently intense to lead the subject to return to regular benzodiazepine usage despite the intention of discontinuing treatment. They can be minimized by using the lowest effective dose of benzodiazepine, avoiding long-term treatment if possible and by then gradually withdrawing treatment rather than suddenly stopping it. This type of physical 'dependency' is distinct from drug addiction in which the subject loses control over the use of the drug, has a compulsive need for it and develops maladaptive drug-seeking behaviour. This type of drug addiction is uncommon with benzodiazepines and is less frequent with them than with barbiturates.

Interaction with other drugs

The sedative and hypnotic effects of benzodiazepines are accentuated if other drugs acting on the $GABA_A$ receptor, especially barbiturates and alcohol, are taken as well. Each drug increases the affinity of the receptor to the others so that the risk of overdose is greatly increased by combined treatment.

Phenobarbitone and spironolactone increase the metabolism of benzodiazepines and reduce their effect, but there is no interaction with oral anticoagulants.

Rebound insomnia

This may occur either during each night of treatment with benzodiazepines or during withdrawal of regular treatment as described above. Rebound insomnia during treatment is associated with short-acting drugs which do not accumulate in the body. The initial hypnotic effect wears off so that towards the end of the night rebound of REM sleep occurs with vivid dreams and frequent awakenings.

Pregnancy

Benzodiazepines cross the placenta and also enter breast milk. It is advisable to avoid benzodiazepines in pregnancy and to discontinue breastfeeding if a benzodiazepine has to be administered.

INDICATIONS IN SLEEP DISORDERS

Insomnia

Benzodiazepines are often considered as first line hypnotic treatment for insomnia, but are similar in many ways to newer drugs such as zopiclone, zolpidem and zaleplon. Their advantages over the older hypnotic drugs are:
1 greater sedation: anxiolysis ratio;
2 less tendency to tolerance and dependency, particularly compared to barbiturates;
3 less abuse potential;
4 safer in overdose, especially compared to barbiturates; and
5 fewer drug interactions since they do not induce hepatic microsomal enzyme production.

Despite these advantages, tolerance and depedency do occur and benzodiazepines should be used in courses of less than four weeks whenever possible. Their indications for insomnia are as follows.

Transient insomnia. Drugs such as diazepam or temazepam may be needed for 2–7 days to consolidate the sleep pattern. They may also be used to relieve jet lag and short-acting drugs may be helpful in rotating shift work.

Chronic insomnia. Their use should be limited to one month or less if possible, and towards the end of the course they should be taken on alternate nights so that their withdrawal is gradual. Occasionally patients require long-term treatment, although tolerance to their effects may reduce their efficacy and psychomotor performance, and mood changes may develop.

The hypnotic effect is only required intermittently and it is important that the blood and cerebrospinal fluid level falls below the threshold for the hypnotic

effect during the daytime, both with single and repeated doses. The exception is if anxiety as well as insomnia requires treatment, in which case symptoms may be helped by a long-acting preparation which retains significant blood levels during the day. In general, short-acting drugs tend to cause more amnesia, rebound insomnia and tolerance than longer-acting preparations, but avoid the difficulties of drug accumulation and daytime sedation.

Details of the choice of benzodiazepine are given in Chapter 5, but in general these drugs should be avoided wherever possible in the elderly. Short-acting drugs should be advised if the patient works with dangerous machinery, has to drive a motor vehicle or be particularly alert at work. Benzodiazepines should be avoided wherever possible in children, in the presence of respiratory impairment, a predisposition to OSAs, liver disease or if there is a history of drug abuse.

Behavioural abnormalities in sleep

Benzodiazepines are effective in treating many of the behavioural abnormalities associated with an increase in motor activity during sleep. These include PLMS, REM sleep behaviour disorder, sleep walking and sleep terrors, although they should be avoided in children whenever possible. Their efficacy is partly due to their muscle relaxant activity and also because they suppress stages 3 and 4 NREM sleep which is when many of these disorders arise. Clonazepam appears to be particularly effective.

Zopiclone

PHARMACOLOGY

Zopiclone is a cyclopyrrolone and has a different structure from the benzodiazepines. The peak plasma level is reached within 2 h. It has a short half-life of 4–6 h and a duration of action of 6–8 h. It is metabolized in the liver and excreted in the urine. The usual dose is 7.5–15 mg nocte, but this should be reduced to 3.75 mg in the elderly and in those with significant liver disease.

MECHANISMS OF ACTION

Zopiclone binds to the $GABA_A$ receptor complex, but at a different site to benzodiazepines.

EFFECTS ON SLEEP

Zopiclone is as effective a hypnotic as the benzodiazepines, but has different effects on sleep architecture. It does not influence REM sleep, but reduces the duration of stage 1 NREM sleep and the number of arousals, and does not significantly alter the duration of stages 3 and 4 NREM sleep.

OTHER ACTIONS AND SIDE-EFFECTS
Zopiclone is short acting, but can cause daytime sedation, particularly at high dose. It has similar anxiolytic, muscle relaxant and anticonvulsant actions to the benzodiazepines. It often causes a metallic or bitter taste in the mouth but does not increase the frequency of OSAs.

PROBLEMS WITH USE

Tolerance
This is probably less than with the benzodiazepines.

Withdrawal symptoms
These may be less than with benzodiazepines.

Interaction with other drugs
There is said to be less interaction with alcohol and other sedatives than with the benzodiazepines.

INDICATIONS IN SLEEP DISORDERS

Insomnia
Zopiclone is similar in its effects to a short acting benzodiazepine although it does have different consequences for sleep architecture. It should be used for up to one month for insomnia, particularly if this is transient and if there is DIS.

To assist with withdrawal from benzodiazepines
Rebound insomnia and other withdrawal symptoms can be reduced by substituting zopiclone.

Zolpidem

PHARMACOLOGY
Zolpidem is an imidazopyridine-derivative which is chemically unrelated to the benzodiazepines. It is rapidly absorbed, has a half-life of only 1.5–2.5 h in healthy adults although this is longer in the elderly and in the presence of liver disease. Its onset of action is detectable within 15–30 min, the peak plasma level is reached within 1–2 h of ingestion and its clinical effect lasts 5–7 h. It is metabolized in the liver. The usual dose is 5–10 mg nocte in adults or 5 mg in the elderly.

MECHANISMS OF ACTION
Zolpidem acts at the $GABA_A$ receptor complex close to but at a different site from the benzodiazepines. Its specificity for the BZ1 receptor may explain its slightly different actions compared to the benzodiazepines which act at both BZ1 and BZ2 receptors.

EFFECTS ON SLEEP
Zolpidem probably has little effect on sleep architecture, in contrast to the benzodiazepines. Its short duration of action occasionally leads to rebound insomnia later in the night.

OTHER ACTIONS AND SIDE-EFFECTS
Zolpidem is not an anxiolytic, muscle relaxant or anticonvulsant, probably because of its different site of action to the benzodiazepines.

It rarely causes daytime sedation because of its short duration of action, but can lead to nausea, vomiting, diarrhoea, headaches and dizziness.

PROBLEMS WITH USE
1 Tolerance. This is said to be less than with benzodiazepines.
2 Withdrawal symptoms. These are unusual.
3 Mild respiratory depression which may induce OSAs.

INDICATIONS IN SLEEP DISORDERS
Zolpidem is as effective as a hypnotic as the benzodiazepines and its indications are similar to this group of drugs. It has less effect on sleep architecture, but the clinical value of this is uncertain. Its short duration of action makes it suitable for treating DIS, in the elderly and in other situations where it is important to avoid daytime sedation.

Zaleplon

PHARMACOLOGY
Zaleplon is a pyrazolopyrimidine compound which is rapidly absorbed. Its peak plasma level is reached 1 h after ingestion and its half-life is half an hour. It has a short duration of action, less than 5 h. It is metabolized in the liver, mainly to inactive compounds, but a small amount of desmethylzaleplon, which has a hypnotic effect, is produced. There is some renal excretion. The usual dose is 5–10 mg.

MECHANISM OF ACTION
Zaleplon binds to BZ1 (omega-1) receptors, in a similar manner to zolpidem.

EFFECTS ON SLEEP

Zaleplon has a dose related effect in reducing sleep latency, but because of its short duration of action it does not increase the total sleep time. In high doses (40–60 mg) it may reduce the duration of REM sleep. Rebound insomnia later in the night is uncommon.

OTHER ACTIONS AND SIDE-EFFECTS

Zaleplon is an anxiolytic with muscle relaxant and anticonvulsant actions. It occasionally causes headaches and dizziness, and may lead to respiratory depression.

It rarely causes daytime sedation because of its short duration of action, and psychomotor impairment is unusual.

PROBLEMS WITH USE

1 Tolerance. The risk of this is unknown.
2 Withdrawal symptoms. These are probably rare.
3 Dependency. This is unlikely.

INDICATIONS IN SLEEP DISORDERS

Zaleplon is a very short acting hypnotic whose main indications are in treating DIS and in promoting naps at times of heightened circadian alertness, for instance in night shift workers who wish to sleep during the day. It may also be of use in the difficulty in maintaining sleep (DMS) type of insomnia when there is a limited time left before the desired awakening time in the morning.

Barbiturates

PHARMACOLOGY

The barbiturates are substituted pyrimidine derivatives with a basic barbituric acid structure. They are well absorbed as sodium salts and have an onset of action of 10–60 min. Their lipid solubility varies and determines how readily they cross the blood–brain barrier. They have a long duration of action, usually 6–8 h, particularly in the elderly and in the presence of liver disease. They are metabolized by hepatic microsomal enzymes and lead to induction of these enzymes which is the basis of the tolerance that develops to them. They are conjugated with glucuronic acid and are excreted in the urine mainly in this form, although some are excreted unchanged.

MECHANISMS OF ACTION

Barbiturates act on the $GABA_A$ receptor complex at a site close to but different from the benzodiazepines. They have a widespread action within the CNS, but particularly in the midbrain reticular formation, and cause generalized CNS depression.

INDIVIDUAL DRUGS

Amylobarbitone: dose 60–200 mg nocte.
Butobarbitone: dose 100–200 mg nocte.
Quinalbarbitone: dose 50–100 mg nocte.

EFFECTS ON SLEEP

Barbiturates may cause sedation, sleep, anaesthesia, and even death according to the dose, age, individual susceptibility and interaction with other drugs. They have a similar effect on sleep to the benzodiazepines in that they reduce the sleep latency and the duration of REM sleep, and REM sleep-latency increases. The duration of stage 2 NREM sleep is increased, but stages 3 and 4 NREM sleep become shorter and the number of arousals is reduced. Withdrawal of barbiturates after prolonged use leads to REM sleep rebound with nightmares and rebound insomnia.

OTHER ACTIONS AND SIDE-EFFECTS

1 Daytime sedation. This is common because of their long duration of action. They reduce psychomotor skills and may cause mood changes.
2 Anxiolytic.
3 Muscle relaxant.
4 Anticonvulsant.
5 Nausea, vomiting and diarrhoea.
6 Respiratory depression. This is dose dependent and is usually fatal at around 10 times the hypnotic dose [6].

PROBLEMS WITH USE

Tolerance
This develops within two weeks of treatment because of induction of hepatic microsomal enzymes.

Withdrawal symptoms
These are more frequently a problem than with benzodiazepines. Withdrawal of barbiturates leads to REM sleep rebound and rebound insomnia.

Drug interactions
The metabolism of barbiturates by microsomal enzymes in the liver underlies most of the drug interactions. The rate of metabolism of warfarin, phenytoin, tricyclic antidepressants and the oral contraceptive pill is increased, and conversely MAOIs inhibit these enzymes and reduce the rate of barbiturate metabolism.

Pregnancy
Barbiturates cross the placenta to reach the fetus and a small quantity enters breast milk. They should be avoided in pregnancy.

Overdose
The barbiturates have a lower toxic : therapeutic ratio than benzodiazepines and much more frequently cause death when an overdose is taken.

INDICATIONS IN SLEEP DISORDERS

Insomnia
Barbiturates are rarely used nowadays because of their disadvantages relative to the benzodiazepines. Their only place is for short-term treatment if benzodiazepines and other modern hypnotics can not be tolerated or are ineffective, as well as in those patients who have been taking barbiturates regularly for many years without any side-effects. When barbiturate treatment is initiated it should be restricted to two weeks because of the risk of tolerance developing.

Chloral and related drugs

PHARMACOLOGY
Chloral is rapidly absorbed and its hypnotic effect is detectable within 30 min. It is widely distributed within the body and has a half-life of 6–8 h. It is metabolized to trichlorethanol by alcohol dehydrogenase, especially in the liver, and this is then conjugated with glucuronic acid and largely excreted in the urine. Trichloroethanol is the active agent of chloral and related drugs and is responsible for their hypnotic effect.

MECHANISMS OF ACTION
These drugs bind to the $GABA_A$ receptor complex.

INDIVIDUAL DRUGS
Chloral hydrate: dose 0.5–2 g in adults; 0.03–0.05 g/kg to a maximum of 1 g in children.
Triclofos sodium: dose 1–2 g nocte.
Dichloralphenazone: dose 0.65–1.3 g nocte.

EFFECTS ON SLEEP
These are similar to benzodiazepines and barbiturates.

OTHER ACTIONS AND SIDE-EFFECTS
Daytime sedation is uncommon because of their short duration of action. These drugs have few cardiovas-cular or respiratory effects except in overdose. They may cause nausea and vomiting.

PROBLEMS WITH USE
1 Tolerance.
2 Withdrawal symptoms.
3 Chloral should be avoided in hepatic and renal failure.
4 Drug interactions. Chloral potentiates the effects of alcohol, barbiturates and other sedatives. Alcohol dehydrogenase is responsible for the metabolism of both chloral and alcohol, and chloral acts as a competitive inhibitor increasing the effects of alcohol.

INDICATIONS IN SLEEP DISORDERS
Chloral is a mild hypnotic and is an alternative to benzodiazepines, particularly in the elderly.

Chlormethiazole (clomethiazole)

PHARMACOLOGY
Chlormethiazole is rapidly absorbed from the gastro-intestinal tract and its peak plasma level is reached within 15–90 min. It has a brief duration of action and is rapidly metabolized in the liver. Dose 192–384 mg nocte.

MECHANISMS OF ACTION
It acts at the GABA receptor complex close to the benzodiazepine receptor site.

EFFECTS ON SLEEP
Its hypnotic effect is dose related.

OTHER ACTIONS AND SIDE-EFFECTS
1 Daytime sedation is rarely a problem because of its short duration of action.
2 Anticonvulsant.
3 Sneezing and conjunctival irritation.
4 Nausea and vomiting.

PROBLEMS WITH USE
Withdrawal symptoms.

INDICATIONS IN SLEEP DISORDERS
Chlormethiazole is a useful hypnotic in the elderly because of its short duration of action. It should be reserved for transient insomnia because of the risk of dependence, but it is also of value in alcohol and narcotic withdrawal.

Paraldehyde

PHARMACOLOGY

This drug is slowly absorbed orally, but is widely distributed and readily crosses the blood–brain barrier. Its half-life is 4–10 h. Eighty per cent is metabolized in the liver to acetaldehyde and then acetic acid, but the remainder is excreted as paraldehyde through the lungs and has a characteristic odour. Dose: 5–10 ml orally, rectally or intramuscularly.

MECHANISMS OF ACTION

Its hypnotic effect is thought to be due to inhibition of the ascending RAS in the brain-stem. It probably acts on the GABA receptor complex.

EFFECTS ON SLEEP

Its effects on sleep are similar to those of the benzodiazepines.

OTHER ACTIONS AND SIDE-EFFECTS

1 Anticonvulsant.
2 Gastric irritation.
3 Hepatitis.
4 Nephrotic syndrome.

PROBLEMS WITH USE

Drug interactions
Its sedative and hypnotic actions are additive to those of other sedative drugs such as alcohol and barbiturates.

INDICATIONS IN SLEEP DISORDERS

Paraldehyde is very rarely used in sleep disorders, but is occasionally indicated in status epilepticus and has been used in acute agitation and alcohol withdrawal.

Alcohol

PHARMACOLOGY

Ethyl alcohol (ethanol) is rapidly absorbed through the mouth, stomach and small intestine, although this absorption is delayed by food, especially fatty food. It is oxidized in the liver to acetaldehyde and then to acetic acid and to carbon dioxide and water. It is also excreted in the urine and to a lesser extent through the lungs.

MECHANISMS OF ACTION

Alcohol acts on the GABA receptor complex in a similar way to benzodiazepines, but at a slightly different site. It influences particularly the RAS and causes generalized CNS depression.

EFFECTS ON SLEEP

Alcohol is an anxiolytic and a weak hypnotic. It increases the total sleep time, reduces sleep latency, reduces the latency before stages 3 and 4 NREM sleep and increases their duration as well as suppressing REM sleep. It is short acting so that as the blood alcohol level falls during the night REM sleep rebound occurs, often with vivid dreams, loss of NREM sleep and frequent awakenings. After a large intake of alcohol these withdrawal features are seen on the next night. High doses may also reduce the duration of stages 3 and 4 NREM sleep and its diuretic effect will cause awakenings from sleep. It also induces OSAs which lead to sleep fragmentation.

Chronic alcohol ingestion disrupts the sleep–wake cycle, possibly through disturbing the pattern of melatonin secretion. Alcohol is often taken initially in order to promote sleep, but tolerance to its hypnotic effect leads to the quantity being increased and often other hypnotics are taken in addition. The pharmacological effects of alcohol are combined with episodes of partial withdrawal and dehydration which lead to DMS. Waking with dreams and headaches is common, especially in older subjects in whom the homeostatic drive to sleep is weaker. The sleep architecture disintegrates with the duration of both stages 3 and 4 NREM and REM sleep being reduced. Frequent sleep-stage shifts and arousals lead to both insomnia and EDS. Periodic limb movements in sleep are common.

EFFECTS ON WAKEFULNESS

Sedation is common if alcohol is taken during the daytime or in large quantity at night. This is partly due to its sedative action and partly to sleep disruption described above. It impairs judgement, attention and concentration.

OTHER ACTIONS AND SIDE-EFFECTS

1 Anxiolytic.
2 Diuretic. Its diuretic action is through inhibition of antidiuretic hormone (ADH).
3 Respiratory depression. Alcohol precipitates OSAs by reducing respiratory drive and upper airway muscle tone, increasing nasal congestion, and it also reduces the threshold for arousal during apnoeas.
4 Drug interactions. Alcohol potentiates the sedative effect of other hypnotics such as benzodiazepines and barbiturates.

PROBLEMS WITH USE

Tolerance
This is due to both enzyme induction in the liver and CNS adaptation to its hypnotic effects.

Withdrawal symptoms
Acute withdrawal of alcohol after long-term consumption causes REM sleep rebound with a short REM sleep latency, a reduction in stages 3 and 4 NREM sleep and sleep fragmentation with an increase in the number of sleep-stage shifts and awakenings. Sympathetic hyperactivity underlies the tachycardia, sweating and headaches and an increase in muscle tone is common. Dreams may be vivid and frightening, and in severe cases merge into delirium tremens. This probably represents intrusion of vivid REM sleep imagery into an alert, but agitated state. Visual hallucinations and paranoid delusions are common. They usually appear around 48 h after withdrawal of alcohol which is at the time that REM sleep rebound would be expected to be most prominent. They may lead to alcohol being restarted, but if abstinence can be maintained for around two weeks these symptoms gradually improve. The sleep pattern may nevertheless remain abnormal with frequent awakenings for up to two years.

INDICATIONS IN SLEEP DISORDERS

Insomnia
Alcohol is commonly taken to treat DIS either on a regular basis or to cope with transient insomnia due to special circumstances such as changes in shift work schedules. It has the disadvantage of causing rebound insomnia later in the night in doses that are sufficient to induce sleep, and can lead to considerable sleep disruption with long-term use.

Tryptophan

L-tryptophan is an essential amino acid which is present in many proteins and particularly in dairy products such as milk, and in meat, eggs and nuts. It is metabolized to 5-hydroxytryptophan and then to 5HT which is thought to mediate its mild hypnotic effect. It has been taken as a food supplement in a dose of 1–2 g three times daily, but in 1989 was recognized to be associated with the eosinophilia–myalgia syndrome which included fatigue and inflammatory changes in the heart, lungs and liver. It was withdrawn from production in 1991 because of this, but subsequent investigation indicated that this syndrome was probably due to a contaminant rather than to tryptophan itself. A limited licence was re-instated in the UK in 1994. 5-hydroxytryptophan is also available.

It is readily absorbed through the gastro-intestinal tract, crosses the blood–brain barrier and is metabolized in the liver. It can cause nausea, vomiting, headaches and Parkinsonism. It reduces sleep latency, prolongs stages 3 and 4 NREM sleep, but has little effect on REM sleep.

It is a weak antidepressant as well as a mild hypnotic, but should not be taken with an SSRI, since this combination may lead to the 'serotonin syndrome' of confusion, agitation, sweating, tachycardia and a fluctuating blood pressure. This syndrome may also develop with other drugs that increase serotonin (5HT) availability within the CNS such as lithium, L-dopa and dopamine agonists, LSD and ecstasy.

Valerian

Valerian is present in many herbal remedies, and is derived from a dried extract of the rhizome, root, and stolon of *Valeriana officinalis*. The active agents have not been precisely identified, but may include valepotriates, volatile oils such as valerenic acid and other compounds. They probably act on $GABA_A$ receptors in the CNS.

The content and purity of the preparations of valerian vary, but a dose of around 200–1000 mg 30–60 min before the desired onset of sleep is usually taken. Valerian has a mild hypnotic action, and particularly reduces the sleep latency. It may be useful in treating DIS, and it also has a muscle relaxant effect. Its long-term safety is uncertain and it has been recognized to lead to liver damage, probably due to a drug induced hepatitis. It may also have cytotoxic effects since valepotriates act as alkylating agents *in vitro* and possibly *in vivo*.

Psychotropic drugs

Introduction

These are primarily prescribed in order to influence mood, thought processes or behaviour, but many of them have important effects on sleep and wakefulness (Table 3.8). They are a heterogeneous group of compounds which for convenience rather than for any pharmacological reason are considered according to their main clinical uses.

Table 3.8 Effects of psychotropic drugs on sleep.

Drug	TST	SL	Arousals	1 and 2 NREM sleep	3 and 4 NREM sleep	REM sleep latency	REM sleep
Antipsychotics	↑	↓	–	–	Slight ↑	–	Variable
Antidepressants	–	–	↓	–	↑	↑	↓
Lithium	–	–	↓	–	↑	↑	↓
Anticonvulsants							
Sodium valproate	↑	↓	–	–	–	–	–
Phenytoin	–	↓	–	–	Transient ↑	–	↓
Carbamazepine	–	–	↓	↑	↑	–	↓

NREM, non-rapid eye movement; REM, rapid eye movement; SL, sleep latency; TST, total sleep time.

Antipsychotics

MECHANISMS OF ACTION

These drugs are dopamine receptor antagonists. Their antipsychotic action is related to D2 and D3 receptors, but most of these drugs are also D1 antagonists. They lead to a general inhibition of the arousal systems in the brain, including the reticular formation, limbic system and cerebral cortex. Many of them also have an anticholinergic, antihistaminic, anti-alpha 1 adrenergic and anti-5HT action.

INDIVIDUAL DRUGS

These are of three main types.
1 Phenothiazines including piperazines (e.g. trifluoperazine and perphenazine), alkylamines (e.g. chlorpromazine) and piperidines (e.g. thioridazine).
2 Butyrophenones (e.g. haloperidol).
3 Atypical antipsychotics (e.g. clozapine, risperidone).

EFFECTS ON SLEEP

These vary considerably. In general the total sleep time increases, there is a reduction in sleep latency, a slight increase in the duration of stages 3 and 4 NREM sleep and usually, but not invariably, an increase in the duration of REM sleep.

Withdrawal of antipsychotic medication shortens the total sleep time and the duration of REM sleep.

OTHER RELEVANT ACTIONS

1 Daytime sedation. This is a problem with many of these drugs but is less prominent with the butyrophenones.
2 Anxiolytic.
3 Mild antidepressant action.

4 Drug interactions. These drugs potentiate the effects of alcohol, hypnotics, narcotics and antihistamines.
5 Movement disorders. These are mainly extra pyramidal and include akinesia, tardive dyskinesia and akathisia which is an unpleasant need to move the limbs associated with anxiety and agitation and which may be confused with the restless legs syndrome.

Antidepressants

MECHANISMS OF ACTION

The MAOIs increase noradrenaline and 5HT activity within the CNS by blocking the activity of monoamine oxidase which normally metabolizes these amines to inactive compounds. The tricyclic antidepressants and venlafaxine block the presynaptic re-uptake of noradrenaline and 5HT and also have an antihistaminic and anticholinergic effect. The SSRIs are more selective in that they reduce 5HT re-uptake, but do not affect noradrenaline. The antidepressants probably also affect the function and number of noradrenaline and 5HT receptors so that the balance between the cholinergic and noradrenergic and 5HT mechanisms, particularly in the pontine reticular formation, is swung in favour of the latter. These effects probably predominate in the hypothalamus, thalamus, limbic system and neocortex and thereby regulate the level of arousal, mood and sensory processing.

INDIVIDUAL DRUGS

These fall into five main groups.
1 Monoamine oxidase inhibitors, e.g. phenelzine and tranylcypromine. These are non-selective drugs with

both type A (noradrenaline metabolizing) and type B (dopamine metabolizing) actions. Moclobemide is a selective, reversible type A inhibitor.
2 Tricyclic and related antidepressants, e.g. amitriptyline, clomipramine, protriptyline.
3 Selective serotonin reuptake inhibitors, e.g. fluoxetine, paroxetine, sertraline.
4 Selective noradrenaline re-uptake inhibitors, e.g. viloxazine.
5 Other drugs, e.g. venlafaxine, trazodone, nefazodone.

EFFECTS ON SLEEP
Almost all the antidepressants increase the REM sleep latency and reduce the duration of REM sleep as well as increasing the duration of stages 3 and 4 NREM [7]. The effects on REM sleep are seen after the first dose of tricyclic and SSRI drugs, but are often delayed with MAOIs. The action is most marked with clomipramine, a 5HT reuptake inhibitor, and is less with trimipramine, and tolerance develops with desipramine. The two antidepressants with different effects on sleep are moclobemide and nefazodone which have different mechanisms of action to the other drugs. They increase the duration of REM sleep and have no effect on stages 3 and 4 NREM sleep. All the sedating antidepressants also reduce the frequency of arousals and awakenings from sleep in depression, and thereby improve sleep efficiency.

Withdrawal of antidepressant treatment usually causes REM sleep rebound which may be prolonged and lead to frightening dreams and insomnia.

OTHER RELEVANT ACTIONS

Daytime sedation
Many of the antidepressants are sedative and this effect often parallels the anticholinergic properties of the drugs which are most marked with trimipramine and amitriptyline, absent with protriptyline and nortriptyline and rarely a problem with SSRIs which may increase alertness and even cause agitation. Sedating tricyclic antidepressants should be taken in the evening while SSRIs can be taken in the morning.

Upper-airway muscle activity
SSRI antidepressants may reduce the degree of loss of tone in upper airway dilator muscle in NREM sleep and thereby reduce the frequency of OSAs. This effect may be due to their action on 5HT release in the dorsal raphe nuclei (DRN).

INDICATIONS IN SLEEP DISORDERS
1 Insomnia associated with depression.
2 Nightmares. The effectiveness of antidepressants is dependent on their REM suppressing action. Clomipramine is probably the most effective.
3 Cataplexy. The anticataplectic effect of antidepressants may be mediated mainly by their 5HT promoting action more than their noradrenergic and anticholinergic effects. Tricyclic antidepressants, particularly clomipramine, imipramine and protriptyline are effective, and although SSRIs are probably slightly less effective, they have fewer side-effects.
4 Obstructive sleep apnoeas, snoring and other motor disorders occurring in REM sleep.

Lithium
Lithium increases the synthesis and concentration of 5HT and reduces noradrenaline and dopamine activity. It competes with mono- and di-valent cations to affect the postsynaptic receptor protein sites and to alter sodium and potassium channel function.

It does not alter the total sleep time but reduces the number of arousals, increases the duration of stages 3 and 4 NREM sleep, increases REM sleep latency and reduces the duration of REM sleep. It also has a small, but consistent effect in delaying circadian rhythms. It interacts with hypnotics, such as alcohol, to cause sedation and confusion.

The main indication for lithium is to stabilize the mood in bipolar (manic-depressive) disorders and in mania.

Anticonvulsants

MECHANISMS OF ACTION
1 Enhancement of GABA activity by altering the function of the GABA receptor complex (e.g. benzodiazepines and barbiturates) or through other actions (e.g. sodium valproate, vigabatrin and tiagabine).
2 Sodium channel blockers (e.g. phenytoin, carbamazepine, lamotrigine and topiramate). This effect inhibits depolarization of the neurones.

INDIVIDUAL DRUGS
These are a heterogeneous group which includes benzodiazepines, barbiturates, phenytoin, sodium valproate, carbamazepine, vigabatrin, lamotrigine, gabapentin, topiramate and tiagabine.

EFFECTS ON SLEEP
1 Benzodiazepines and barbiturates—see hypnotics section.

2 Sodium valproate increases total sleep time, reduces sleep latency and reduces the number of sleep-stage shifts, but has little effect on sleep architecture.

3 Phenytoin reduces sleep latency, may reduce the duration of REM sleep and causes a transient increase in the duration of stages 3 and 4 NREM sleep.

4 Carbamazepine reduces the frequency of arousals, reduces the duration of REM sleep and increases the duration of stages 1, 3 and 4 NREM sleep.

OTHER RELEVANT ACTIONS

Most of these drugs cause sedation, especially when used in combination. The sedative effect of carbamazepine is usually transient and can be minimized by slowly increasing the dose. Lamotrigine and clobazepam cause little sedation.

INDICATIONS IN SLEEP DISORDERS

1 Nocturnal epilepsy.

2 Restless legs syndrome and periodic limb movements in sleep. These respond to clonazepam and occasionally to other anticonvulsants such as carbamazepine, gabapentin and sodium valproate.

Other drugs influencing neurotransmitters

Introduction

An increasingly wide range of compounds are now recognized to act as neurotransmitters, cotransmitters or sleep factors, and to influence sleep and wakefulness. In this section the effects of agonist and antagonist drugs on the main types of these chemicals are considered (Table 3.9).

Amines

NORADRENERGIC AND ADRENERGIC DRUGS AND BLOCKERS

Agnoist drugs tend to suppress REM sleep and increase wakefulness. They may have both alpha and beta effects.

Alpha agonists

Clonidine is an alpha-2 agonist as well as an H1 antagonist and an anticholinergic drug which causes sedation, increases total sleep time, increases REM sleep latency, reduces the duration of REM sleep, causes vivid dreams and an increase in stages 3 and 4 NREM sleep.

Methyldopa is also a sedative leading to lethargy,

drowsiness and fatigue. It increases REM sleep and reduces the duration of stages 3 and 4 NREM sleep and predisposes to nightmares.

Alpha blockers

These include prazosin and indoramin both of which can cause daytime sedation, and thymoxamine which increases REM sleep.

Beta agonists

Isoprenaline stimulates both beta-1 and beta-2 receptors, dobutamine is a selective beta-1 stimulant and salbutamol a selective beta-2 stimulant. There has been little study of their effects on sleep, but, in general, their actions are potentiated by xanthines and amphetamines.

Beta blockers

These drugs reduce the duration of REM sleep, increase the number of arousals from REM sleep and of nightmares, and cause visual hallucinations. They also cause tiredness, at least partly through peripheral effects on skeletal muscle. The lipophilic drugs such as propranolol, metoprolol, labetalol and pindolol have more effects on sleep than lipophobic drugs such as sotalol and atenolol. Withdrawal of beta blockers leads to an increase in REM sleep and nightmares.

CHOLINERGIC DRUGS AND ANTAGONISTS

Acetylcholine is a neurotransmitter which has muscarinic effects at post ganglionic parasympathetic synapses and nicotinic effects in the CNS and at preganglionic synapses. It promotes REM sleep and wakefulness.

1 Muscarinic agonists (e.g. carbachol and pilocarpine). These increase the duration of REM sleep.

2 Nicotinic agonists (e.g. nicotine).

3 Anti-muscarinic agents (e.g. atropine and hyoscine). Both these drugs are CNS stimulants, delay the onset of REM sleep, may lead to agitation and excitement and reduce the motor inhibition during REM sleep.

4 Nicotinic antagonists (e.g. succinylcholine, atracurium and tubocurarine).

5 Anticholinesterases (e.g. pyridostigmine and neostigmine). These inhibit the enzymes responsible for the metabolism of acetylcholine and thereby prolong its neurotransmitter action. They reduce REM sleep latency, increase REM sleep duration, are associated with dreams and nightmares and increase the number of arousals from sleep.

Table 3.9 Drugs that influence NREM and REM sleep.

	Promoter	Suppressant
Stages 1 & 2 NREM sleep	Glucocorticoids (slight) Hypnotics Carbamazepine (stage 1) Baclofen	Zopiclone (stage 1)
Stages 3 & 4 NREM sleep	Tryptophan Antipsychotics (slight) Antidepressants Lithium Phenytoin (transient) Carbamazepine Clonidine Cyproheptadine Cimetidine Cannabis	Caffeine and other xanthines Amphetamines and related drugs Hypnotics Methyldopa Opiates Aspirin

REM sleep	Antipsychotics
	Methyldopa
	Thymoxamine
	Muscarinic agonists, e.g. pilocarpine
	Anticholinesterases, e.g. neostigmine
	LSD
	Reserpine
	Baclofen
	Withdrawal of:
	  Amphetamines and related drugs
	  Hypnotics
	  Antidepressants
	  Beta blockers
	  Opiates
	  Cannabis
		Caffeine and other xanthines
		Glucocorticoids (slight)
		Mazindol
		Amphetamines and related drugs
		Hypnotics
		Antidepressants
		Lithium
		Phenytoin (slight)
		Carbamazepine
		Clonidine
		Beta blockers
		Opiates
		Cannabis
		Withdrawal of antipsychotics

LSD, lysergic acid diethylamide.

5HT AND ANTI-5HT DRUGS

The release of 5HT enhances NREM and suppresses REM sleep through action at 5HT 1, 2 and 3 receptors within the CNS. The action of 5HT can be increased slightly by oral administration of L-tryptophan which is its precursor. It has a mild sedative effect and increases the total sleep time. 5HT release is increased by amphetamines and its action is also enhanced by tricyclic and SSRI antidepressants which reduce its re-uptake and alter the characteristics of its receptors.

Cyproheptadine is a 5HT antagonist which increases stages 3 and 4 NREM sleep. The action of 5HT at type 2 receptors is antagonized by LSD which is also a dopamine (D1 and D2) agonist. It increases the duration of the early REM sleep episodes and interrupts stages 3 and 4 NREM sleep with short bursts of REM. These are associated with frequent body movements and arousals from sleep. Use of LSD may lead to an agitated psychosis with severe sleep disruption which can last for several days.

DOPAMINE AGONISTS AND ANTAGONISTS

Dopamine does not have direct effects on sleep and wakefulness, but interacts with other neurotransmitter systems involved in physiological functions during sleep.

Dopamine agonists

L-dopa is a precursor of dopamine and synthetic dopamine receptor agonists include bromocriptine, ropinirole and pergolide. Amphetamines and aman-tadine also cause release of preformed dopamine and are therefore indirectly acting dopamine agonists.

These drugs have a variable effect on sleep and wake-fulness, but may cause vivid dreams and nightmares.

Dopamine antagonists
These include antipsychotics and reserpine which reduces dopamine storage, increases REM sleep, and causes nightmares. Domperidone is a D2 blocker which does not cross the blood–brain barrier and causes little daytime sedation.

HISTAMINERGIC DRUGS AND ANTAGONISTS
H1, H2 and H3 receptors are present within the CNS and their stimulation has a role in arousal from sleep, in increasing vigilance while awake and in inhibiting REM sleep.

The earlier H1 antihistaminic drugs, e.g. prometh-azine, chlorpheniramine and diphenhydramine also had antinoradrenaline, anti-5HT and anticholinergic activity. The latter caused their sedative and hypnotic effects, with an increase in stages 3 and 4 NREM sleep. They have been widely used as hypnotics, par-ticularly in children, but may cause daytime sedation, psychomotor impairment and anticholinergic side-effects. More selective and less hypnotic drugs have now been developed. These include the H1 antagon-ists astemizole and terfenadine which do not cross the blood–brain barrier and are non-sedating.

The H2 antagonist, cimetidine, increases the dura-tion of stages 3 and 4 NREM sleep, but ranitidine has no effect on sleep.

Amino acids

GAMMA AMINOBUTYRIC ACID AGONISTS AND ANTAGONISTS
Gamma aminobutyric acid is a widespread inhibitory neuro transmitter. Its action is potentiated by many hypnotic drugs and some anticonvulsants which act at the $GABA_A$ receptor. Baclofen is a $GABA_B$ agonist. It increases the total sleep time and the duration of stages 1 and 2 NREM sleep and of REM sleep, but does not alter stages 3 and 4 NREM sleep.

The effects of GABA are antagonized by tetanus toxin.

Peptides
Administration of peptide hormones and their ana-logues can influence sleep and it is likely that more

drugs of this type which interact with sleep-control-ling peptides will be developed.

OPIATES
Most of the older opiates act on all three types of CNS opioid receptor (Mu, Delta, and Kappa). Their sedat-ive effect is mainly due to kappa- and to a lesser extent Mu-activity. Opioids reduce total sleep time, increase sleep latency, increase the number of arousals and lead to sleep fragmentation, reduce the duration of REM sleep and increase stage 2, but decrease stages 3 and 4 NREM sleep. The sleep disturbance is about twice as great with diamorphine as with morphine.

Withdrawal of opioid drugs leads to rebound insomnia, rebound increase in REM sleep and, to a lesser extent, a rebound increase in stages 3 and 4 NREM sleep for up to several days.

Opioids lead to a relaxed wakefulness, reducing anxiety and distress. They impair cognitive and psy-chomotor performance, and in overdose they lead to sedation, respiratory depression, coma and death. Their main use in sleep medicine is in the treatment of periodic limb movements.

Other drugs

ASPIRIN
Aspirin (acetyl salicylic acid) inhibits prostaglandin synthesis and release and, probably through this mechanism, reduces the duration of stages 3 and 4 NREM sleep.

CANNABIS
The active component of cannabis preparations is delta-9-tetrahydrocannabinol (THC) [8]. Marijuana is made from the flowering top and leaves of *Cannabis sativa* and hashish, which is more concentrated, is derived from a dried exudate from the flowers. Around 50% of THC is absorbed into the blood when cannabis is smoked and a subjective effect is detect-able within 10 min but disappears after around 2–4 h. Delta-9-tetrahydrocannabinol is metabolized in the liver. It acts at specific CNS receptors which also respond to an endogenous compound, anandamide, whose metabolism is blocked by interleukin-1.

The duration of REM sleep is reduced by THC, which is a sedative, and it disproportionately reduces the number of rapid eye movements. It slightly increases the duration of stages 3 and 4 NREM sleep, but these effects become less marked with long-term THC use. Withdrawal leads to REM sleep rebound and a reduction in REM latency, as well as anxiety and anorexia.

Delta-9-tetrahydrocannabinol causes euphoria and is a mild anxiolytic which may help to induce sleep. In low doses it improves memory, but in higher doses psychomotor and cognitive skills and reaction times are impaired. It is frequently abused and dependency is common. Its effects are potentiated by alcohol and chronic use leads to increased duration of sleep and lassitude.

References

1 Zhdanova IV, Lynch HJ, Wurtman RJ. Melatonin. A sleep-promoting hormone. *Sleep* 1997; 20: 899–907.
2 Roehrs T, Merlotti L, Halpin D, Rosenthal L, Roth T. Effects of theophylline on nocturnal sleep and daytime sleepiness/alertness. *Chest* 1995; 108: 382–7.
3 Buguet A, Montmayeur A, Pigeau R, Naithoh P. Modafinil, d-amphetamine and placebo during 64 hours of sustained mental work. II. Effects on two nights of recovery sleep. *J Sleep Res,* 1995; 4: 229–41.
4 Brun J, Chamba G, Khalfallah Y *et al.* Effect of modafinil on plasma melatonin, cortisol and growth hormone rhythms, rectal temperature and performance in healthy subjects during a 36h sleep deprivation. *J Sleep Res* 1998; 7: 105–14.
5 Gillin JC. The long and the short of sleeping pills. *N Engl J Med* 1991; 324: 1735–6.
6 Launois S, Similowski T, Fleury B *et al.* The transition between apnoea and spontaneous ventilation in patients with coma due to voluntary intoxication with barbiturates and carbamates. *Eur Respir J* 1990; 1: 573–8.
7 Sharpley AL, Cowen PJ. Effect of pharmacologic treatments on the sleep of depressed patients. *Biol Psychiatry* 1995; 37: 85–98.
8 Hall W, Solowij N. Adverse effects of cannabis. *Lancet* 1998; 352: 1611–16.

4 Assessment of Sleep Disorders

Introduction

The assessment of sleep disorders requires an understanding of normal sleep and how it may alter in abnormal circumstances, such as following sleep deprivation; and with disorders that affect the nature of sleep. The details of the history obtained at interview with the patient, and often with a member of the family, partner, friend or carer, should be supplemented by a physical examination where this is applicable. The expanding range of investigative techniques are often invaluable, but these should only be used with clear aims. This chapter assesses the use of the sleep history and examination, and examines the principles underlying the most important investigations. The precise indications for each group of sleep disorders are described in Chapters 5–10.

History

Aims

It can be more difficult to take a history of a sleep disorder than to enquire about a complaint that occurs during wakefulness. The patient often has little or no awareness of the problem and it is important to obtain the bed partner's view of the events during sleep, and where appropriate, during wakefulness as well. The aim is to establish whether or not there is a sleep disorder and to assess the relative contribution

of psychological, medical and social factors to the complaint. The exact nature of the symptoms and the sequence of the appearance of the complaints should be recorded. Details of their onset and the nature of any progression of the complaints should be obtained. Some sleep disorders resolve, others fluctuate or progress.

Content

Detailed sleep questionnaires have been developed to cover the most important questions that need to be asked. They can supplement a conventional history and may even substitute for this if a history is unavailable. A detailed history is, however, preferable and the first step is to assess the patient's complaint or the reason for seeking attention. It should be established whether this is primarily insomnia, excessive daytime sleepiness or abnormal experiences or movements during sleep. The next step is to establish when the sleep problem began and whether there was any relationship to an external factor which may be physical, such as a head injury, or more subtle and psychological.

These initial questions should enable the more detailed history to remain focused on the patient's problem (Table 4.1). It is often useful to consider the details of events during sleep and wakefulness as a 24-h cycle, and to follow them around the clock (Fig. 4.1). The most important aspects of the sleep history are detailed below.

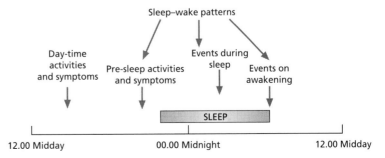

Fig. 4.1 Timing of sleep–wake events and symptoms.

Table 4.1 Important sleep symptoms and their possible implications.

Symptom	Implications
Short sleep time	Short sleeper; sleep deprivation; depression; DSPS; ASPS
Irregular sleep times	Social- or work-induced; circadian rhythm disorder
Delay in falling asleep	DIS—look for cause
Difficult to wake in the morning	Sleep deprivation; sleep inertia; ICNSH
Restlessness at night	Frequent arousals; OSA; PLMS; other behavioural disorder including epilepsy
Complex movements at night	Behavioural disorder including epilepsy
Snoring	Simple snorer; UARS; OSA
Nocturnal choking	OSA; gastro-oesophageal reflux; vocal cord adduction; panic attacks
Unrefreshing sleep	Sleep restriction; poor quality sleep, e.g. OSA, PLMS; circadian rhythm disorder, hyperarousal disorder, e.g. fibromyalgia
Early morning headaches	CO_2 retention; insomnia
Daytime naps	Sleep restriction; poor quality sleep, e.g. OSA, PLMS; narcolepsy; ICNSH ; depression
Loss of strength with emotion	Cataplexy
Pre-sleep apprehension	Anxiety; psycho-physiological insomnia; fear of event during sleep
Pre-sleep leg ache and movements	RLS and PLMS

ASPS, advanced sleep phase syndrome; DIS, difficulty in initiating sleep; DSPS, delayed sleep phase syndrome; ICNSH, idiopathic central nervous system hypersomnia; OSA, obstructive sleep apnoea; PLMS, periodic limb movements in sleep; RLS, restless legs syndrome; UARS, upper airway resistance syndrome.

SLEEP–WAKE PATTERNS

What time does the patient go to bed? What time does he or she go to sleep, wake up in the morning and get out of bed? The regularity or lack of regularity of these schedules and patterns should be noted, for instance during the working week, at weekends, or holidays. Do shift work or travel influence these sleep schedules?

Is there a reason for any delay in the initiation of sleep and if so what is this? Is the sleep environment satisfactory? Is the bedroom used for other activities, such as work? Is the bed comfortable and is the bedroom quiet, dark and neither too hot nor too cold?

If the patient finally wakes early in the morning, why is this? Is depression a feature or is there pain or discomfort? Is there any difficulty in awakening in the morning? Is an alarm clock needed?

The sleep pattern before the onset of the sleep disorder should also be noted. Was the patient a long sleeper, more alert in the evenings or early in the mornings? Was there any history of insomnia, sleep walking, etc?

EVENTS DURING SLEEP

Does the patient wake during the night? Is he or she aware of this or is it the partner who notices that an awakening has taken place, for instance because of the subject speaking or moving? Why does the awaken-

ing happen? Is there any sensation of pain, anxiety, panic, intrusive thoughts or nightmares? What happens when awakening occurs and how long is it before sleep is re-entered?

The frequency, time during the night (or more precisely during the sleep episode), and awareness of any mental or physical activity should be noted. Is there any relationship to other events? For instance, are any limb movements related to snoring and what is the patient's condition after an event such as sleep walking? Is he or she awake or confused, and is there any recall of the episode?

Does the subject dream or are there any nightmares? Is there any significance in the content of the dreams, and are any of these repetitive? Are there either intrusive thoughts or an awareness of thinking for much of the night? Does pain or discomfort lead to arousal from sleep? This may, for instance, be backache whose onset may not be directly related to sleep, or heartburn due to gastro-oesophageal reflux which is exacerbated by sleep.

Are there any abnormal movements, such as sleep walking, periodic limb movements, or nocturnal epileptic fits? Do any of these movements suggest that violence is being directed towards the bed partner?

Does the patient snore, appear to stop breathing, or make snorting noises at the end of an apnoea? These may be associated with jerking movements, suggesting an arousal from sleep. Are there any trigger factors for these problems such as the position of the patient or alcohol consumption? Is there a sensation of choking during sleep which may be related to obstructive sleep apnoeas (OSAs), gastro-oesophageal reflux, vocal cord adduction or panic attacks?

Does the subject have nocturia, nocturnal wheeze, sweating or episodes of being unable to move while awake (sleep paralysis)?

EVENTS ON AWAKENING
Is sleep refreshing? Are there any symptoms such as frontal headaches which might be due to carbon dioxide retention caused by hypoventilation during sleep? What is the level of alertness on waking and is there a history of confusional arousals? Has this led to any accidents? How does the subject feel emotionally on waking?

DAYTIME ACTIVITIES
Are naps taken during the day, and if so when and for how long? Are they refreshing? Is there adequate exposure to light during the day? Is exercise taken and what is the timing and size of meals? Does the type and timing of social activity promote or prevent sleep?

DAYTIME SYMPTOMS

Sensory
Does the subject have any hallucinations which might suggest narcolepsy, schizophrenia, amphetamine-induced psychosis, severe sleep deprivation or what is an extreme form of this, delirium tremens due to alcohol withdrawal. Is there any problem with concentration or memory?

Is there any pain or unpleasant sensations in the legs in the evenings which are relieved by movement, suggesting the restless legs syndrome?

Motor
Are there any abnormal movements to indicate epilepsy or cataplexy or a primary movement disorder which may be related to unusual movements during sleep, e.g. Parkinsonism?

Excessive daytime sleepiness
True hypersomnia in which the subject sleeps for an abnormally long duration during each 24-h cycle should be distinguished from hypersomnolence which is the sensation of sleepiness. These two symptoms should also be distinguished from mental fatigue with

poor concentration or motivation, physical weariness or fatigue which usually has an organic cause or may be related to insomnia, and the feeling of subalertness which may be due to a reduced wakefulness drive or an increased drive to sleep, as in narcolepsy. The duration, frequency and timing of naps should be noted, and whether or not these are refreshing. Many patients with narcolepsy feel refreshed after a nap of 10–30 min, whereas in idiopathic central nervous hypersomnia naps are longer but are unrefreshing.

The severity of daytime sleepiness can be gauged by its frequency and the type of situation in which the subject falls asleep. If it is mild, it only occurs infrequently, at times of day when sleep would be expected, e.g. 2.00–4.00 PM or late in the evening, or at rest or in a monotonous or passive environment, e.g. as a passenger in a car, bus or train, while sitting watching television or reading, or in a meeting. It is likely to be more severe if sleep occurs despite stimulating circumstances, for instance while talking, eating or on exertion, such as walking, and if it occurs frequently and at any time of the day.

Cyclical sleepiness may be due to intermittent sleep deprivation. Patients often sleep too little during the week and catch up their sleep debt at the weekends. This leads to a weekly cycle of sleepiness and recovery. Longer cycles of sleepiness are characteristic of other disorders, such as the monthly cycles in premenstrual sleepiness and even longer cycles in the Kleine–Levin syndrome. Elimination of sleepiness when sufficient sleep is allowed, for instance during holidays, indicates that sleep deprivation rather than a primary sleep disorder is the cause.

PRE-SLEEP ACTIVITIES AND SYMPTOMS
Is there apprehension about obtaining a poor night's sleep, or of waking, for instance with pain or discomfort? Has he or she been able to wind down mentally prior to the intended time of falling asleep or is mental over-activity and worry about the next day a problem? Are there any physical symptoms preventing sleep or features to suggest the restless legs syndrome, such as an inability to keep the legs still or an unpleasant sensation within the legs?

OTHER RELATED PROBLEMS
Symptoms that may be associated with sleep abnormalities should be enquired. These include, for instance, muscle aches and pains which are a feature of the chronic fatigue syndrome and fibromyalgia, and headaches which may indicate carbon dioxide retention. Poor concentration, reduction in short-

term memory and irritability are psychological consequences of sleep deprivation and hypnotic treatment.

Medical disorders which may be relevant to the sleep problem should be noted. These include depression, head injuries, Parkinsonism, nocturnal asthma, angina, prostatic symptoms and arthritis. The symptoms of nocturnal breathlessness, pain or nocturia that these conditions lead to may significantly disrupt sleep.

SOCIAL HISTORY

Does the patient work regular hours or shift work? Does he or she cross time zones frequently through international travel? Is there any history of foreign travel which might have predisposed to a sleep disorder, such as trypanosomiasis? What are the patient's housing and sleeping arrangements? Is the bedroom a suitable environment for sleep? Do any pet animals disturb sleep?

GENERAL HEALTH

Has there been a change in the patient's weight or collar size which might predispose to snoring and OSAs? Is the subject depressed?

MEDICAL HISTORY

Is there any history of disorders such as acromegaly or hypothyroidism? Is there a history of heart failure, which may cause Cheyne–Stokes respiration and nocturnal pulmonary oedema? Has the patient undergone any relevant surgery, such as a tonsillectomy or palatal surgery for snoring? A developmental history is important in children.

FAMILY HISTORY

Is there a family history of any sleep disorders such as narcolepsy, snoring, OSAs or periodic limb movements? Does the bed partner have a sleep problem which may be disturbing the patient? What is the partner's attitude to the patient's complaint? Do the patient and partner still sleep in the same bed, or same bedroom, and has the sleep disorder caused this to change?

DRUG HISTORY

Does the patient take any drugs for medical or recreational use which might affect sleep? What are the doses and when are they taken? Could the sleep symptoms be due to withdrawal of one of the drugs or to previous excessive alcohol consumption? What is the caffeine intake in total in each day and what is the tim-

ing of this? A stimulant such as caffeine taken shortly before the intended sleep time may cause insomnia, whereas the same amount taken in the morning may not have any effect on night-time sleep. What is the subject's alcohol and nicotine intake, and is he or she taking any 'alternative' or non-prescription medicines which may have effects on sleep which are unknown or at least uncertain?

Physical examination

A general physical examination is often not required to assess the patient with a sleep disorder, but there are specific aspects which should be noted in certain situations (Table 4.2). The degree of sleepiness or alertness, depression or anxiety should be recorded as well as any psychiatric features, for instance, schizophrenia or a personality disorder. The attitudes of the patient and the partner to the sleep complaint are important. The physical appearance may suggest a condition such as hypothyroidism or acromegaly which may be the cause of the sleep disorder.

The weight and collar size, examination of the nose and pharynx and the presence of retrognathia are relevant to snoring and OSAs. Ground down teeth are a feature of bruxism and evidence of physical injuries which might be the result of a behavioural abnormality in sleep, or the cause of the sleep disorder, should be sought. A neurological examination may be required to assess the cause of daytime sleepiness or a behavioural disorder, and any evidence of a movement disorder such as Parkinsonism should be noted. Examination of other systems such as the respiratory or cardiovascular system is indicated if the clinical picture suggests that these may be implicated in the sleep disorder.

Investigations

Investigation is required to assess the cause, nature and severity of the sleep disorder (Table 4.3), as well as its response to treatment.

Blood and urine tests

HAEMOGLOBIN CONCENTRATION

This may rise in hypoxic respiratory failure and fall in association with periodic limb movements in sleep, either because of iron deficiency or renal failure. The urea and electrolytes should be estimated if the latter is suspected.

Table 4.2 When to examine the patient.

	Situation	Examination
Insomnia	CNS disorder unlikely	Little value
	CNS disorder likely	CNS
EDS	Snoring	Weight, neck, upper airway, jaw
	Features of REM sleep while awake	Little value
	General medical disorder	Relevant system
Behavioural disorder	Epilepsy	CNS
	Disorder of arousal	Little value
	Features of REM sleep	CNS
	Cataplexy	Little value
	Daytime movement disorder	CNS
Respiratory disorder	Breathlessness	Respiratory and cardiovascular systems
	Irregular breathing pattern	CNS, respiratory and cardiovascular systems including upper airway

CNS, central nervous system.

ARTERIAL BLOOD GASES

These are required if nocturnal respiratory failure due to chronic lung disease or neuromuscular and skeletal disorders is suspected, or if there are central sleep apnoeas or frequent and severe OSAs.

HUMAN LEUCOCYTE ANTIGEN TYPING

Human leucocyte antigen (HLA) typing is of value in diagnosing or, more accurately, excluding narcolepsy.

DRUG LEVELS

Both therapeutic and recreational drug levels can be assessed in the blood or urine.

MELATONIN

The melatonin profile during the day and night can be obtained from plasma, urine or saliva, although the levels are delayed by at least 40 min in the latter, and it may be difficult to sleep when these samples are being acquired. The salivary concentrations are only around one third of those in plasma and diurnal changes may be difficult to detect. The pattern of secretion can be more precisely assessed if hourly samples, usually of blood, are obtained, but two- or four-hourly samples are adequate for most clinical purposes.

CORTISOL LEVELS

Frequent cortisol estimations can be used to assess the amplitude and timing of circadian rhythms, often in conjunction with continuous temperature recording, usually using a rectal probe.

Imaging and endoscopy techniques

1 A chest radiograph may be indicated if a pulmonary or cardiac cause of the sleep problems is suspected.
2 A skull radiograph, head computerized tomograph (CT) or magnetic resonance imaging (MRI) scan may be indicated to assess whether there is an organic cause for excessive daytime sleepiness (EDS), insomnia, abnormal movements, or other events occurring during sleep. MRI which utilizes changes in the extent of oxygenation of haemoglobin in the blood (functional MRI) can indicate areas of neuronal activity. Positron emission tomograph (PET) scans detect the decay of radioisotopically labelled molecules which are functionally important, such as glucose, and can provide 'metabolic imaging' [1]. Single photon emission tomography (SPET) is a similar technique and both may give information about the activity of various regions of the brain during sleep.
3 Radiographic examination of the upper airway (cephalometry) is occasionally useful in OSAs.
4 Upper airway endoscopy is used to localize the site of origin of snoring and OSAs, and abnormalities of the larynx and tracheobronchial tree can be visualized. Upper gastro-intestinal endoscopy may be required if, for instance, gastro-oesophageal reflux is thought to be related to the sleep disorder.

Table 4.3 Important investigations for sleep disorders.

Symptom	Probable diagnosis	Test
EDS		
– All	Any	Self-assessment scale
+ Snoring	OSA	Respiratory sleep monitoring
+ REM sleep features	Narcolepsy	HLA, polysomnography, MSLT
+ Restlessness	PLMS	Blood tests, actigraphy, polysomnography
+ Complex movements	Neurological disorder	Head CT or MRI, polysomnography
Insomnia		
– All	Any	Sleep diary
– DSPS, ASPS features	Circadian rhythm disorder	Sleep diary, actigraphy, blood and urine tests
– Neurological symptoms	Neurological disorder	Head CT or MRI, polysomnography
– Restlessness	PLMS	Blood tests, actigraphy, polysomnography
Behavioural disorders		
Limb jerks	Hypnic jerks	Nil
Walking	Sleep walking	Nil
Complex movements	Epilepsy, etc.	Polysomnography
Vocalization	Frontal lobe epilepsy, etc.	Polysomnography
Uncertain nature	Unknown	Polysomnography
Violence	REM behaviour disorder	Polysomnography
Dream related	PTSD, REM behaviour disorder	Polysomnography
Autonomic disorders		Disease-specific investigations
Respiratory disorder	Central sleep apnoeas	EDS self-assessment scale, arterial blood gases
	Cheyne–Stokes respiration	Chest X-ray, ECG lung function tests, respiratory sleep study
	Obstructive sleep apnoeas	EDS self-assessment scale, respiratory sleep study or polysomnography, arterial blood gases if severe
	Snoring	EDS self-assessment scale, respiratory sleep study, localization test, e.g. endoscopy
Combination of 1–5	Any combination	Polysomnography

ASPS, advanced sleep phase syndrome; CT, computed tomography; DSPS, delayed sleep phase syndrome; EDS, excessive daytime sleepiness; HLA, human leucocyte antigen; MRI, magnetic resonance imaging; MSLT, multiple sleep latency test; OSA, obstructive sleep apnoeas; PLMS, periodic limb movements in sleep; PTSD, post-traumatic stress disorder.

Daytime physiological tests

An electrocardiogram (ECG) or lung function tests help evaluate cardiopulmonary disorders and obstructive and central sleep apnoeas. Maximal inspiratory and expiratory mouth pressures and a flow volume loop assess respiratory muscle strength, and large airway function. An electro-encephalogram (EEG) during wakefulness may be indicated if epilepsy is suspected. Actigraphy during the day as well as the night is an indirect indicator of sleep–wake patterns.

Assessment of severity of daytime sleepiness

The severity, but not the cause, of EDS can be assessed by several techniques. They all have disadvantages and none is applicable to all situations. They measure different aspects of sleepiness and consequently the correlation between the results of the different tests is, in general, poor. The most widely used methods are described below.

SLEEP DIARIES

These are usually completed for two weeks, and the subject should record all episodes of sleep, whether these are during the day or at night, together with any other relevant events, such as taking caffeinated drinks, alcohol, meals and exercise (Fig. 4.2). They are of value in patients with irregular sleep–wake patterns and in assessing circadian rhythm disorders and the cause of EDS and insomnia.

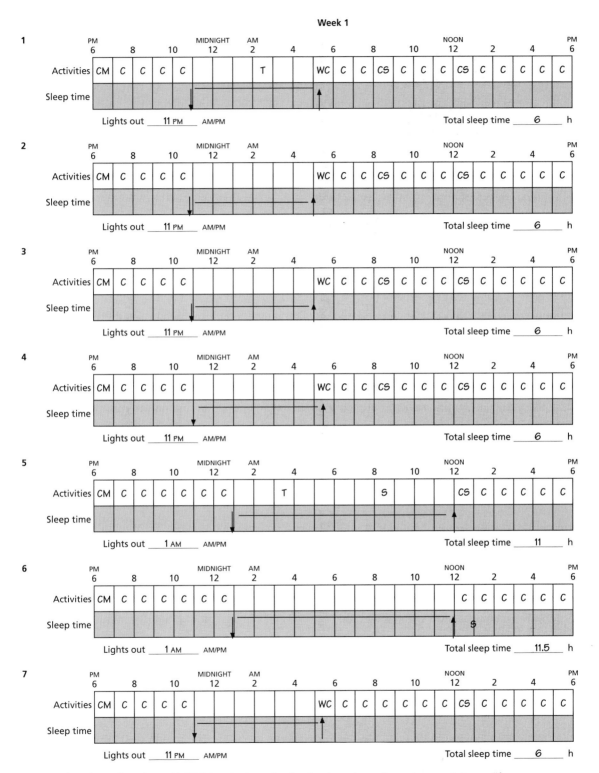

Fig. 4.2 Sleep diary of a patient with EDS showing irregular sleeping times, intermittent sleep restriction and frequent caffeinated drinks, as indicated by 'C' in activities line. M, meals; S, snacks; T, use of toilet in sleep time; W, wake-up time.

SELF ASSESSMENT SCALES

These are subjective or introspective tests which depend on the accuracy of the subject's perception of sleepiness and the ability to record this precisely. The attitude can influence whether the sleep problem is denied or exaggerated, and the degree of motivation to stay awake may affect the results. Some of the tests, such as the Epworth Sleepiness Scale (ESS), involve commenting on particular situations of which the subject may have no experience, but these are simple tests which should be regularly used in the assessment of EDS and insomnia. There are two types of these scales, discussed below.

Generic questionnaires

These focus on general health and may thereby give an indication of the impact of any sleep disorder on the quality of life. The Short Form 36 Health Survey (SF36) has been most widely used. Normal values are available for males and females and different age groups and social classes in the USA and UK. The SF36 is sensitive to some sleep disorders, such as OSAs, but is probably less so than the sleep-specific questionnaires.

Sleep-specific questionnaires

Most of these assess the individual's perception of how sleepy they feel, but the ESS enquires about the probability of actually falling asleep in certain situations. The simplest test is a Visual Analogue Scale in which the degree of sleepiness or alertness is scored from 0 to 10. This test is repeatable, easy to administer and is best used to assess the degree of sleepiness at the moment that the test is undertaken.

Other sleepiness scales such as the Stanford Sleepiness Scale (SSS) and Karolinska Sleepiness Scale (KSS) have been used, but the most satisfactory is the ESS (Table 4.4) [2]. This has eight items which the subject grades from 0 to 3 according to the likelihood of falling asleep in everyday situations, some of which are passive and some active. It has been validated for patients with OSA and has been shown to change when effective treatment is applied, but it may not be as useful in other conditions such as narcolepsy.

BEHAVIOURAL TESTS

Laboratory tests of performance do not have a wide application because of the lack of normal values, the improvement in the results with practice and their uncertain sensitivity and specificity for detecting sleepiness. The best recognized tests are described below.

Reaction times

The principle of these tests is that patients who are sleepy have a reduced ability to maintain attention.

Table 4.4 Epworth Sleepiness Scale. How likely are you to doze off or fall asleep in the following situations, in contrast to just feeling tired? This refers to your usual way of life in the last few weeks. Even if you have not done some of these things recently, try to work out how they would have affected you. Use the following scale to choose the most appropriate number for each situation.

Please tick one box on each line.

0 = Would never doze
1 = Slight chance of dozing
2 = Moderate chance of dozing
3 = High chance of dozing

Situation	0	1	2	3
Sitting and reading				
Watching television				
Sitting inactive in a public place (e.g. a theatre or a meeting)				
As a passenger in a car for an hour without a break				
Lying down in the afternoon, when circumstances permit				
Sitting and talking to someone				
Sitting quietly after lunch without alcohol				
In a car, while stopped for a few minutes in the traffic				

Their main value is in assessing responses to treatment by serial testing. Repetitive and unpredictable stimuli, such as flashing lights, are presented to the subject who has to respond as rapidly as possible. Delays or failure to respond to these stimuli are recorded. These tests require the subject's cooperation and are influenced by the degree of motivation.

Driving simulators

These have been used extensively, particularly in the USA, in order to assess the risk of the subject causing a road traffic accident. The most widely used is the Steer Clear Test. These tests are, however, as much a computer game as an estimate of sleepiness or safety while driving and the results depend on the aptitude and interest of the subject.

PSYCHOLOGICAL TESTS

Simple tracking tests and tests of higher cognitive function, such as decision making, have been used to assess the degree of daytime sleepiness and ability to maintain attention.

PUPILLOMETRY (PUPILLOGRAPHY)

This test depends on the principle that the pupil diameter is determined by the balance of sympathetic and parasympathetic tone and this is influenced by the state of arousal. The test measures the degree of sleepiness or the presence of sleep, and not its cause. During sleep the parasympathetic discharge dominates and the pupil constricts, whereas it dilates if the subject is alert, especially in a darkened environment.

During pupillometry the subject is kept in the dark for at least 10 min and if he or she is alert the diameter of the pupil should be stable and greater than 7 mm diameter. During sleepiness the pupil fluctuates in size and when the subject falls asleep it becomes smaller.

The problems with this test include difficulties in the subject collaborating, closure of the eyelids when he or she becomes sleepy, darkness of the iris which may make it difficult to determine the pupil size (although the use of infra red pupillography has reduced this difficulty), and ocular and neurological disorders particularly affecting the autonomic nervous system which may hinder interpretation of the test.

Pupillometry is being increasingly used but requires carefully controlled conditions, technical skill and better defined normal values.

BLINK FREQUENCY

Blinking becomes less frequent as sleepiness increases and is absent during micro sleeps. This simple observation has been used to assess the degree of acute sleepiness, but is best used in conjunction with other tests.

MULTIPLE SLEEP LATENCY TEST

This is an objective test which assesses the ease with which the subject can fall asleep during the day in the artificial environment of a sleep laboratory. Subjects should ideally have been following a normal sleep–wake routine for two weeks, without night or shift work and without taking any medication that might affect sleep. Polysomnography is carried out during the night before the Multiple Sleep Latency Test (MSLT) to establish that the duration of sleep is adequate and to look for any signs of sleep deprivation or a sleep disorder. The first MSLT begins either 2 h after waking or at around 09.00 AM and the test is repeated at 2-h intervals. Four tests are carried out during the day, plus a fifth if one of the first four has shown sleep-onset rapid eye movement (REM) and the possibility of narcolepsy is being considered. During each MSLT the subject is asked to lie down in a quiet, darkened room and to try to fall asleep. The test is terminated after 20 min if sleep has not been documented electrophysiologically or at 15 min after the first appearance of sleep. The onset of sleep is the interval from the time that the lights are switched off until the appearance of stage 1 non-rapid eye movement (NREM) sleep for a single epoch of 30 s. This differs from the criterion for sleep onset during polysomnography. Rapid eye movement sleep arising within 15 min of sleep onset is scored as sleep-onset REM (SOREM).

Exact normal values have not been determined for the MSLT. They are longer in prepubertal children and vary during the day according to fluctuations in the circadian rhythm and sleep and wake drives. The mean of the four or five MSLTs is taken as the value of the test. In general this is greater than 10 min in normal subjects. A mean MSLT of 8–10 min is indeterminate, but 5–8 min is probably mildly abnormal, and less than 5 min is definitely abnormal. An MSLT of less than 5 min is seen in 80% of subjects with narcolepsy, and less than 8 min in 95%, but the feature which distinguishes this most clearly from other causes of excessive daytime sleepiness is the presence of sleep-onset REM in two out of four or five of the MSLTs. If one SOREM period is documented in the first four tests, a fifth MSLT should be performed. Sleep-onset REM may also occasionally be seen in severe obstructive apnoeas, depression, severe sleep deprivation and in infants.

Multiple sleep latency tests are based on the assumption that the degree of sleepiness is related to the time that it takes to enter sleep as judged by EEG criteria. This has not been demonstrated and MSLTs do not correlate closely with other measures of sleepiness. They are insensitive at documenting serial changes with, for instance, drug treatment and may not give an accurate representation of the degree of sleepiness in daily life, let alone in a sleep laboratory [3].

Multiple sleep latency tests have the advantage that they are quantitative, objective and repeatable tests, but are difficult to standardize, time consuming and require technical experience and expensive equipment. They need careful interpretation if the subject has not been able to follow the ideal sleep–wake routines before the test or has remained on drugs that may influence the results. Micro sleeps are not scored in MSLTs and normal values are hard to establish, particularly because of the changing phases of the circadian rhythm during the test. It is common for REM sleep to appear during the first MSLT and for anxiety about the need for the patient to leave hospital at the time of the last test to cause them to stay awake.

MAINTENANCE OF WAKEFULNESS TEST
The Maintenance of Wakefulness Test (MWT) is similar to the MSLT except that the subject is asked to sit in a comfortable chair in a quiet darkened room for 20–40 min and to resist falling asleep. It is a measure of the ability to remain awake in a non-stimulating environment and more closely simulates real life situations than the MSLT which measures the ease with which the subject can fall asleep. The onset of sleep is assessed as in an MSLT. The mean of 4 MWTs is taken as the value for each subject. A normal MWT is greater than around 18 min, although precise normal values have not been established. The mean MWT for untreated patients with narcolepsy is around 10 min.

The MWT can detect acute and severe sleep deprivation, but it is as much a test of will power as of sleepiness. Its role in the assessment of EDS is unclear, but it may be useful in monitoring changes after, for example, drug treatment [4].

EVOKED POTENTIALS
The degree of sleepiness influences the EEG evoked potential that can be detected after various stimuli, particularly auditory [5]. This technique has been used mainly in research rather than clinical practice.

Physiological tests during sleep
The choice of which sleep study to use depends on the questions that need to be answered. In general it is best to start with the simplest type of study and then to proceed to more complicated, expensive and time consuming investigations if the initial test does not provide the required information. The specificity and sensitivity of more complex tests in identifying the possible causes of the sleep problem and in providing information that contributes to decision making about further treatment should guide their use.

These important issues have hardly been addressed and as a result of this lack of data there is wide variation between different sleep centres in the way in which sleep studies are used. Studies may need to be extended into wakefulness during the day to identify possible episodes of epilepsy or cataplexy or to document the type, duration and timing of sleep during the day time. The detailed indications for the different types of sleep study are discussed in Chapters 5–10.

There are several uses of sleep studies, detailed below.

ASSESS SLEEP STATE AND STAGES
The electrophysiological assessment of sleep enables it to be differentiated from wakefulness, the stage of sleep to be identified, the details of arousals and awakenings recorded, and, when it is combined with other physiological measurements, for the cause of the sleep disturbance to be investigated. Three signals are required to assess sleep accurately: an EEG, an electro-oculogram (EOG) and an electro-myogram (EMG). Polysomnography (PSG) (or, more accurately, somnopolygraphy) is the simultaneous acquisition and coordinated analysis of these and other physiological signals during sleep (Fig. 4.3). It has the advantages of being able to determine sleep onset and offset, the stages of sleep, and to correlate these with simultaneous physiological, video and other findings. It does, however, require the patient to sleep in an unnatural environment, is dependent on skilled technician time and is expensive. Portable polysomnography which can be used in the home can now provide good quality signals and may be useful, not only in avoiding the problems of sleeping in an unfamiliar room, but also in enabling the disabled and those living far from hospital to be investigated [6].

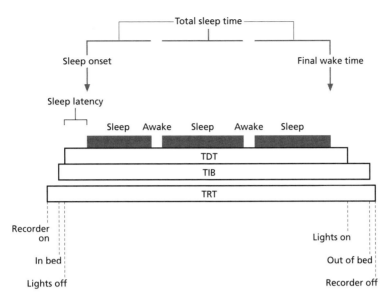

Fig. 4.3 Polysomnography definitions. TRT: total recording time, time from switching on to switching off recording equipment. TIB: time in bed, time from lights out to time of getting out of bed. TSP: total sleep period, (SPT: sleep period time) time from sleep onset to end of sleep. TDT: total dark time, time from lights out to lights on in the morning. SO: sleep onset, time of sleep onset. SL: sleep latency, time from lights out until sleep onset. Final wake time: time of final wakening. TST: total sleep time, time from sleep onset to the end of sleep, minus time awake. WT: wake time, time awake between sleep onset and end of sleep. Sleep efficiency: total sleep time divided by time in bed, as a percentage.

Duration of each sleep stage or state in minutes or as a percentage of TST. REM latency: time from sleep onset to onset of REM sleep. REM cycle duration: interval between onset of consecutive REM periods. REM density: percentage of REM epochs containing rapid eye movements. MT: movement time, total time of sleep epochs obscured for greater than 50% by movements or muscle artefact. Awakenings: episodes of longer than 15 s in any 30 s epoch with abrupt changes in EEG frequency and other related features. Arousal: episodes of longer than 3 s with abrupt changes in EEG frequency and other related features.

Practical aspects

The EEG, EOG and EMG electrodes are usually silver–silver electrodes and the signals are filtered and amplified before being either recorded on paper by a polygraph or stored and displayed by computer. A recording speed of 10–15 mm/s is most suitable for paper recordings.

Patients are often daunted by the thought or sight of the electrodes and other equipment, and reassurance is important in order to try to help them fall asleep naturally during the study. The quality of sleep is often poor initially ('first night effect') and the study may need to be repeated. Checks of the adequacy of the signals should be made once the electrodes are applied and before the subject falls asleep. Artefacts may arise during the study due to movement, poor contact of the electrodes, either due to displacement or sweating, electrical interference or other problems with the recording system.

Electro-encephalogram recording

The electrical potentials that are recorded on the scalp reflect the overall activity of the neurones in the underlying regions of the brain, particularly the cerebral cortex. They provide a continuous and non-invasive monitor of the electrical activity and its oscillation during sleep. The activity of the cortex is, however, only sampled at the locations where the electrodes are applied (Fig. 4.4). A full 10–20 montage is only required to diagnose nocturnal epilepsy or to assess other focal abnormalities. In practice it is usual for only two electrodes to be used and these monitor the central regions of the brain. Two occipital electrodes can be added to evaluate alpha activity in detail since this is most prominent in this region. Sampling of cortical activity by only two electrodes is probably valid because of the coherence of the whole of its activity due to the widespread projections of the thalamo-cortical fibres which cause synchronized

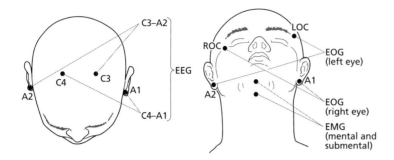

Fig. 4.4 Electrode positions for polysomnography. The left-hand side of the figure indicates the EEG position, and the right-hand side indicates the EOG and EMG. EEG, electro-encephalogram; EMG, electromyogram; EOG, electro-oculogram; LOC, outer canthus of the left eye; ROC, outer canthus of the right eye.

waves of depolarization and hyperpolarization. There is a slight time lag across the cerebral cortex as this wave of activity is propagated, and during NREM sleep the site of maximum activity drifts forwards from the occipital towards the frontal cortex.

Electro-oculogram recording
Movements of the eyes are important in diagnosing whether the subject is falling asleep and particularly whether REM sleep or wakefulness is present. The potential difference between the cornea and the retina is measured and it is movement of this electrical dipole, and not the activity of the extra-ocular muscles, that is recorded. One electrode is applied one centimetre above, but close to the outer canthus of the right eye (ROC) and another electrode one centimetre below the outer canthus of the left eye (LOC). Reference (neutral) electrodes are connected to the contralateral ear (see Fig. 4.4).

Electro-myogram recordings
The presence or absence of muscle activity ('tone') is important in establishing whether the subject is awake, or in NREM or REM sleep. It is usually identified by electrodes on the chin (mentalis) and under the chin (submentalis; see Fig. 4.4).

Sleep staging
Sleep stages are conventionally scored according to recommendations set out in 1968 (Fig. 4.5) [7]. These have proved useful, but only characterize the dominant sleep stage at any one time and do not show the dynamic structure of sleep adequately. The criteria have been validated for healthy young adults, but not in other situations. The recording is divided into units (epochs) of 20 or 30 s. The sleep stage during each epoch is designated according to which one is present for over half of the time. This makes it insensitive to

rapid changes in sleep state and ignores the microstructure of sleep. The criteria for diagnosing events during sleep are inflexible and no attention is paid to differences in, for instance, the alpha frequency or types of sleep spindle. There is considerable inter-observer variation in the conventional reporting of sleep staging, although this is more accurate than the computerized reporting systems that have been developed. Newer approaches using computerized analysis of the continuous trends in frequency and amplitude, and the analysis of sleep microstructure are being developed, but are not yet in general use [8].

Wakefulness, NREM and REM sleep can be distinguished by a combination of their EEG, EOG and EMG features. The EEG rhythms are identified and classified primarily by their frequency, but also by their amplitude (Tables 4.5 and 4.6, Fig. 4.6). As sleep is entered the frequency of the EEG slows, with a loss of alpha, increase in theta and then of delta waves. Patterns of electrical activity specific to sleep appear. These include K-complexes, spindles, vertex sharp waves and transients, both spikes (< 70 ms duration) and sharp waves (> 70 ms duration). The characteristic electrophysiological features of each of these states of consciousness in adults are as follows.

Alert wakefulness. With the eyes open and when the subject is alert, the EEG tracings show a dominant rhythm of up to 30–50 Hz with a low amplitude. There is a high level of muscle tone and blinking is detectable in the EOG channel.

Relaxed wakefulness. When relaxed with the eyes closed the frequency of the dominant rhythm falls to around 8–13 Hz (alpha rhythm), although this can be abolished by opening the eyes. The alpha rhythm is most easily detected in the occipital region. Muscle tone is less prominent than during alertness.

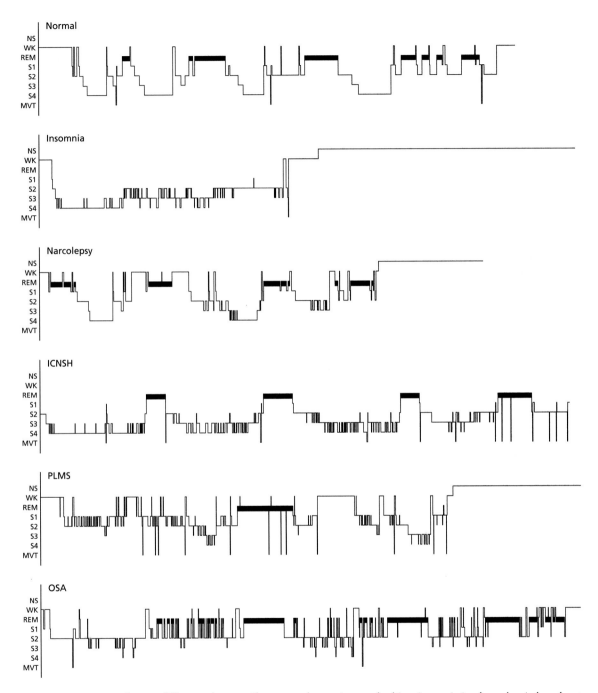

Fig. 4.5 Hypnograms showing differences between (from top to bottom): normal subject; insomnia (prolonged period awake at the end of the night); narcolepsy (sleep onset REM and frequent sleep stage shifts); ICNSH (prolonged episodes of stages 3 and 4 NREM sleep); periodic limb movement syndrome (frequent arousals early in the night with difficulty in establishing stages 3 and 4 NREM sleep); and OSAs (frequent arousals and lack of stages 3 and 4 NREM sleep). ICNSH, idiopathic central nervous system hypersomnia; MVT, movement artefact; NREM, non-rapid eye movement; NS, no signal; OSA, obstructive sleep apnoea; REM, rapid eye movement; S1–4, stages 1–4 NREM sleep; WK, wakefulness.

Table 4.5 EEG waveforms during sleep and wakefulness.

Waveform	Frequency or duration	Amplitude	Location	Main sleep–wake state and stage
Beta	Unstable frequency, > 13 Hz	10–20 μV	Frontal and prefrontal	Alert wakefulness, stage 1 NREM and REM
Alpha	8–13 Hz	20–50 μV	Occipital	Relaxed wakefulness
Theta	4–8 Hz	10–30 μV	Generalized	Wakefulness, stage 1 NREM
Delta	0.5–4 Hz	> 75 μV	Generalized	Stages 2, 3 and 4 NREM
Vertex sharp waves	0.05–0.2 s duration	30–200 μV	Vertex	Stage 1 NREM
K-complexes	1 Hz, > 0.5 s duration	> 75 μV	Generalized, maximum at vertex	Stage 2 NREM
Sleep spindles	12–16 Hz, > 0.5 s duration	20–40 μV	Generalized	Stage 2 NREM
Sawtooth waves	2–5 Hz, > 0.25 s duration	20–100 μV	Generalized, especially vertex	REM

Table 4.6 Common causes of sleep-stage abnormalities on polysomnography.

Sleep state and stage	Increased	Reduced
NREM stages 3 and 4	Sleep deprivation Drugs ICNSH Neurological hypersomnias Thyrotoxicosis Fever	First night effect Old age Sleep fragmentation, e.g. OSA, ventilatory failure, PLMS, pain Drugs Degenerative cerebral disorders Depression
REM latency	REM suppressant drugs ICNSH PLMS CSA and CSR	REM sleep deprivation Infancy REM sleep fragmentation, e.g. OSA, pain Drugs Narcolepsy Depression Mania Circadian rhythm disorders
REM	Infancy After REM sleep deprivation Drugs	REM sleep deprivation REM sleep fragmentation, e.g. OSA, ventilatory failure, pain Drugs Degenerative cerebral disorders

CSA, central sleep apnoea; CSR, Cheyne–Stokes respiration; ICNSH, idiopathic central nervous system hypersomnia; OSA, obstructive sleep apnoeas; PLMS, periodic limb movements in sleep; REM, rapid eye movement.

Non-rapid eye movement sleep. In stage 1 of NREM sleep alpha activity diminishes and is replaced by 2–3 s runs of slower waves at a frequency of 4–8 Hz (theta rhythm) and vertex sharp waves. These are seen particularly in children and young adults. Muscle tone is reduced further and slow rolling eye movements lasting 2–4 s are detectable.

In stage 2 NREM sleep, spindles appear often at a rate of 3–8 per minute, with K-complexes (often 1–3 per minute). High-amplitude slow-frequency delta waves appear, but occupy less than 20% of each epoch. The spindle frequency of 12–14 Hz is determined by the duration of hyper-polarization in the thalamo-cortical neurones. They are related to the blocking of sensory stimulus transmission. K-complexes consist of two negative waves followed by a positive wave and have a frequency of only around 1 Hz. They are bilaterally symmetrical, predominantly

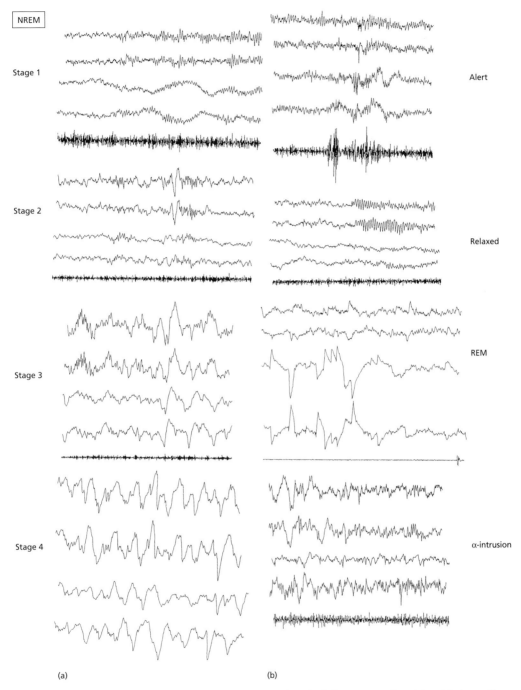

Fig. 4.6 The EEG, EMG and EOG appearances. (a) Stage 1 NREM sleep: high-frequency EEG activity with slow rolling eye movements. Stage 2 NREM: K-complex with spindles. Stage 3 NREM: delta waves present in EEG for 20–50% of tracing and conducted to the EOG tracings, less chin EMG activity than in stages 1 and 2 NREM. Stage 4 NREM: the EEG shows slow high-amplitude delta waves throughout with no chin EMG activity. (b) Alert wakefulness: high-frequency EEG recording with eye movements and considerable chin EMG activity. Relaxed wakefulness: conspicuous alpha rhythm (8–13 Hz) on EEG tracing and chin EMG activity present. REM sleep: irregular mixed frequency EEG with frequent eye movements and absence of chin EMG activity. Alpha intrusion into stage 3 NREM: alpha waves, superimposed on delta waves in EEG tracing and conducted to EOG recordings. EEG, electro-encephalogram; EMG, electro-myogram; EOG, electro-oculogram; NREM, non-rapid eye movement; REM, rapid eye movement.

fronto-parietal, and result from increasing synchro-nization of the cerebral cortex as NREM sleep deep-ens. They probably represent a partial response of the cortex to sensory stimuli, some of which are external (usually auditory) and easily identified, and others internal and often cryptic and not sufficient to gener-ate a full arousal from sleep [9]. There is less muscle tone than in stage 1 and no eye movements.

The deeper stages of NREM sleep (stages 3 and 4) are characterized by the presence of delta waves. They are known as slow waves because of their low frequency (0.5–4 Hz) and at least some of the delta waves are due to the low firing frequency of the thalamo-cortical projection fibres. These waves occupy 20–50% of each epoch in stage 3 and over 50% of the epochs in stage 4 NREM. Their amplitude is greater than 75 mV in young adults, but this falls in the elderly. Sleep spindles and K-complexes may also be present and may be difficult to distinguish from, and may be masked by, the delta waves. There is some 30–50 Hz activity, but this is much less prominent than in REM sleep. Muscle tone is less than in stages 1 and 2 and eye movements are absent.

Rapid eye movement sleep. The EEG of REM sleep is very similar to that of relaxed wakefulness with a wide range of frequencies of low and irregular amplitude. These largely reflect the 30–50 Hz (gamma band) activity in the cerebral cortex which is characteristic of REM sleep, and which is thought to be a feature of attention in the cerebral cortex, whether this is occur-ring during sleep or while the subject is awake. Interestingly, this high frequency is also seen in the basal ganglia when they are focusing attention on a movement and this 30–50 Hz activity is driven by the burst frequency in the thalamo-cortical projection neurones. This high-frequency activity in REM sleep is more localized than the projection of electrical activity during NREM sleep so that the surface EEG appears to be 'desynchronized'. The vertex sharp waves of stage 2 are replaced in REM by sawtooth waves of 2–5 Hz, which often precede rapid eye movements.

In REM sleep the EMG recording appears flat because of lack of muscle activity, except for sporadic bursts of phasic muscle twitches, especially in the facial and limb electrodes. The EOG shows absence of eye movements (tonic REM sleep), except for intermittent bursts of rapid eye movements (phasic REM sleep). The frequency of epochs which contain these movements is termed the 'density' of REM

sleep. Ponto-geniculo-occipital (PGO) waves can be detected in some animals, especially cats, and when deep, rather than surface, electrodes are used. They are said to be characteristic of REM sleep but are usually not detectable with surface electrodes in humans.

MONITOR MOVEMENTS
This is particularly valuable in assessing whether the patient is awake or asleep on behavioural grounds and in conjunction with other monitoring in assessing abnormal movemenzts during sleep. Micro arousals from any cause can be detected, but the value of mon-itoring is limited, especially in the elderly, in whom movements during sleep occur as a result of disorders such as the periodic limb movement syndrome and OSAs, and conversely immobility is frequent during wakefulness.

There are various methods of recording movements, detailed below.

Video and examination
This is usually used in conjunction with an audio recording and sleep-stage monitoring. It can detect not only movements of the limbs and respiratory movements, but also the position of the patient. The movements may be difficult to quantify by video recordings, but a combination of video and audio recordings can be useful in assessing the frequency of OSAs and hypopnoeas.

Electromyogram electrodes
These are conventionally applied to the anterior tib-ialis muscle of both legs and ideally these are recorded separately, although often they are combined to give a single EMG input to the recording system. This technique is particularly useful for diagnosing periodic limb movements (Fig. 4.7) and arousals from sleep, but EMG recordings from other muscles can be used in certain circumstances.

Actigraphy
This alternative to EMG uses an accelerometer in which small movements are transduced into electrical signals which can be recorded and analysed. It identi-fies small accelerations in contrast to the EMG which records electrical activity of the muscles. Actigraphy can be used on a domiciliary basis and modern acti-graphs can record and store data from several nights. They can be used as an indirect indicator of whether the subject is awake or asleep which may be useful in

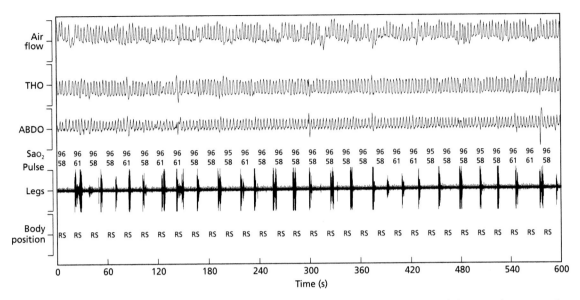

Fig. 4.7 EMG monitoring to show periodic limb movements in sleep. Regular leg movements recorded at around 20 s intervals throughout the tracing. ABDO, abdominal movement; RS, right side; Sao₂, arterial oxygen saturation; THO, thoracic movement.

insomnia and excessive daytime sleepiness, as well as to identify, for instance, the degree of suppression of OSAs and periodic limb movements with treatment.

MONITOR RESPIRATION

The normal noises of respiration and those of snoring, OSAs, snorting, grunting, wheezing and stridor can be sensed by a microphone placed either close to the upper airway or over the trachea. Frequency analysis and estimation of the loudness of the noise can be carried out. Air flow can be measured using oral, nasal or oro-nasal thermistors which detect changes in temperature between the inspired and expired air (Fig. 4.8). These give a semiquantitative estimate of airflow, but can become displaced. An end tidal Pco₂ monitor is an alternative, but nasal pressure transducers can be better quantified than these other techniques. The pressure profile during each breath indicates whether there is flow limitation due to upper-airway narrowing, but a blocked nose, mouth breathing or dislodgement of the cannulae can make interpretation difficult. The forced oscillation technique may also detect upper airway flow limitation. High-frequency, low-amplitude pressure waves are applied to the airway and, if this narrows, the amplitude of the pressure oscillation falls. Air leaks through the mouth may produce similar findings but this technique is useful in detecting upper airway narrowing or temporary

occlusion in the titration of continuous positive airway pressure (CPAP) treatment for OSA.

Respiratory movements can be measured by inductance, impedance or magnetometry methods, or by using mercury strain gauges. These are all semiquantitative and together with recording of airflow can be used to distinguish between central and obstructive sleep apnoeas. Respiratory effort can be estimated by measuring the oesophageal pressure which reflects the intrapleural pressure. This is an indicator of the activity of the chest wall muscles. The pressure swings increase during, for instance, OSAs, and the upper airway resistance syndrome in order to overcome the high airflow resistance. This technique is invasive in that it requires swallowing a balloon or catheter into the oesophagus. An indirect estimate of pleural pressure swings can be obtained from continuous monitoring of the blood pressure by deriving the pulse transit time. This is the time taken for the arterial pulse to travel through the peripheral circulation. It is usually measured as the interval between the R wave of the ECG, which corresponds to the aortic valve opening, and the onset of the pulse wave on a pulse oximeter applied to the finger. The pulse transit time is reduced if the blood pressure rises, for instance, in response to changes in the intrathoracic pressure during OSAs. It is, in effect, a non-invasive equivalent of measuring the oesophageal pressure, and has the

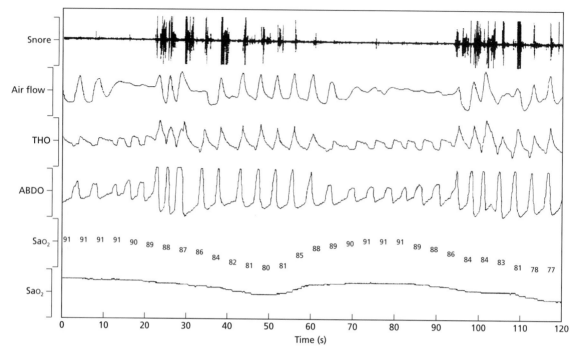

Fig. 4.8 Respiratory monitoring in OSA. Obstructive sleeps apnoeas demonstrated by cessation of airflow associated with paradoxical thoracic and abdominal movement and terminated with snoring sounds, followed by an increase in oxygen saturation. ABDO, abdominal movement; Sao_2, arterial oxygen saturation; THO, thoriacic movement.

additional advantage of detecting 'autonomic arousals' at the end of each apnoea at which time the pulse transit time increases suddenly. Interpretation is difficult in the presence of cardiac dysrhythmias, left ventricular dysfunction or with beta blockers. Electromyogram recordings of the diaphragm and other respiritory muscles show whether they are active during respiration, but do not give an indication of the force that they develop.

The arterial blood gases can be measured non-invasively during sleep. A transcutaneous Pco_2 or end tidal Pco_2 monitor can be used and pulse oximetry can also give a continuous non-invasive record of oxygen saturation. This uses a spectroscopic technique identifying oxyhaemoglobin in the wave band of 660 nm and reduced haemoglobin at the 940 nm wave band. Most oximeters are accurate to within 3% when the saturation is above 70%. Visual inspection of the oximetry tracing during sleep may be of more value than using unvalidated indices. Pulse oximetry also gives a continuous recording of the heart rate which may be useful in identifying whether the patient is awake or asleep and whether OSAs or other organic sleep disorders such as periodic limb movements are present.

MONITOR CARDIOVASCULAR CHANGES

The heart rate can be identified using a pulse oximeter and an ECG gives more detail about the nature of electrical conduction of the cardiac impulse. A three-lead ECG is conventionally used in polysomnography but this may be inadequate to define dysrrhythmias accurately in which case conventional 24 h cardiac monitoring may be required. Blood pressure can be monitored at home using the techniques described above and a continuously recording pulmonary artery pressure catheter is now available.

MONITOR OESOPHAGEAL PH

This can be recorded from a sensor in the oesophagus and is used particularly to identify episodes of gastro-oesophageal reflux. Their significance depends on the frequency, duration and extent of the fall in pH, which relate to the degree of acid reflux and the ease with which it is cleared from the oesophagus.

MONITOR PENILE ERECTION

This has been used to distinguish organic from psychogenic causes of impotence. In the latter, erections during sleep are retained, in contrast to organic disorders, but they may be impaired if REM sleep fragmentation is severe as in OSAs and with PLMS. The increase in penile circumference can be measured with a mercury-filled strain gauge whose electrical resistance is proportional to the length of the gauge. The rigidity of the penis is recorded by assessing the force that is needed to cause it to buckle. Normal values have been obtained for the frequency of erections during sleep, the total duration of the erections and the increase in penile circumference. Knowledge of the sleep structure is required to interpret these findings and these investigations should be carried out as part of polysomnography.

References

1 Maquet P, Phillips C. Functional brain imaging of human sleep. *J Sleep Res* 1998; 7 (Suppl. 1): 42–7.
2 Johns MW. Daytime sleepiness, snoring and obstructive sleep apnea. The Epworth Sleepiness Scale. *Chest* 1993; 103: 30–6.
3 Sangal RB, Thomas L, Mitler MM. Maintenance of Wakefulness Test and Multiple Sleep Latency Test. Measurement of different abilities in patients with sleep disorders. *Chest* 1992; 101: 898–902.
4 Poceta JS, Timms RM, Jeong D-U, Ho S-L, Erman MK, Mitler MM. Maintenance of Wakefulness Test in Obstructive Sleep Apnea Syndrome. *Chest* 1992; 101: 893–7.
5 Bastuji H, Garcia-Larrea L. Evoked potentials as a tool for the investigation of human sleep. *Sleep Med Rev* 1999; 3: 23–45.
6 Mykytyn IJ, Sajkov D, Neill AM, McEvoy RD. Portable computerized polysomnography in attended and unattended settings. *Chest* 1999; 115: 114–22.
7 Rechtschaffen A, Kales A, eds. *A Manual of Standardized Terminology, Techniques and Scoring System for Sleep Stages of Human Subjects*. Los Angeles: Brain Information Service/Brain Research Institute, 1968.
8 McKeown MJ, Humphries C, Achermann P, Borbely AA, Sejnowski TJ. A new method for detecting state changes in the EEG. Exploratory application to sleep data. *J Sleep Res* 1998; 7 (Suppl 1): 48–56.
9 Davies RJO, Bennett LS, Stradling JR. What is an arousal and how should it be quantified? *Sleep Med Rev* 1997; 2: 87–95.

5 Insomnia

Introduction

Insomnia (agrypnia) is not a diagnosis, but a symptom, or more usually a symptom complex or syndrome. It is commonly defined as a perception of insufficient or poor quality sleep, leading to a feeling of being unrefreshed, either on waking, during wakefulness or in both of these situations. The relative importance of the two components of the syndrome, poor sleep at night and tiredness during the day, varies considerably. Most insomniacs find it difficult to fall asleep during the day despite feeling tired, and therefore do not have true excessive daytime sleepiness (EDS), although 'sleep reversal' is characterized by severe insomnia at night with prominent episodes of sleep during the day. It usually indicates severe disorganization of the sleep controlling mechanisms as in Alzheimer's disease, African sleeping sickness and after encephalitis lethargica, but may occur in depression and schizophrenia. Insomniacs can be distinguished from short sleepers in that the latter, although they may sleep for no longer, wake feeling refreshed, function normally during the day, and do not complain about their sleep at night.

The large number of physiological factors that influence sleep often combine to cause a poor night's sleep. This is usually recognized as a natural response to the circumstances. A mild degree of insomnia merges into normality on the one hand, and into what can be a severe disability on the other, but the complaint of insomnia depends very much on the subject's expectations of the quality and length of sleep and of daytime tiredness. The correlation between the subjective reporting of sleep quality and objective findings at polysomnography is poor, although as a group those with insomnia tend to sleep less and wake more frequently than the general population. Anxiety and frustration may lead the degree of wakefulness to be overestimated during the night. The extreme form of this is sleep state misperception when the subject complains of insomnia, but has completely normal sleep as assessed at polysomnography. The mood, degree of boredom and medical disorders, both physical and psychological, also influence how severe insomnia is perceived to be. It therefore represents the degree of dissatisfaction with sleep or the mismatch between the expectation and reality rather than reflecting an absolute degree of sleep disturbance. It is less frequently due to organic disease than EDS, but, similarly, its origin is often multifactorial.

Prevalence

Insomnia is the commonest sleep complaint. Almost every adult suffers from it at some stage in their life. Surveys have indicated that around one third of adults in westernized societies have some degree of insomnia each year, and 10–15% of the population have insomnia at any one time. It becomes more common in middle age and is probably five times as frequent at 70 years as at 40 years [1]. Difficulty in initiating sleep (DIS) is twice as common in women as men, but there is less gender difference in difficulty in maintaining sleep (DMS), and early morning awakening (EMW) is equally common in men and women.

The high prevalence figures need to be interpreted cautiously because of the subjective nature of the complaint and differences in the definitions of insomnia. Its commonness may reflect the pressure in westernized societies to function effectively during the day, particularly at work, while restricting sleeping time because of social activities and leisure opportunities, combined with an increasing preoccupation with medical problems. The complaint of insomnia is commoner in those who are anxious or depressed, and those who drink excessive quantities of alcohol or take drugs which affect the quality of sleep. In about half of these it is felt to be severe enough to require medical care, although this is surprisingly often not obtained. The reasons for this are uncertain, but the lack of attention directed to insomnia by the medical profession, the failure to develop coherent management plans and the perception that there is a lack of effective treatments probably all contribute.

Effects of insomnia

Psychological disturbances

These are common during the episode of insomnia, but are completely reversible once it is relieved.
1 Loss of concentration and deterioration of memory.
2 Irritability and mood disturbance including anxiety and depression. Anxiety and depression are present in more than 50% of those with chronic insomnia and may be either a cause or a result of the insomnia. A vicious cycle of insomnia and worsening anxiety and depression often develops.
3 Loss of motivation.
4 Fear regarding long-term health effects of insomnia.
5 Intrusive ruminating thoughts at bedtime. These are often related to a fear of not sleeping or frustration or anger at the degree of insomnia and of not being able to function effectively, either at work or in family or social life.

Physical effects

These are also common and reversible once the insomnia is relieved. They include:
1 A sensation of physical weariness, fatigue or tiredness. This is distinct from EDS which mainly occurs in the minority of patients with insomnia in whom there is an organic cause.
2 Muscle aches. These are usually worse in the limbs, but may be diffuse and cause headaches and neckache; they are probably due to muscle tension associated with a lack of the normal inhibition of

motor activity during sleep with the result that the muscles are contracting throughout sleep as well as wakefulness.

Social effects

Insomnia is more common in lower socio-economic groups and is said to be associated with fewer episodes of promotion at work than in those without insomnia. This may be due to tiredness and poor work performance, but, equally, anxiety about the latter could be the cause of the insomnia. An excessive concern about responsibilities is thought to contribute to the insomnia of ambitious, high-achieving personalities.

Mortality

Individuals who sleep for less than 6 h per night have a shorter life expectancy than those who report sleeping for 7–8 h per night. This may be because diseases causing the sleep disturbance also shorten life expectancy, or because of the high arousal state which is often present in insomnia. Insomnia itself may also induce or perpetuate physiological dysfunctioning which may increase morbidity, reduce the rate of recovery from other medical disorders and shorten the life expectancy.

Patterns of insomnia

Insomnia can be separated into the following three patterns (Table 5.1).
1 Difficulty in initiating sleep (sleep onset insomnia). This is defined as a sleep latency of greater than 30 min and is often due to a high level of arousal associated with anxiety, and other factors.

Table 5.1 Causes of patterns of insomnia.

Difficulty in initiating sleep	Difficulty in maintaining sleep	Early morning waking
Poor sleep hygiene	Pain, discomfort	Old age
Poor sleep environment	Poor sleep environment	Poor sleep environment
Drugs	Drugs	Drugs
Anxiety	Medical problem, e.g. asthma, nocturia	Depression
Psychophysiological insomnia	PLMS	Mania
PLMS	OSA, CSA, CSR	ASPS
DSPS	Dementia	
	Psychophysiological insomnia	

ASPS, advanced sleep phase syndrome; CSA, central sleep apnoeas; CSR, Cheyne–Stokes respiration; DSPS, delayed sleep phase syndrome; OSA, obstructive sleep apnoeas; PLMS, periodic limb movements in sleep.

2 Difficulty in maintaining sleep (sleep maintenance insomnia). Waking may occur irregularly during the night, or at specific times as in cluster headaches occurring during rapid eye movement (REM) sleep and the 90-min cycles of REM sleep behaviour disorder episodes.

3 Early morning waking without further sleep. This is common in the elderly and in the conditions listed in Table 5.1.

Time course of insomnia

Insomnia may be a temporary phase, may fluctuate or be a long-term problem. The causes and perpetuation of these three patterns are different.

Transient insomnia (adjustment sleep disorder, acute insomnia)

The diagnosis of transient insomnia can only be firmly made retrospectively after it has been relieved. It is usually defined as insomnia that lasts for less than 3 weeks, and very often has a close temporal association to an event which is clearly recognized by the patient and is often stressful. It is equally common in males and females and is more likely if there is a history of previous poor sleep, or if there is a low threshold for emotional arousal. Recurrent episodes of transient insomnia are also common.

Transient insomnia is usually triggered by one of the following factors.

CHANGES IN SLEEP ENVIRONMENT

These may be physical stimuli such as noise or bright lights, or movements or noises such as snoring made by the bed partner. Sleeping in unfamiliar environments such as a hotel or in hospital, including a sleep laboratory, may also impair sleep.

HIGH AROUSAL STATES

These may be due to emotional events which increase the level of alertness and physiological arousal. They include bereavement, apprehension before an examination, excitement before a holiday, anxiety about job insecurity, brief illnesses or pain.

POOR SLEEP HYGIENE

Transient insomnia may result from temporary adoption of an irregular sleep–wake cycle. Drinking excess coffee or alcohol in the evenings or other central nervous system (CNS) stimulants or drugs which can impair sleep, either while being taken or during the withdrawal phase, may be responsible.

SHORT-TERM CIRCADIAN RHYTHM DISORDERS INDUCED PARTICULARLY BY JET LAG AND ROTATING SHIFT WORK

This type of transient insomnia may be severe, but resolves once the trigger factor is removed or the patient adjusts to the new circumstances. It may evolve into chronic insomnia if this adjustment fails to take place.

Cyclical insomnia

Cyclical insomnia is less common than transient insomnia and implies an unstable balance between the sleep and wake drives. This instability may be temporary or life-long. The insomnia may recur in phase with physiological changes as in circadian rhythm disorders and premenstrual insomnia, psychological changes such as manic depression, and anorexia nervosa or with recurring behavioural changes such as in drug addicts and alcoholics who binge drink.

Chronic insomnia (persistent insomnia)

Chronic insomnia is due to a heterogeneous group of conditions that have been investigated less than most other sleep disorders. Insomnia is usually related to a hyperarousal state which persists during wakefulness as well as sleep. This probably represents an accentuation of the adaptive drive to wakefulness and facilitates the awakening effect of the reticular activating system (RAS). Abnormalities in the homeostatic drive to sleep less commonly lead to insomnia, but may cause idiopathic insomnia. Circadian rhythm disorders leading to an irregular sleep–wake cycle cause a combination of insomnia and EDS, whereas the delayed sleep phase syndrome (DSPS) leads to DIS and the advanced sleep phase syndrome (ASPS) to EMW. Insomnia may also result from frequent arousals from sleep, for instance due to periodic limb movements in sleep (PLMS) and narcolepsy in which REM sleep is abnormal and the sleep–wake state is unstable.

Assessment

History

A careful history is essential to accurately assess insomnia (Chapter 4) (Table 5.2). The issues that should be considered are described below.

1 What is the nature of the insomnia? Is the complaint mainly about poor sleep, or feeling tired during the day? Is the insomnia at night due to a difficulty in initiating or maintaining sleep, or to EMW, and is there a pattern of sleep reversal?

Table 5.2 Diagnosis of the cause of insomnia from the history.

Dignosis	History
Poor sleep hygiene	Erratic sleeping times, especially wake-up times Poor sleep environment, e.g. uncomfortable bed, noisy or light bedroom Shift worker High caffeine or other stimulant intake, especially in the evening
Hyperarousal state	Identifiable cause of onset of insomnia Excessive concern about sleep Rarely falls asleep in the day May show generalized anxiety features May have other disorder specific symptoms, e.g. muscle pain and stiffness
Depression	EMW Early onset of sleep, often with daytime naps Other symptoms of depression
Neurological disorders	Insomnia may be profound Other neurological symptoms often present Sleep reversal in dementia Restless legs symptoms in evenings suggest PLMS Daytime sleepiness and cataplexy suggest narcolepsy
Non-neurological medical disorders	Awakenings associated with recognizable symptom, e.g. angina, wheeze, nocturia Other symptoms of the underlying disorder Daytime sleepiness often accompanies insomnia
Circadian rhythm disorders	Regular pattern of DSPS or ASPS Irregular but recognizable pattern of non-24-h sleep–wake cycles Risk factor, e.g. shift work, transmeridian travel, blind, CNS lesion

ASPS, advanced sleep phase syndrome; CNS, central nervous system; DSPS, delayed sleep phase syndrome; EMW, early morning awakening; PLMS, periodic limb movements in sleep.

2 What are the subject's sleep–wake routines and sleep hygiene? The timing of sleep onset and waking up, and the regularity of these is particularly important.
3 Why does the subject wake up? What is it that he or she is aware of on waking? Is there awareness of snoring, choking, vivid dreams, panicking or symptoms such as headache, wheezing, a need to micturate, pain or discomfort? What does the subject do after waking? Are there any intrusive thoughts or does environmental noise prevent sleep from starting again? How long does the awakening last?
4 What is the time course of the insomnia? Is it acute or long-term, and if so at what age did it start? Is there any identifiable cause for the initiation of insomnia? Has it been cyclical since its onset and, if so, are these fluctuations associated with any identifiable factors? Are there features to suggest a circadian rhythm disorder?
5 Are there any factors that are perpetuating the insomnia? These include environmental noise or light, poor sleep hygiene, anxiety, depression, inappropriate drugs such as caffeine or excess alcohol before going to sleep, or medical disorders such as circadian rhythm disorders, dementia, organic midbrain, hypothalamic or thalamic lesions.
6 What is the patient's attitude to the insomnia and what are the expectations of sleep? Are there any fears regarding its effects or psychological reactions to it such as a sense of loss of control?

Physical examination

Physical examination is usually normal in those with insomnia and contributes little to the assessment of its severity and causes, except in the minority with an underlying neurological disorder.

Investigations

A factor such as depression, anxiety, inappropriate drug treatment or poor sleep hygiene can often be identified and treated without further investigation.

Cause	Polysomnography Findings
Organic causes: circadian rhythm disorder	Abnormal sleep onset and wake up times ± sleep architecture
PLMS	Limb movements and arousals
CSA and CSR	Abnormal respiratory patterns
thalamic lesions	Abnormal sleep architecture
Sleep-state misperception	Normal sleep demonstrated
Multifactorial origin: e.g. combination of drug effects and a hyperarousal state, or poor sleep hygiene and chronic fatigue syndrome	Relative contributions of each factor

Table 5.3 Causes of insomnia requiring polysomnography.

CSA, central sleep apnoea; CSR, Cheyne–Stokes respiration; PLMS, periodic limb movements in sleep.

Investigation in a specialist centre is required if insomnia persists despite treatment interventions or if there is doubt about its cause. Investigations may be needed to investigate either the degree or the causes of insomnia.

DEMONSTRATE THE DEGREE OF INSOMNIA
A sleep diary and actigraphy in the home may be of value, but polysomnography may be needed, particularly to diagnose sleep state misperception.

INVESTIGATE THE CAUSES OF THE INSOMNIA
This includes the following.
1 Questionnaires regarding anxiety and depression.
2 Polysomnography. This shows the extent and stages of sleep, and helps to elucidate the cause of insomnia (Table 5.3). It can be combined with temperature recording and melatonin and cortisol estimations to assess circadian rhythm disorders;
3 Imaging of brain. Computerized tomography (CT) and magnetic resonance imaging (MRI) scans are indicated if organic brain-stem disorders and dementia are being considered.

Principles of treatment

Explanation, optimization of sleep hygiene and treatment of the causes of the insomnia are almost always required, but if these are insufficient additional treatments should be considered (see Fig. 5.2).

Explain, reassure and advise
Explain, reassure and give advice about modification of lifestyle and about accepting a degree of long-term insomnia if necessary.

Optimize sleep hygiene
The quantity, quality and timing of sleep are affected by many everyday activities and attitudes (Table 5.4). The importance of these in assisting or interfering with sleep is generally underestimated. In westernized societies sleep is being increasingly squeezed into the time left over after family, social, work and recreational activities with the result that insomnia, EDS and other sleep symptoms are becoming increasingly common. The aim of sleep hygiene is to translate an understanding of the nature and the control of sleep into practical advice about how to promote this. It is especially important that the elderly counteract the loss of consolidation of the sleep pattern and the ASPS. Sleep hygiene is useful in a wide range of sleep disorders and combines advice about homeostatic, adaptive and circadian aspects of sleep control, how to avoid sleep deprivation and sleep fragmentation, and how to respond to awakenings from sleep if these occur. Some aspects of sleep hygiene fall into more than one of these categories, but in general it entails the following.
1 Altering the sleep environment so that the bed is comfortable and the bedroom warm, dark and quiet.
2 Improving sleep–wake patterns. This is required for most subjects with insomnia. Attention to increasing physical activity during the day; preparation for sleep (for instance by mentally winding down and taking a hot bath); regular meals and sleep and wake times; and avoiding daytime naps may all be of help.

Table 5.4 Sleep hygiene in the treatment of insomnia.

Good practice	Time	Bad practice
Wake up at same time	Awakening	
Take exercise	Daytime	Take more than 6 caffeinated drinks per day
		Take a nap in the day
Set aside time to deal with tomorrow's stresses	Early evening	
Set aside time to unwind		
Establish regular patterns, e.g. hot bath	Late evening	Take exercise within 3 h of desired sleep time
Relaxation routines		Take caffeine in the evening
Take a light snack and a milky drink		Go to sleep hungry
Go to bed when drowsy		Have a heavy meal within 3 h of desired sleep time
		Drink excess fluid in the evenings
		Drink alcohol late in the evenings
		Continue to work within 1.5 h of desired sleep time
		Watch exciting videos or TV late in the evening
Ensure your bed is comfortable	In bed	Use bedroom for watching TV or as an office
Ensure bedroom is quiet, dark and neither too hot nor too cold		Read stimulating books in bed before sleeping
Put the light out soon after going to bed		Try too hard to fall asleep
Ignore intrusive ideas and thoughts		Lie in bed feeling angry if you are unable to sleep

3 Changing drug intake. Avoiding caffeinated drinks in the evenings and discontinuing other stimulants, such as glucocorticoids, and altering the timing of diuretics in order to minimize nocturia may all be of benefit.

Treat the cause of insomnia

Medical disorders and symptoms due to, for instance, thyrotoxicosis, nocturnal asthma or angina should be treated, and it is important to treat depression and anxiety which can both be either causes of insomnia or responses to it, before more complex aspects of management are considered. Antidepressants should only be used if features of depression are present and not as a routine treatment. Sedating tricyclic antidepressants, such as imipramine and doxepin, are particularly effective. Selective serotonin re-uptake inhibitors (SSRIs) may worsen insomnia even if it is due to depression (Fig. 5.1, Table 5.5).

Insomnia associated with the menopause often responds to oestrogen replacement treatment and the duration of stages 3 and 4 non-rapid eye movement (NREM) sleep is increased. Symptomatic improvement is most likely if hot flushes are also relieved by the oestrogen.

Some sleep disorders such as PLMS require specialist investigation and assessment before initiating treatment.

Hypnotic treatment

The aim of hypnotic treatment is not only to improve the quality and duration of sleep, but also to increase the degree of alertness during the day. Unfortunately, the doses of many hypnotics which are required to improve sleep at night also cause sedation during the day. Short-acting benzodiazepines, zaleplon, zolpidem and zopiclone avoid this complication. They are of particular value in the elderly, in whom the metabolism of benzodiazepines is slowed and sedation during wakefulness may lead to confusion, amnesia and ataxia leading to falls. Long-acting hypnotics may also impair psychomotor performance during the day in younger subjects and lead to accidents related to driving and handling moving machinery.

Tolerance develops to most hypnotics with prolonged use and because of this it is usually recommended that treatment should not exceed one month in duration. This is often sufficient to break the pattern of insomnia, especially when hypnotic treatment is used in conjunction with other measures. This is also

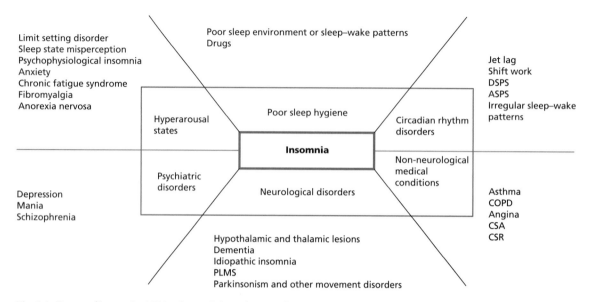

Fig. 5.1 Causes of insomnia. ASPS, advanced sleep phase syndrome; COPD, chronic obstructive pulmonary disease; CSA, central sleep apnoea; CSR, Cheyne–Stokes respiration; DSPS, delayed sleep phase syndrome; PLMS, periodic limb movements in sleep.

Table 5.5 Age and insomnia.

Childhood	Adolescence	Young and middle-aged adults	Old age
Limit-setting disorders			
Anxiety			
Idiopathic insomnia			
Drugs			
Poor sleep hygiene			
DSPS			
PLMS			
Hyperarousal states			
Depression			
			Menopause
Dementia			
Medical disorders			
Neurological disorders			
Narcolepsy			

DSPS, delayed sleep phase syndrome; PLMS, periodic limb movements in sleep.

sufficiently long to cope with temporary exacerbations of chronic insomnia and with transient and cyclical insomnia. Occasionally, however, longerterm treatment is required, in which case the benefits of treatment have to be weighed against the risks of tolerance, dependence and withdrawal symptoms. These may be reduced by giving the hypnotic for only 3–5 days each week.

Hypnotics should be avoided wherever possible in children, and during pregnancy and breastfeeding since, for instance, benzodiazepines cross the placenta and enter breast milk. Most hypnotics interact with

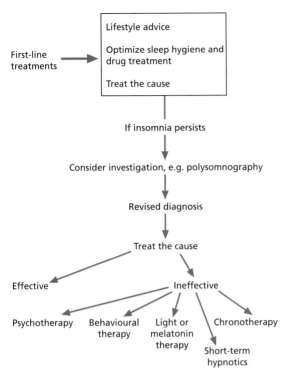

First-line treatments →

Lifestyle advice

Optimize sleep hygiene and drug treatment

Treat the cause

↓

If insomnia persists

↓

Consider investigation, e.g. polysomnography

↓

Revised diagnosis

↓

Treat the cause

Effective   Ineffective

Psychotherapy   Behavioural   Light or   Chronotherapy
                 therapy   melatonin
                                therapy
                                            Short-term
                                            hypnotics

Fig. 5.2 Management of insomnia.

Table 5.6 Choice of benzodiazepine and related types of hypnotic.

other similar drugs and alcohol to accentuate their hypnotic effect and daytime sedation. There is a risk of respiratory depression and induction of obstructive sleep apnoea (OSA), and wherever possible hypnotics should be avoided in the presence of risk factors for these conditions.

The most effective drugs for transient insomnia are quick acting hypnotics, such as diazepam, zopiclone and zolpidem. The most suitable drugs for treating chronic DIS, DMS, EMW with and without anxiety are shown in Tables 3.6 and 5.6. Older drugs, such as barbiturates, are rarely used because of their low toxic : therapeutic ratio and the risk of tolerance and dependence. Valerian may be useful in DIS, but its long-term safety has not been established. Chloral is a mild hypnotic which may be useful in the elderly. Alcohol is frequently used to facilitate sleep, but causes problems, including REM sleep rebound late in the night. Sedating antihistamines such as chlorpheniramine lead to daytime sleepiness as well as anticholinergic side-effects. Melatonin is only a mild hypnotic; this effect is only apparent if it is taken during the day, but it may be useful in relieving insomnia where this is associated with jet lag or shift work. It can also alter the sleep phase (page 87).

Indication	Drug property	Drugs
DIS	Rapid onset	Triazolam Flunitrazepam Zaleplon Zolpidem Zopiclone
DMS	Intermediate duration	Temazepam Lormetazepam Oxazepam Zopiclone Zolpidem
EMW	Moderately long-acting	Temazepam Lormetazepam Flurazepam Nitrazepam
EMW with anxiety	Long-acting	Nitrazepam Diazepam Clorazepate Clonazepam Oxazepam

DIS, difficulty in initiating sleep; DMS, difficulty in maintaining sleep, EMW, early morning awakening.

Behavioural therapy

Behavioural therapy differs from treatment with hypnotics in that it aims to reverse the maladaptive thought and behaviour patterns that perpetuate insomnia. It particularly influences the adaptive drive but can also increase the homeostatic sleep drive and modify circadian rhythms. The techniques of behavioural therapy are, however, time consuming, expensive and require a skilled therapist. The treatments should be individualized for each patient, but the optimum duration and frequency of treatment has yet to be established. It is also uncertain which modes of behavioural therapy are most effective for the different types of insomnia. It may be best to combine behavioural therapy with a course of up to one month of hypnotic treatment in order to break the established patterns of thoughts and behaviour, as well as to give rapid relief of insomnia which can then be maintained by the behavioural therapy.

Sleep hygiene can be considered as the simplest form of behavioural therapy, but there are other more specialist techniques which have been developed.

PHYSICAL RELAXATION

Physical tension, particularly shortly before bedtime, is common in insomnia. A programme of relaxation exercises shortly before attempting to fall asleep may be effective, especially in DIS. Meditation, deep breathing and bio-feedback techniques may be useful.

STIMULUS CONTROL THERAPY

The principle of this treatment is to condition the patient to associate being in bed with successful attempts at falling asleep and maintaining sleep. It aims to interrupt the negative link between the patient's thoughts about sleep by encouraging sleep-promoting behaviour. The subject should only go to bed when they feel sleepy and should get out of bed if they remain awake for 15–30 min, or wake for this duration during the night. It is best to leave the bedroom and carry out a non-stimulating activity such as reading or listening to music before returning when feeling sleepy again. A consistent awakening time should be adopted regardless of the amount of sleep that has been obtained.

No other activity should be allowed in the bedroom, except for sexual activity, and in particular watching television, working and eating should not take place in the bedroom. This should become associated in the subject's mind with the need for sleep. These techniques enable control to be exerted over the problem which then becomes more manageable, although a degree of sleep restriction may be induced.

SLEEP RESTRICTION

This technique assumes that sleep deprivation will lead to deeper and more continuous sleep which, in turn, will reverse the negative conditioning which perpetuates insomnia. Too much time in bed leads to an increase in the time lying awake. Sleep restriction techniques reduce the time in bed in order to increase sleep efficiency.

A sleep–wake diary is kept and the initial time spent in bed should represent the average time asleep or felt to be asleep. This is gradually increased as long as the subjective sleep efficiency remains above 75% for 5 nights in every 7. A constant awakening time is adhered to irrespective of the time of going to bed. Fifteen to thirty minute increments of sleep time are usual and no daytime naps are allowed. There may be an initial worsening of daytime sleepiness but this gradually improves over a period of months.

Psychotherapy

MENTAL RELAXATION

Many insomniacs have intrusive thoughts before falling asleep or during the night if they are awake, and they often become preoccupied with these, or with the difficulty of falling asleep. These thoughts may be concerned with activities of the previous day or the next day, and it is important that they are minimized by allowing time before going to bed to sort out problems that have arisen or may arise. Encouragement to relax, to ignore irrelevant thoughts and to visualize a reassuring or pleasant scene are important.

COGNITIVE THERAPY

This includes techniques which enhance the ability to cope with stresses which may be contributing to insomnia, and aims to change the assumptions and perceptions about insomnia. It is important to identify the main problem with sleep and to modify both thoughts and behaviour. Cognitive therapy requires a good relationship between the patient and the therapist and is most effective if the patient has an active and coping style.

Chronotherapy

Chronotherapy is the manipulation of sleep and waking times by resetting the sleep cycle and then maintaining the change. It is in effect similar to a time zone transition but changes in the sleep cycle are made gradually in order to avoid symptoms similar to jet lag.

Many insomniacs regularly go to bed too early and this contributes to DIS. A regular waking time helps to establish a regular circadian pattern and this should be continued even at weekends.

The indications for chronotherapy are as follows.
1 To prevent and minimize the effects of jet lag. Chronotherapy induces a progressive adjustment to the new environmental time before and after arrival at the destination.
2 Delayed sleep phase syndrome. Putting the bedtime back 3 h each night, and waking up 3 h later until the desired sleep and waking times are reached is often effective. This requires a motivated patient and determination to maintain the rhythm.
3 Advanced sleep phase syndrome.

Light therapy (phototherapy, luminotherapy)
Exposure to bright light has an alerting effect and also leads to sleep phase changes. The latter are influenced by the timing of the light, its brightness and the duration for which it is applied. From a source 1 m from the patient at eye level, 2500 lux for 2 h, 5000 lux for 1 h or 10 000 lux for 30 min have equal effects, but high intensities of light exposure can cause eye damage. There is little evidence that any particular wavelength of light is preferable to ordinary white light. Ultraviolet light is not required and should be filtered out because it can cause cataracts and skin cancer.

Light therapy is usually delivered from a fluorescent light, which is best situated on a white or light coloured surface to increase reflection, or from a visor which can be worn on the head. Fluorescent bulbs are more energy-efficient and produce less heat, but are noisy and flicker. They have diffusers which enable the light to reach a wide area of the retina in contrast to incandescent light bulbs which tend to give a point source which stimulates a smaller area of the retina and has less effect. The optimal distance of the light source from the patient varies with its intensity, but, by the inverse square law, doubling the distance reduces the light that is received to one quarter. It should be unnecessary to look directly at the light intentionally, but it is important to keep the eyes open. Excessive light exposure can cause headaches, dizziness, hyperactivity and insomnia.

A response rate of 50–60% is usually obtained with light therapy. Its indications are:
1 jet lag;
2 shift work;
3 DSPS;
4 ASPS; and
5 EMW.

Melatonin
Exogenous melatonin has the opposite effects to light therapy and induces early endogenous melatonin secretion and sleep-phase advance, especially if it is given in the evening. Long-term treatment entrains the circadian sleep rhythm.

Melatonin should be considered in:
1 jet lag;
2 shift work;
3 irregular sleep–wake rhythms;
4 DSPS;
5 ASPS.

Poor sleep hygiene

Poor sleep hygiene is probably the most important cause of insomnia. It is often combined with other factors that promote poor quality sleep. Some of the factors affecting sleep hygiene are outlined below.
1 Sleep environment. An uncomfortable bed, or a hot, cold, noisy or light bedroom may all disturb sleep.
2 Sleep patterns. Irregular sleep and waking times and naps in the daytime can disrupt nocturnal sleep.
3 Daytime activities. Too little physical activity during the day, going to bed hungry or after mentally stimulating activities can impair nocturnal sleep.
4 Drugs. Caffeinated drinks or alcohol in the evening, and drugs taken for medical purposes (such as diuretics and glucocorticoids), can lead to insomnia.

Apart from a careful history, a sleep diary occasionally combined with actigraphy to assess the pattern of activity during each 24-h cycle, may be indicated. Treatment includes explanation of the ways in which poor sleep hygiene is impeding sleep and the provision of a practical personalized plan. Regular follow-up to monitor progress and to maintain motivation is important.

Hyperarousal states

Overview
Hyperarousal states are the second commonest causes of chronic insomnia [2], but may coexist with other conditions and the relative contribution of each needs to be assessed. The hyperarousal state is usually present throughout wakefulness as well as during sleep, and represents an exaggeration of the normal adaptive drive to wakefulness which allows alertness to continue

even when the homeostatic and circa dian influences are promoting sleep. Increased sympathetic activity is probably responsible for the faster heart rate during sleep in those with insomnia than in normal subjects.

Intrusion of alpha waves into sleep is a common feature of hyperarousal states. The alpha rhythm is characteristic of relaxed wakefulness and usually disappears at sleep onset. When it does occur during sleep, it is most prominent in the fronto-central rather than occipital areas and is usually 1–2 Hz slower than during wakefulness. It is most commonly present in stages 1 and 2 NREM sleep, but may also intrude into stages 3 and 4 (alpha–delta rhythm). This is thought to be related to arousals, or a lowered threshold for arousal to stimuli such as pain or sounds. It is associated with awareness of thoughts during sleep and with the perception that sleep is unrefreshing. It may be related to the establishment of explicit memory of which the subject is aware, but not implicit memory which takes place subliminally. It may, therefore, represent an abnormal form of information processing during sleep which is associated with a low threshold for arousal from other internal or external stimuli. It may represent a failure of the thalamo-cortical projections to modify the activity of the cerebral cortex in the usual way during sleep, and while it may be seen in any of the hyperarousal states, it is a feature particularly of fibromyalgia.

Causes

This large group of chronic insomnias has three main components, which vary in relative importance in each condition and each individual (Table 5.7).

PREDISPOSING FACTORS

1 Constitutional factors. These probably have a genetic basis.
2 Abnormal circadian rhythms, e.g. shift work or a DSPS which predisposes to DIS.
3 Personality differences. A personality pattern with intrusive and ruminating thoughts and internalization or somatization of stress and a tendency to depression is present in around 75% of those with chronic insomnia.
4 Age. Elderly subjects are more vulnerable to develop disturbed sleep and also have an ASPS pattern.
5 Susceptibility to specific diseases. Disorders whose symptoms are exacerbated by sleep such as peptic ulcer, rheumatoid arthritis or asthma predispose to insomnia.

PRECIPITATING FACTORS

Seventy five per cent of those with chronic insomnia link the onset of their sleep disorder to a stressful event. This may be a difficulty in a close relationship, bereavement, a change in school or employment, or the onset of a medical disorder. The stress leads to

Table 5.7 Comparison of hyperarousal states.

Characteristic	Psychophysiological insomnia	Anxiety states	Chronic fatigue syndrome	Fibromyalgia
Age of onset (years)	20–40	Any age	Young adults	Young adults
Gender	M < F	M < F	M < F	M < F
Trigger	Stressful event	Nil or stress	Often infection	Nil
Psychological effects	Anxiety about sleep	Generalized anxiety	Poor concentration and memory	Generalized anxiety
Somatization of symptoms	++	±	Fatigue	Muscle aches, point tenderness
Polysomnography				
–TST	↓	↓	↓	↓
–SL	↑	↑	↑	↑
–1 and 2 NREM sleep	↑	NAD	?	↑
–REM sleep		NAD	↑	
–Alpha intrusion	+	−	+	+
–Awakenings	↓	↑	?	↑

F, Female; M, Male; NAD, normal; NREM, non-rapid eye movement; REM, rapid eye movement; SL, sleep latency; TST, total sleep time.

both physiological and psychological arousal which is more likely to precipitate insomnia if the predisposing factors listed above are present. If they are absent, or if the patient adapts to the stress, insomnia may only be transient.

PERPETUATING FACTORS

These become more important than the predisposing and precipitating factors once chronic insomnia has become established. They are mainly aspects of sleep hygiene. An excessive concern about a lack of sleep may lead to anxiety with intrusive thoughts which initiate a vicious cycle of insomnia, hyperarousal, and an inability to relax. This may develop into an introspective obsession with the difficulty in sleeping (psychophysiological insomnia).

Secondary behavioural changes may be adopted. Fear of not being able to sleep may lead to an earlier bedtime or an attempt to reduce 'overstimulation' by avoiding social contact. An excess of caffeine or alcohol in the evenings may contribute to insomnia. Irregular sleep–wake habits and naps during the day may worsen the night-time sleep pattern. The inability to sleep at night may lead to a conditioned reflex whereby going to bed is associated with the anticipation of staying awake rather than falling asleep.

The disability resulting from insomnia may provide a secondary gain by helping to avoid work, family responsibilities, or interactions with other people. It may also attract an increased level of care from others which may tend to perpetuate the insomnia.

Clinical types of hyperarousal insomnia

A variety of clinical patterns of insomnia have been identified and given distinct names. There is, however, considerable overlap and their classification is unsatisfactory, at least partly due to the lack of clear definitions (Table 5.7). The most important of these disorders are discussed below.

LIMIT SETTING DISORDER

This occurs in children over the age of 2 years and may occur in 5–10% of the childhood population. It is due to inadequate enforcement of bedtime by parents or other carers, who may give in to repeated requests for drinks or stories. Refusal to go to bed at a normal time perpetuates this problem. The child may become irritable, with poor attention and poor school performance during the day, and this may lead to family tension with the parents complaining about the child's sleep. This may improve in

adolescence as control of the sleep patterns passes to the patient who may choose to return to normal sleeping hours. Quite commonly, however, the pattern of DSPS, or of a short sleeper is adopted. Children who have a predisposition to the 'owl' or DSPS patterns may be more likely to have the limit setting disorder early in life.

This disorder should be distinguished from DSPS, in which sleep onset occurs at a constant time each night, and anxiety, in which the child seeks company to enable sleep to occur rather than for wakefulness to continue.

Education of the parents or carers and adoption of regular sleep times is often effective.

SLEEP-STATE MISPERCEPTION
(PSEUDO-INSOMNIA)

Sleep-state misperception may be due to an abnormal expectation of sleep, difficulty in assessing the duration of sleep accurately or to a pathologically low threshold for perceiving any inadequacy of sleep. It usually occurs in young adults, especially females. Their complaint is of a difficulty in sleeping at night, especially DIS and DMS, or occasionally even of not sleeping at all. This may be associated with daytime fatigue and mood changes. Investigations do not reveal any sleep abnormality. Polysomnography shows a normal sleep duration, sleep latency and architecture, with few arousals. A similar degree of poor sleep is usually reported during the study as during sleep at home. MSLTs are normal.

The diagnosis is made by a combination of the history of insomnia with normal polysomnography and the absence of any other cause of a sleep disorder. The condition should be distinguished from short sleepers, DSPS, psychophysiological insomnia and malingering, in which the subject is aware that there is no true insomnia. The demonstration of a normal sleep pattern and treatment of any associated anxiety or depression may improve or relieve the symptoms.

PSYCHOPHYSIOLOGICAL INSOMNIA
(CONDITIONED INSOMNIA)

Overview

An apprehensive over concern about sleep perpetuates insomnia.

Occurrence

This is common, and probably accounts for around 15% of chronic insomnias. It is more common in women than in men, and the usual age of onset is 20–40 years.

Pathogenesis
The cardinal feature is an emotional trigger or precipitating event which may be stressful and which initiates the insomnia. Even after the stress abates the insomnia persists and a specific anxiety develops regarding sleep. Confidence about the ability to fall asleep deteriorates and in effect a specific sleep neurosis or somatized anxiety develops. Negative conditioning develops which increases the anxiety and the level of arousal, making sleep more difficult.

Pre-sleep rituals such as brushing the teeth become associated mentally with the failure to fall asleep. This becomes extended to anything associated with sleep, particularly the bedroom. Sleep is better elsewhere, for instance in a hotel room, during holidays, or even in a sleep laboratory or while watching television in the living room, where the expectations regarding sleep are lower. The continual application of excessive efforts to try to fall asleep raises the state of arousal, reinforces the apprehension about sleep, and the sense of difficulty about sleeping. Secondary sleep hygiene maladaptations may also develop.

Clinical features
These patients have often been poor sleepers before the initiating event, which is usually recalled as focusing their attention on their sleep problem. They often minimize any emotional response to their sleep difficulty. They do not become excessively sleepy during the day, but complain of daytime fatigue, lack of energy, poor memory, poor concentration and physical symptoms such as tension headaches and dizziness. During the night they lie awake with intrusive thoughts and a sensation of restlessness. Psychophysiological insomnia usually remains stable for long periods but improves on holiday. It may lead to depression, loss of motivation and concentration.

Investigations
Polysomnography shows a prolonged sleep latency with a short total sleep time, increased stage 1 and 2 NREM sleep with alpha intrusion, frequent awakenings and positional shifts during the night. There is a reversed first night effect in that sleep is better in the sleep laboratory than at home, but unlike sleep state misperception this satisfactory sleep is acknowledged.

Multiple sleep latency tests are normal.

Differential diagnosis
Psychiatric disorders, circadian rhythm disorders, poor sleep hygiene and insomnia due to other causes should be excluded. Psychophysiological insomnia differs from generalized anxiety states, in which anxiety pervades all aspects of life, since in psychophysiological insomnia it is focused only on the sleep problem.

Treatment
Excessive alcohol is often taken regularly, but is of little value. Hypnotics may have a place in short courses to try to break the pattern of the insomnia. Sleep hygiene advice may help and behavioural therapy, including relaxation, stimulus control and sleep restriction treatments may be of value.

ANXIETY STATES

Clinical features
These are characterized by excessive worrying, fear or guilt and an unrealistic apprehension about common life situations. Generalized anxiety may be somatized causing muscle tension, palpitations, breathlessness, fatigue, sweating and loss of concentration. There is no change in circadian rhythms but DIS with intrusive thoughts is common.

Investigations
Polysomnography is rarely required, but reveals a short total sleep time, increased sleep latency, reduced sleep efficiency, an increased number of arousals from sleep, and normal NREM and REM sleep proportions.

Treatment
Long-acting benzodiazepines are often effective in improving insomnia and relieving daytime anxiety.

POST-TRAUMATIC STRESS DISORDER

Clinical features
This causes repetitive re-experiencing of the traumatic event through thoughts, flashbacks and nightmares which trigger awakening with anxiety attacks. Awakening usually occurs from REM sleep and both insomnia and EDS may develop. There may be an increase in motor activity around the time of awakening and this may be sufficient for the subject to fall out of bed.

Investigations
The diagnosis is usually made clinically, but poly-

somnography shows a prolonged sleep latency, low sleep efficiency due to long awakenings during the night as well as to micro arousals, an increase in stage 1 NREM and reduced stages 3 and 4 NREM sleep with a normal or prolonged REM sleep latency and a short duration of REM sleep. There may be an increase in the ratio of phasic to tonic REM sleep and PLMS may be more common in NREM sleep than in normal subjects.

Treatment

Behavioural therapy and psychotherapy may be of help, especially when combined with antidepressants, particularly the SSRIs, venlafaxine or nefazodone.

CHRONIC FATIGUE SYNDROME

Chronic fatigue syndrome (CFS), post-viral fatigue syndrome, myalgic encephalomyelitis (ME).

Clinical features

This condition is commonest in young adults and is characterized by unexplained fatigue which lasts for more than six months. This is often associated with insomnia, unrefreshing sleep, daytime fatigue and lack of energy which is not relieved by sleep or rest and which is worsened by exercise. Memory, concentration and attention span deteriorate.

There may be a genetic factor or personality type which predisposes to CFS in the presence of an initiating event, which may be a viral infection such as the Epstein–Barr virus or emotional stress. The characteristic response in CFS is a hyperarousal state with abnormalities of pituitary and other aspects of endocrine function. It may be complicated by depression and anxiety.

Investigations

Polysomnography may be required to establish the cause of the sleep symptoms. It shows a prolonged sleep latency with reduced sleep efficiency and often alpha intrusion into NREM sleep. Rapid eye movement sleep latency is normal, but the duration of REM sleep is reduced, and there is an increased frequency of arousals and awakenings from sleep. Multiple sleep latency tests are normal.

These changes occur even in the absence of depression and anxiety, but these can cause sleep disturbances which are superimposed on those of CFS. The sleep abnormalities of CFS may be related to changes in immune function, such as increases in IL-1, which frequently occur.

Treatment

There is no specific treatment to reverse the sleep abnormalities of CFS, but it is important to treat any depression and anxiety, and to recognize and treat problems with sleep hygiene which are common and which may contribute to the sleep disturbance. Frequent naps are often taken during the day, together with a lack of exercise and little exposure to light. These maladaptations may be the most important factors in the sleep disturbance. Cognitive therapy may help in gradually increasing the level of activity and in achieving carefully structured goals. Tricyclic antidepressants may be of benefit and the condition usually improves gradually over months or years.

FIBROMYALGIA

Clinical features

This is a poorly defined syndrome which is commoner in females than males and usually develops in young adults. Its characteristic features are fatigue with tenderness over various points, particularly in the chest and abdomen, and diffuse musculo-skeletal pain and stiffness. This is usually worst around the neck and shoulders on waking. Sleep is usually felt to be light and unrefreshing. Tiredness is common during the day, but it is unusual for sleep to be entered. Fibromyalgia may have a similar pathogenesis to the chronic fatigue syndrome with hyperarousal, changes in endocrine function and in autonomic responses, abnormal reactions to stress, and a particularly increased sensitivity to pain.

Investigations

Polysomnography may be required to elucidate the cause of the sleep symptoms. It shows a prolonged sleep latency, an increased number of arousals from sleep, prolonged stage 1, but reduced stages 3 and 4 NREM sleep and alpha intrusion, particularly into stages 3 and 4 NREM sleep. The duration of REM sleep is reduced. The extent of alpha activity is related to the severity of the musculo-skeletal pains and to the awareness of sleeping lightly.

Treatment

Pain relief and improvement in sleep hygiene often help to relieve symptoms, but low-dose tricyclic antidepressants and cognitive therapy may be of benefit.

ANOREXIA NERVOSA

Anorexic patients rarely complain of insomnia but

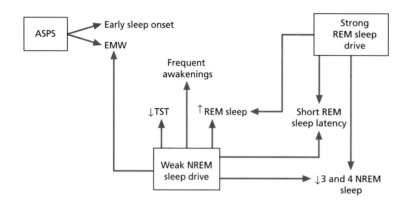

Fig. 5.3 Changes in sleep control in depression. ASPS, advanced sleep phase syndrome; EMW, early morning awakening; NREM, non-rapid eye movement; REM, rapid eye movement; TST, total sleep time.

often wake early in the morning. Psychiatric problems may contribute to the changes in sleep pattern, but weight loss is associated with polysomnographic findings of a short total sleep-time, reduced sleep efficiency, frequent awakenings and to a variable extent with lengthening of stages 1 and 2 and shortening of stages 3 and 4 NREM sleep. These abnormalities improve as weight is regained.

Psychiatric disorders

Depression

Clinical features
Insomnia is a common and occasionally the initial symptom of depression. It is not related to the number of depressive episodes or to the duration of the depression, but is more common in older subjects. There is usually little difficulty in initiating sleep, but there are frequent awakenings during the night and EMW, often after an unpleasant dream, especially in endogenous depression. Sleep is often unrefreshing and frequent naps may be taken during the day.

There is a tendency towards an ASPS in depression (Fig. 5.3) which may contribute to early morning awakening. In contrast, depression in the seasonal affective disorder causes EDS and a DSPS. Changes in circadian rhythms such as cortisol secretion are common in depression and a reduction in melatonin secretion may contribute to early morning awakening.

Investigations
Polysomnography is occasionally required to establish the relative contributions of depression and other conditions that may contribute to the sleep symptoms. Polysomnography is usually normal in depression occurring before puberty and may only be slightly

Table 5.8 Effects of dementia and depression on sleep.

Characteristic	Dementia	Depression
TST	↓	↓
Awakenings	↑↑	↑
EMW	+	+
Sleep latency	–	↑
1 and 2 NREM sleep	↑	↑
3 and 4 NREM sleep	↓	↓
REM sleep latency	↑	↓
REM sleep	↓	↑
Daytime naps	++	±

EMW, early morning awakening; NREM, non-rapid eye movement; REM, rapid eye movement; TST, total sleep time.

abnormal in adolescence. In adults, especially the elderly, it characteristically reveals a short total sleep time, increased sleep latency with a short REM sleep latency (usually 20–40 min), an increase in the duration of REM sleep, particularly in the first half of the night, and a reduction in stages 3 and 4 NREM sleep with an increase in stages 1 and 2, and frequent awakenings (Table 5.8).

These abnormalities are most obvious during an episode of depression, but they rarely disappear completely even between these, and the REM sleep latency in particular usually remains short. Similar findings are often seen in close relatives who have not been and are not depressed. They may represent a 'trait' for depression rather than the state of depression.

The increase in REM sleep is due to both an increase in the drive to REM sleep and to a weak NREM sleep drive. The REM sleep drive appears to be proportional to the severity of the depression. The NREM sleep drive becomes weaker with age and this may underlie the increased frequency of sleep abnormalities in older subjects with depression. It also leads to a shorter sleep time and briefer NREM sleep episodes with an increase in the number of awakenings from sleep, although some of these may be related to anxiety. Interestingly, sleep deprivation leads to mood elevation in depression and even to mania in bipolar disorders. Sleep deprivation increases the homeostatic drive to NREM sleep and reduces the duration of REM sleep, particularly if sleep is lost towards the end of the night. Loss of REM sleep is also a feature of all antidepressant drugs, except moclobemide and nefazodone, and of electroconvulsive treatment (ECT), suggesting that REM sleep generation is closely linked to the development of depression.

Treatment

The main pharmacological agents used for treating depression are the tricyclic antidepressants and related drugs, and the SSRIs. Older drugs such as the mono-amine oxidase inhibitors (MAOIs) and newer preparations unrelated to these groups are also of value. The neurotransmitter basis of depression is uncertain, but probably relates to the balance between the REM sleep-promoting influence of the cholinergic mechanisms in the pons, particularly those related to the pedunculopontine and laterodorsal tegmental (PPN/LDT) nuclei, and the REM sleep inhibiting influence of other centres, particularly the noradrenergic locus coeruleus and the dorsal raphe nuclei which produce 5HT at their synapses. The theory that depression is due to a deficiency of these two latter chemicals (the monoaminergic theory of depression) may explain why tricyclic and SSRI antidepressants improve the sleep pattern in depression during the first night, but changes in mood may take around two weeks and be due to alterations in the function of the receptors for these neurotransmitters.

Early morning wakening may respond to light therapy in the evening and possibly to melatonin.

Mania and manic depression (bipolar disorder)

Mania may prevent sleep for several days until the subject is exhausted. The total sleep time is shortened, sleep latency is prolonged, there is a short REM sleep latency and often a gross alteration in the sleep architecture. Abnormalities of circadian rhythms include changes in the diurnal cortisol secretion pattern. Sleep deprivation tends to elevate the mood as in depres-

sion and this may worsen the mania and lead to further sleep restriction. Excessive daytime sleepiness only occurs in the depressive phase of bipolar illnesses.

Obsessive–compulsive disorders

Patients often complain of insomnia and frequent awakenings at night, and the rituals that they need to carry out before sleep may disturb the quality of sleep. The total sleep time is reduced, the duration of stage 4 NREM sleep is shortened, REM sleep latency is reduced and awakenings are frequent.

Schizophrenia

Schizophrenia may cause insomnia, especially before and during acute exacerbations. This may be associated with sleep reversal, but there are no changes in circadian rhythms. Daytime sleepiness is, however, more commonly related to psychotropic drugs used for symptom control. Bizarre thoughts and distortions of reality during wakefulness may resemble dreams. This led to the theory that schizophrenia was due to REM sleep intrusion into wakefulness and that it was similar to narcolepsy, but this is unlikely. The dreams of schizophrenics during sleep often feature strangers.

Polysomnography has shown variable results, but in general the total sleep time is reduced, sleep latency is increased, sleep efficiency is low and the number of arousals is increased. Rapid eye movement sleep latency is occasionally shortened and the duration of stages 3 and 4 NREM sleep is reduced, especially during psychotic episodes.

Neurological disorders

Insomnia is particularly associated with lesions of the anterior hypothalamus, thalamus and cerebral cortex, which are responsible for integrating the afferent information and brain-stem activity that controls sleep and wakefulness. Normal functioning of these areas enables sleep to take place and lesions affecting them cause insomnia, probably due to the unopposed action of the RAS.

Hypothalamic disorders

Lesions such as tumours in the anterior hypothalamus may cause insomnia. They probably derange the function of the suprachiasmatic nuclei (SCN) as well as reduce the homeostatic drive to sleep. Head CT and MRI scans may be required.

Thalamic lesions

INFARCTION

This is the commonest thalamic lesion and like tumours and trauma, more commonly causes insomnia than EDS. This is probably due to a loss of the ability of the thalamus to synchronize the cortical activity which is required to enter NREM sleep. Anencephalic infants without a thalamus appear to sleep, probably because they have little cerebral cortex, and so do not require organized thalamic activity to regulate its activity.

FATAL FAMILIAL INSOMNIA

Pathogenesis

This autosomal dominant disorder is due to a mutation at codon 178 of the prion protein gene, in which asparagine is substituted for aspartate coupled with the presence of methionine rather than valine at position 129 [3]. This leads to production of an abnormal form of a glycoprotein (prion protein) which is resistant to proteases and leads to neuronal death. Progression of the disease is more rapid in methionine homozygotes than methionine-valine heterozygotes.

Clinical features

This condition is characterized by degeneration in the dorsomedial and anterior thalamic nuclei so that the thalamus can no longer initiate and maintain sleep. It is equally common in males and females, is usually familial but occasionally sporadic, and usually appears between the ages of 40–70 years. Progressively worsening insomnia is associated with vivid dreams and motor activity characteristic of the REM behaviour disorder. The fall in total sleep time is associated with disintegration of the sleep structure with no discernible NREM or REM sleep. The normal 24-h rest–activity cycle is lost and the circadian cortisol rhythm disappears. Autonomic and motor abnormalities appear, but cognitive function is retained until stupor and eventually coma develop shortly before death. This usually occurs 6–24 months after the onset of the condition.

Differential diagnosis

The differential diagnosis includes REM behaviour disorder, although this does not have any autonomic abnormalities, dementia particularly due to Alzheimer's disease, Creutzfeldt–Jakob disease and occasionally schizophrenia.

Treatment

There is no effective treatment.

CREUTZFELDT–JAKOB DISEASE

This is usually sporadic, but is occasionally familial. It is due to the same codon 178 mutation as in fatal familial insomnia, but polymorphism at other codons, such as 129, leads to a different phenotypic expression of the genetic abnormality. The cerebral cortex is usually predominantly affected, but in a subtype of the disease there is extensive thalamic atrophy. In these subjects insomnia is a prominent feature, in addition to the dementia and motor abnormalities. There is a progressive loss of both NREM and REM sleep with absence of spindles and K-complexes, and eventually there is no recognizable NREM or REM sleep.

Basal forebrain lesions

Lesions in the basal forebrain may cause insomnia although this is only temporary after leucotomy (frontal lobotomy) and after around 10 years there is an increase in the duration of stages 3 and 4 NREM sleep.

Dementia

Clinical features

Insomnia is common in the elderly, probably due to degeneration of the sleep-regulating mechanisms, but these effects are exaggerated in dementia due to degenerative disorders such as Alzheimer's disease [4] and multi-infarct dementia. The clinical features vary according to the distribution of the degeneration, and in particular whether the SCN, homeostatic sleep control mechanisms or other regions of the brain are mainly involved. There is a loss of the sleep–wake cycle and of the normal sleep architecture (see Table 5.8). Nocturnal restlessness, agitation, confusion and frequent awakenings and wanderings occur ('sundown syndrome') and may alternate with periods of sleep during the day (sleep reversal) giving a polyphasic sleep pattern. These abnormalities may be worse in winter when there is less exposure to light.

Investigations

Polysomnography is rarely required, but shows that the sleep efficiency may be reduced to around 60% by the frequent awakenings, which are often prolonged. The duration of stage 1 NREM sleep is lengthened and stages 3 and 4 are shortened. Sleep spindles are few in number, and slow in frequency and there are few K-complexes. There is an increase in REM sleep latency and the duration of REM sleep is reduced. Periodic limb movements are common, possibly due to a reduction in dopamine and acetylcholine as neurotransmitters, and obstructive and central sleep apnoeas and Cheyne–Stokes respiration are frequently seen.

Treatment

Improvement in sleep hygiene is the most important aspect of management. Regular sleep–wake patterns, exposure to light during the day, encouragement to take exercise and avoidance of stimulants such as caffeine may be of help. Short-acting hypnotics such as chloral or zopiclone in low dose may be indicated, but drugs which induce daytime sedation should be avoided.

Head injury

Excessive daytime sleepiness is more common than insomnia after head injuries (Chapter 6), but this is a feature of the postconcussion syndrome. Difficulty in initiating sleep and DMS are more prominent than EMW and may be associated with EDS.

Movement disorders

Many of the movement disorders of wakefulness cause insomnia. The most important are idiopathic Parkinsonism, multiple system atrophy, progressive supranuclear palsy, Huntington's disease, torsion dystonia and Gilles de la Tourette syndrome (Chapter 7).

Narcolepsy

Insomnia is a common but under recognized symptom of narcolepsy (Chapter 6).

Encephalitis

Encephalitis usually leads to EDS, but may cause insomnia if it damages the mechanisms that are involved in sleep initiation or maintenance. Encephalitis lethargica has been recognized to cause insomnia (page 134) and encephalitis due to cerebral involvement in Whipple's disease can cause severe insomnia without any recognizable stages 3 and 4 NREM or REM sleep.

Periodic limb movements in sleep

These may cause insomnia and excessive daytime sleepiness (Chapter 7). Insomnia is unusual in other behavioural abnormalities during sleep (parasomnias) unless they are very frequent.

Idiopathic insomnia (primary insomnia)

Overview

This condition is characterized by the early onset of insomnia without any underlying psychological or psychiatric abnormalities or other detectable cause (Table 5.9).

Occurrence

It is uncommon but occasionally familial. The onset is usually in early childhood and it persists throughout adult life without remission.

Pathogenesis

No physical or psychological cause has been detected, but idiopathic insomnia may represent the wakeful end of the range of normal subjects. It may be due to a chronic hyperarousal state, or to a reduction in one of the drives to sleep. It is probably heterogeneous and in some patients minor organic neurological abnor-

Table 5.9 Comparison of idiopathic insomnia, limit setting disorder and DSPS.

Characteristic	Idiopathic insomnia	Limit setting disorder	Delayed sleep phase syndrome
Age of onset	Childhood	Childhood	Adolescence
Trigger	Nil	Poor sleep hygiene enforcement	Nil or poor sleep hygiene enforcement
Sleep onset time	Variable	Variable	Constant and late
Poor sleep hygiene	Follows insomnia	Alters in adolescence	May improve in adult life
Natural history	Constant and lifelong	Alters in adolescence	May improve in adult life
Psychological changes	Secondary anxiety and depression	Attention seeking	Nil

malities such as dyslexia or hyperkinesis have been detected. A reduction in 5HT turnover has been found in some patients.

Clinical features
Insomnia may be severe with as little as 3–4 h sleep being obtained each night and with frequent awakenings. The subject awakes feeling unrefreshed and feels tired and irritable during the day, but EDS is not a feature. Poor attention, mood disorders, lack of motivation and secondary anxiety occur, often with somatic symptoms and depression. Attention deficit hyperactivity disorder (ADHD) is associated with idiopathic insomnia in children. Secondary maladaptive sleep hygiene patterns are common, but follow, rather than predate, the insomnia.

Investigations
The waking EEG may show a diffuse abnormality such as ragged rather than sinusoidal alpha waves at night. The sleep latency may be markedly prolonged with a reduction in total sleep time and sleep efficiency, often with poor definition of individual sleep stages. Sleep spindles are poorly formed and there are few eye movements in REM sleep which is often prolonged. The duration of stages 3 and 4 NREM sleep is often markedly reduced and there is alpha intrusion.

Differential diagnosis
Diagnosis requires the establishment of a childhood onset of insomnia prior to any detectable cause or psychological changes. Insomnia is chronic and stable and independent of any sleep hygiene abnormalities. It should be distinguished from short sleepers, who do not complain of any sleep problem or daytime fatigue, anxiety states, limit-setting disorder and psychophysiological insomnia.

Treatment
Alcohol and other hypnotics are often taken to assist sleep and caffeine to keep awake during the day, but none of these treatments are very effective. Behavioural therapy may be of some help.

Non-neurological medical conditions

These are an important, but heterogeneous, group of conditions which frequently contribute to insomnia. Many of them are further discussed in Chapter 8. Sleep can be prevented, fragmented or terminated by symptoms such as: pain, for instance from rheumatoid arthritis; discomfort, which is common, for example, in Parkinsonism at night; and nocturia. Symptoms due to autonomic changes during sleep, such as those related to nocturnal angina, asthma and peptic ulceration may cause insomnia, although the complaint may be primarily of the specific symptom rather than of insomnia. Sleep can also be disrupted by disorders that occur only during sleep, such as central and obstructive sleep apnoeas.

Of these organic causes, the most important are discussed below.

Respiratory disorders
Examples of respiratory disorders that may lead to insomnia are: obstructive and central sleep apnoeas, Cheyne–Stokes respiration, asthma, chronic bronchitis and emphysema (Chapters 8, 9 and 10). These more commonly cause EDS than insomnia.

Musculo-skeletal disorders
Any musculo-skeletal disorder that causes pain, stiffness, or limited mobility during sleep may lead to insomnia. This may be DIS but is more commonly DMS. Insomnia in fibromyalgia is accentuated by a hyperarousal state and rheumatoid arthritis may be complicated by the restless legs and periodic limb movement syndromes, possibly because of its associated iron-deficiency anaemia.

Excessive daytime sleepiness may also develop in rheumatoid arthritis as a result of OSA due to crico-arytenoid arthritis or obesity caused by glucocorticoid treatment, opiate analgesics or poor sleep hygiene induced by the lifestyle limitations imposed by the arthritis. Excessive daytime sleepiness in musculo-skeletal disorders should be distinguished from depression and physical tiredness due to the underlying disorder.

Autonomic disorders
Examples of these are angina and peptic ulcer (Chapter 8).

Metabolic disorders
An example of a metabolic disorder that may lead to insomnia is chronic renal failure. Insomnia is a frequent problem with a short total sleep time with disorganized sleep architecture and frequent arousals. The sleep architecture improves following dialysis and renal transplantation, suggesting that most of the abnormalities are due to a metabolic disturbance.

This may underlie the association between chronic renal failure and PLMS, but nocturia also causes arousal from sleep.

Endocrine disorders

THYROTOXICOSIS
This causes DIS and EMW with a reduction in total sleep time and an increase in the duration of stages 3 and 4 NREM sleep. Hyperactivity with a high level of arousal is usual and EDS is not a feature.

DIABETES MELLITUS
Polyuria, paraesthesia from a peripheral neuropathy, and nocturnal cramps all cause awakenings from sleep.

CUSHING'S SYNDROME
This is manifested by DMS and EMW insomnia which are similar to the effects of administered glucocorticoids. The insomnia may be mediated by interactions with cytokines.

PREMENSTRUAL INSOMNIA
This commonly occurs in the week before each menstrual period, and is often partly due to physical symptoms such as abdominal pain. Polysomnography premenstrually shows frequent sleep stage transitions and arousals and a reduced sleep efficiency.

PREGNANCY INSOMNIA
This usually worsens as the pregnancy progresses. Pregnancy insomnia may be due to nausea, backache, urinary frequency, heartburn, cramps, discomfort and fetal movements. Vivid dreams and nightmares are common. The postnatal need to respond to and care for the child at night, and occasionally postnatal depression, may perpetuate the insomnia so that it becomes established as a long-term difficulty.

MENOPAUSAL INSOMNIA
Spontaneous awakenings from sleep are often associated with night sweats or hot flushes which respond to oestrogen replacement treatment. The condition usually resolves after several months but occasionally only after a few years. Depression may contribute to the insomnia.

Circadian rhythm disorders

The endogenous circadian rhythm has a cycle of around 24.2 h (Chapter 2), but its fine tuning to the environment is achieved through the influence of external time givers of which the most important is light. The fluctuations in the circadian sleep rhythm alter the threshold of the homeostatic and adaptive drives to initiate sleep. Disturbances in circadian sleep rhythms can therefore cause either insomnia, excessive daytime sleepiness or both.

The sleep, temperature and hormonal circadian rhythms are usually synchronized and are synergistic in promoting sleep and wakefulness at different points in each circadian cycle. This synchrony can break down in certain situations because each rhythm adapts to changes in external factors at different rates and to different degrees. The circadian sleep rhythm could, for instance, be promoting sleep at a time when the temperature is rising instead of falling as is usual late in the evening, and when catabolic rather anabolic hormones are being secreted. The conflicting effects of this 'internal desynchronization' probably disturb sleep and reduce the level of alertness during wakefulness.

Causes
The causes of circadian rhythm disorders fall into three groups according to whether the disturbance is due to an endogenous (intrinsic) abnormality, unusual environmental (exogenous) conditions which disturb them, or to a disorder of the linkage between the circadian rhythms and their environmental control. In practice, however, there is considerable overlap between the 3 groups. Endogenous disorders may modify the influence of the environmental factors on sleep and the latter may accentuate endogenous disorders.

ENDOGENOUS FACTORS
Both the amplitude and timing of the circadian sleep rhythm can become abnormal. It may become completely irregular with no discernible relationship to time, or may show a regular 24 h cycle which is set at a different point to normal. The onset of sleep and the natural waking time can both be delayed while the quality and duration of sleep remain normal and without any EDS if the patient is allowed to sleep as desired (DSPS). In contrast, a pattern of early sleep onset and waking-up time with a normal sleep quality and duration and no excessive daytime sleepiness can also develop (ASPS).

These two patterns are usually thought to be due to an abnormality in the timing of the circadian sleep rhythm. A circadian rhythm that is too long to be entrained to a 24 h cycle by light and other stimuli, an insensitivity to light as a sleep phase modifier, or an asymmetry in the response to light so that exposure in the evening causes a longer phase-delay than the phase-advance in response to early morning light could all cause DSPS. The converse may lead to ASPS but these patterns could equally well be due to alterations in the amplitude of the circadian sleep rhythm. A high amplitude rhythm would tend to delay the onset of sleep since it would oppose the homeostatic drive to sleep more effectively in the evening and delay the wake-up time in the morning. In contrast, a low amplitude circadian rhythm enables the increasing homeostatic drive in the evening to initiate sleep at an earlier time. When this drive wanes in the morning there is little circadian sleep tendency to oppose waking up.

The circadian sleep rhythms are probably under genetic control, and there is a wide variation among normal subjects. The so-called 'larks' prefer to go to sleep early and wake early, in contrast to 'owls' who tend to go to sleep later and wake later in the morning. Sleep patterns are also influenced by age. In adolescence the circadian rhythm causes a tendency towards DSPS, but in the elderly, when either its timing changes or its amplitude falls, an ASPS tendency is common.

These sleep patterns should be distinguished from 'short sleepers' who have a normal sleep quality and are not excessively sleepy during the day but have a short sleep duration, and 'long sleepers' who require a prolonged time asleep, even when this is of normal quality, to remain alert during the day. These patterns may be due to a low and high intensity, respectively, of the homeostatic drive to sleep, and long sleepers may merge into the category of idiopathic CNS hypersomnia (Chapter 6). Their sleep-onset and wake-up times are appropriate for the duration of sleep in contrast to the DSPS and ASPS patterns.

Most of these disorders are uncommon, but involve dysfunction of the SCN or the pathways leading to and from this which control circadian rhythms, particularly those in the hypothalamus and pineal gland. The most important disorders in this group are outlined below.

Head injuries

The irregular sleep–wake pattern may be either temporary or permanent and probably reflects damage to the circadian and other control mechanisms.

Degenerative disorders

The irregular sleep–wake pattern in these conditions reflects the extensive disorganization of sleep controlling mechanisms. It is a feature of Alzheimer's disease, fatal familial insomnia and African sleeping sickness.

Tumours

Tumours of the pinealocytes, but not the pineal glia, hypothalamic and pituitary tumours and craniopharyngiomas cause this type of disorder. Other hypothalamic disturbances such as endocrine abnormalities and weight gain, which may induce sleep disorders such as OSA, are common.

ENDOGENOUS AND EXOGENOUS LINKAGE

These disorders lead to alterations in the timing of sleep so that there is a complaint of either insomnia, EDS or both. The connection between the endogenous circadian rhythms and time givers, particularly light, is reduced or absent. The most common causes are:
1 blindness;
2 damage to the retinohypothalamic tract; and
3 hypothalamic disorders.

The sleep rhythm usually approximates to a free-running cycle of around 24.2 h, but in most societies, cultural and social factors entrain this cycle at least partially and intermittently. This pattern is most common if there is no light perception, but is also present in around 70% of those with unilateral blindness. Insomnia and EDS fluctuate from day to day according to the degree of mismatch of the endogenous cycle and environmental time. The failure to link the circadian rhythms to the external environment also leads to internal desynchronization of the sleep, temperature and endocrine rhythms which may contribute to the sleep disorder.

Occasionally, a sleep rhythm of the DSPS, ASPS or irregular type results from these disorders of endogenous and exogenous linkage.

EXOGENOUS FACTORS

The imposition of unusual or artificial changes in the environment induces physiological responses in the circadian rhythms which may cause symptoms, usually insomnia, EDS or both. These may be due to social factors, jet lag or shift work. The most important environmental factor is a change in the exposure to light which often leads to alterations in sleeping times. A mismatch between the circadian time and environmental time develops, to which the circadian rhythms adjust slowly and internal desynchronization of sleep, temperature and endocrine rhythms may arise. A DSPS, ASPS or irregular sleep–wake rhythm may be seen.

Delayed sleep phase syndrome

Clinical features

This syndrome is characterized by a stable sleep rhythm in which sleep onset and time of awakening occur later than normal, but with a normal total sleep time and sleep architecture unless sleep is curtailed early in the morning. It causes difficulty in initiating sleep and in waking at conventional times. The latter in particular may be very disruptive and may lead to recurrent episodes of lateness for school or work which may be interpreted as laziness or a lack of motivation. Sleepiness often continues through the morning, especially if the subject has been prematurely woken up, but excessive sleepiness later in the day is not a problem. Alertness is maximal later in the afternoon, evening and even after midnight, and sleep is often only initiated at around 3.00 AM. The natural waking time is usually 10–12 AM so it is predominantly REM rather than NREM sleep that is lost if the subject is woken prematurely (Fig. 5.4).

Delayed sleep phase syndrome is by definition characterized by an unusually late time of sleep onset and of waking. It may be worse in the winter, particularly in northern latitudes when the intensity of light exposure is reduced in the mornings, compared to the summer when the earlier dawn promotes a phase advance. The prevalence of DSPS depends on the conventional sleeping times of society. In warmer climates a late bed time is common and DSPS is less frequently diagnosed than in northern climates where sleep onset is usually earlier and where individuals with this disorder are more conspicuous.

Causes

NORMAL ADOLESCENCE

A mild DSPS is normal in adolescence from the age of around 16–18 years into the early twenties. This tendency is often accentuated by social pressures, for instance late night parties, watching television or videos. Students without fixed class times find it easier to adapt to their DSPS, but this situation may also encourage the maintenance of this sleep pattern.

INTRINSIC DELAYED SLEEP PHASE SYNDROME

This disorder is familial. It may be due to a genetic abnormality causing a delay in melatonin secretion or in the response of the SCN to melatonin, but the exact mechanism has not been established. Its onset is usually in childhood or adolescence and it usually worsens from the age of 16–18 for a few years. It may simply be an exaggeration of the normal changes in adolescence and also appears to merge into the group of subjects known as 'owls' or 'evening types', who prefer to stay awake late, wake up late and are most alert in the evenings.

EXTRINSIC DELAYED SLEEP PHASE SYNDROME

This is due to psychosocial factors which promote the DSPS pattern. It often begins in childhood or as a teenager with staying up late on holidays, at weekends or other special occasions but may be triggered as a single major event. The habit of choosing to remain up late or being encouraged to do so then persists and this may come to have secondary gains such as avoiding school on the following morning. Light exposure late in the evening tends to delay the sleep phase and perpetuate the DSPS.

The complaint usually comes from the parent rather than the child and this condition is unlikely to respond to treatment unless the priorities and motivation of both parents and child can be altered.

SEASONAL AFFECTIVE DISORDER

This is a seasonal circadian rhythm disorder which is four times more common in women than in men, is occasionally familial and is most frequent between the ages of 20–40 years. It is most prevalent in high latitudes where there is a greater seasonal change in the intensity and duration of exposure to light. The seasonal affective disorder (SAD) develops during autumn and winter and remits in spring and summer, at which time there may even be mild hypomania. In the winter a DSPS pattern develops associated with depression, an increase in appetite, particularly for carbohydrates, weight gain, fatigue and reduction in physical activity. The total sleep time increases, unlike other forms of depression, and the duration of both REM and NREM sleep increases. The rhythm of cortisol secretion is also phase delayed.

Seasonal affective disorder may be the extreme end of the normal range of seasonal variation in mood and behaviour and may be related to an alteration in the control of sleep by melatonin. The lengthening duration of the melatonin signal overnight as winter

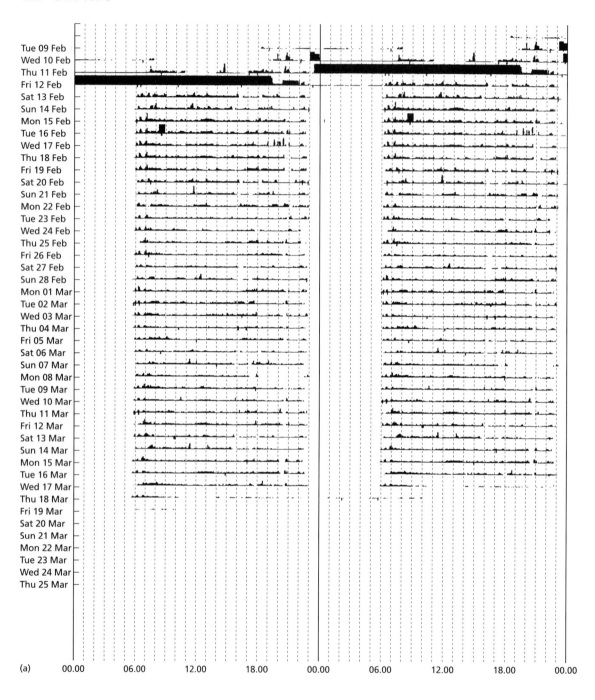

(a)

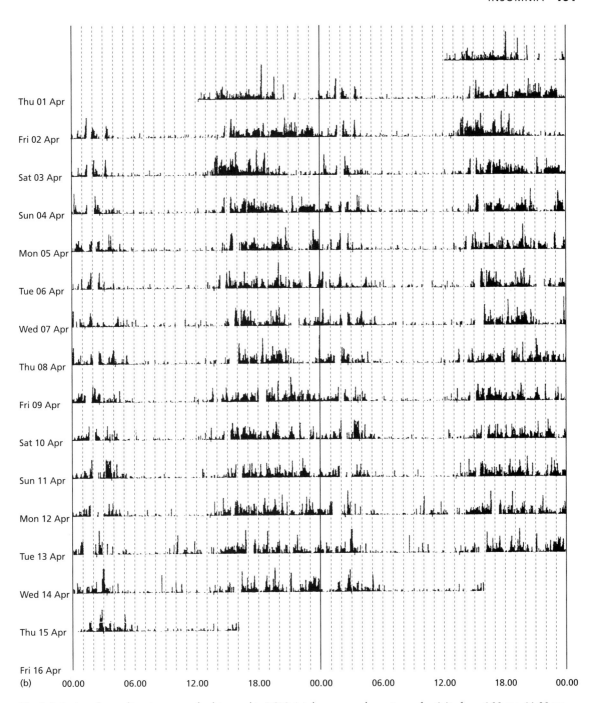

Fig. 5.4 Actigraphy readings in a normal subject and in DSPS. (a) shows a regular pattern of activity from 6.00 AM–11.30 PM with inactivity at night corresponding to sleep. (b) the actigraphy tracing shows that inactivity starts around 3.00–4.00 AM and lasts until around midday, corresponding to the delayed sleep phase. The subject is then active later in the day and into the first part of the night.

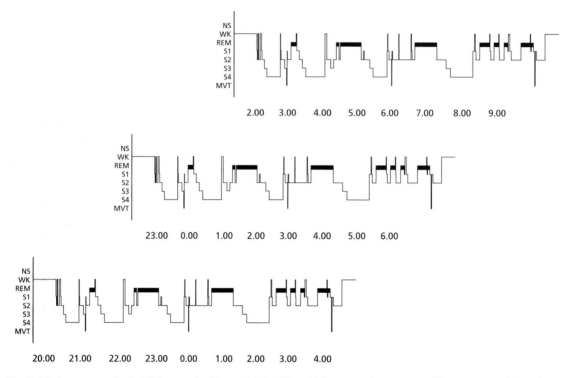

Fig. 5.5 Polysomnography in ASPS, normal subject and DSPS. The middle tracing shows a normal hypnogram with the subject asleep from around 11.00 PM–7.00 AM. In the top tracing the same normal hypnogram does not start until around 2.00 AM because of the delayed sleep phase syndrome (DSPS) and in the lower line the same sleep pattern is initiated at around 8.00 PM due to an advanced sleep phase syndrome (ASPS).

approaches identifies the seasonal change and may initiate the DSPS and other changes. Seasonal affective disorder responds to light therapy, particularly if it is given on waking in the morning, as well as tricyclic and SSRI antidepressants.

HEAD AND NECK INJURIES
These may impair the secretion of melatonin from the pineal gland or more commonly cause damage to its connections, especially the tortuous path between it and the SCN through the cervical spinal cord. Cervical cord transection and whiplash injuries to the neck are particularly associated with DSPS.

Diagnosis

The diagnosis of DSPS depends on the presence of the clinical features, especially a stable phase delay of the major sleep episode in relation to the desired time for sleep. This introduces a subjective element into the diagnosis according to the patient's perception of the impact of the disorder in addition to the difficulties in

diagnosis due to the differing sleep times that are prevalent in individual societies. Delayed sleep phase syndrome should be distinguished from psychophysiological insomnia, and other causes of difficulty in initiating sleep, and other causes of EDS, particularly idiopathic central nervous system hypersomnia.

Polysomnography excludes other causes for the symptoms and reveals a normal sleep structure if it is carried out at the subject's usual sleeping time (Fig. 5.5). If it is carried out at normal hours there may be a long sleep latency, low sleep efficiency, difficulty in waking the subject and a short duration of REM sleep which is truncated by the early time of ending the study in relation to the subject's normal sleep time. Sleep diaries and actigraphy recordings may confirm the sleep pattern of DSPS and secretion of melatonin is delayed. The distinction between intrinsic and extrinsic DSPS can be difficult, but patients with the latter may assume more normal sleep times when removed from their usual environment if they are motivated to do so.

Treatment

The aims of treatment are to reset the sleep phase and to maintain this. This can be achieved by the following methods.

SLEEP HYGIENE

Application of sleep hygiene principles may enable sleep to be initiated earlier and improve the sleep architecture. This is particularly important if early awakening from sleep is essential because of school or work attendance. These measures may need to be combined with the other treatments listed below in order to maintain resetting of the sleep phase. The success of this type of treatment depends very much on the motivation of the patient.

CHRONOTHERAPY

The aim of this, as with light therapy and melatonin, is to reset the circadian rhythm. Over a period of days or weeks the sleep–wake cycle is shifted by gradually introducing a phase delay and avoiding naps during the day. The time of sleep onset should be retarded in 3 h steps each night until it reaches the desired or socially acceptable sleep time. The sleep cycle is in effect lengthened to 26–27 h and kept constant until it has been realigned. Hypnotics may help to reduce sleep during the 'forbidden zone' and the changes should be supported by careful sleep hygiene. Once the new pattern has been established it is important to maintain a constant time of going to bed and of waking up in the morning. Less than 1 h deviation from the intended time should be the aim, and this should be maintained at weekends as well as during weekdays. It is important to avoid naps during the day, and particularly during the 2 h preceding sleep. Sleeping late in the morning should be avoided, even after going to sleep late on the previous night.

These routines should be combined with other aspects of sleep hygiene, especially taking physical activity during the day and, if necessary, with light therapy.

LIGHT THERAPY

Exposure to bright light early in the morning leads to a phase advance with an earlier onset of sleep and of subsequent waking up times. Light therapy is most effective if it is given between 6.00 and 10.00 AM. As the wake-up time becomes earlier so the timing of the light therapy can be moved earlier to further advance the phase shift. Bright lights in the bathroom, bedroom and kitchen and the encouragement to walk to work may help, but treatment with a light box or visor may be required. Sitting by a window and exposure to ordinary indoor electric light are insufficient. If it is not possible for light therapy to be provided early in the morning a light box installed on the desk at work throughout the morning may be effective.

Once the syndrome has been controlled, the maintenance dose of light may be reduced or the frequency of light therapy decreased to 2–3 times per week. Light therapy should be combined with sleep hygiene, particularly with regular sleep-onset and wake-up times and can be used in conjunction with chronotherapy. It is particularly effective in SADS.

MELATONIN

Exogenous melatonin can be used to induce earlier secretion of endogenous melatonin and thereby to advance the sleep phase to a more nearly normal time [8]. Melatonin administration in the evening is able to advance the onset of endogenous secretion and sleep by 1.5 h per day, but does not alter sleep architecture. It acts in effect as an early night replacement treatment for endogenous melatonin, and it is often, but not always, effective in the long term.

Advanced sleep phase syndrome

Clinical features

This syndrome is characterized by a stable sleep rhythm which is offset relative to normal, so that the sleep-onset and waking-up times occur earlier than is conventional and desired. Sleep often begins around 9.00 PM and ends between 3.00 and 5.00 AM. The total sleep time and sleep architecture are normal and daytime sleepiness is not a problem, unless going to sleep early in the evening is prevented. Advanced sleep phase syndrome causes fewer problems than DSPS although it is common for subjects to fall asleep in the evening and to have to be woken in order to go to bed. The early awakening time can disrupt the partner and family, but occurs even if sleep onset is delayed, in which case sleepiness is worse during the day because of sleep restriction. Alertness is maximal in the mornings and sleepiness develops early in the evening.

Like DSPS, the criteria for the diagnosis depend on the normal sleep patterns within each society. It is more frequent and more troublesome when the conventional sleep times are late as in most warmer climates. Advanced sleep phase syndrome has probably become more prominent since the introduction of the electric light bulb since it was previously usual to fall asleep by around 9.00 PM or soon after sundown. The

ASPS may be a biological adaptation to the natural light–dark cycles.

Causes

OLD AGE
The amplitude of the circadian rhythm is reduced in the elderly and its timing may change so that it fails to combat the homeostatic drive to enter sleep early in the evening. This tendency is compounded by a variety of behavioural and other factors (Chapter 1).

INTRINSIC ADVANCED SLEEP PHASE SYNDROME
This syndrome is less common than intrinsic DSPS. It is often familial and it usually appears in late middle age or in the elderly. It may be due to a genetic defect in the circadian sleep rhythms, or in the way in which they control the release of or respond to melatonin. It may simply be an exaggeration of the ASPS of the elderly and it merges into the group of subjects known as 'larks' or 'morning types,' who are least alert in the evenings, tend to go to sleep early and awaken early in the mornings.

EXTRINSIC ADVANCED SLEEP PHASE SYNDROME
This may be socially induced, for instance by tiredness following early awakening for a morning shift or to commute to work, especially when this is associated with factors which promote sleep early in the evening, such as a large meal, dim lighting and watching unstimulating television. Early morning waking with exposure to light also leads to a sleep phase advance and this may perpetuate, and even in some people initiate, the ASPS.

DEPRESSION
This frequently causes mild ASPS.

Diagnosis
Advanced sleep phase syndrome needs to be distinguished from causes of EDS and EMW. Polysomnography carried out at the patient's normal sleep time shows a normal sleep architecture and duration, but if this is carried out at more conventional times, the duration of NREM sleep, particularly stages 3 and 4, is reduced (Fig. 5.5). The pattern of sleep and wake can be confirmed by sleep diaries and actigraphy, and melatonin secretion occurs earlier than in normal subjects. Intrinsic ASPS may be difficult to distinguish from extrinsic ASPS unless

modification of the factors responsible for the latter cause it to resolve.

Treatment

SLEEP HYGIENE
This is as important as in DSPS. Sleep onset should be delayed, a regular wake-up time adopted, and naps avoided during the day.

CHRONOTHERAPY
A gradual delay in the sleep phase may realign it with environmental conditions based on similar principles to the treatment of DSPS, but there is little evidence regarding its effectiveness.

LIGHT THERAPY
The sleep phase can be delayed by exposure to bright light in the evening, but not within 1 h of the intended time of going to sleep. A bright light bulb used while eating, reading or watching television may be of some help, but formal light therapy with a light box or visor is preferable. The duration and intensity of the light therapy needed vary between individuals, but 1–3 h treatment is commonly given. Exposure to bright light early in the morning may cause a phase advance and should be avoided either by staying indoors or by wearing dark glasses in bright sunlight. The effects of light therapy may take 1–8 weeks to appear. Advanced sleep phase syndrome often relapses within a month of stopping treatment, which may need to be maintained in the long term to prevent relapses.

MELATONIN
Exogenous melatonin taken in the morning delays endogenous melatonin secretion and may help to postpone the onset of sleep.

Non-24 h sleep–wake rhythm

Clinical features
This results from a failure of environmental factors to control the circadian sleep rhythm and melatonin secretion. The rhythm has an intrinsic cycle of around 24.2 h and if it remains independent of the environment (free running), its relationship with it changes each day. At one point in the cycle the two are in phase, but the sleep rhythm then moves progressively forward, leading initially to what appears to be a DSPS and then through sleep reversal with insomnia at night and sleepiness during the day to an ASPS

before returning temporarily to synchrony with the environment again. The rhythm may be partially entrained by cultural and social factors to an extent which depends on their intensity and the entrainability of the individual's circadian rhythm. The fluctuating insomnia and daytime sleepiness can be difficult to cope with and while the same symptoms arise in partially entrained subjects as in free-running cycles, they are milder. Daytime naps tend to occur at the times of melatonin secretion.

Causes

A reduction in the variation of light intensity as in cave dwellers, residents at polar latitudes, and space travellers diminishes the influence of the environment on the circadian sleep rhythm and predisposes to a non-24 h sleep–wake rhythm. An extreme example is space travel in which exposure to the sun rising and setting may occur several times in each 24 h period. The unusual pattern of activity and sleeping position in an environment with little gravitational force, and the imposed and restricted social interactions, all combine to alter circadian rhythms and sleep. A non-24 h sleep–wake rhythm may also be due to blindness, damage to the retinohypothalamic tract and disorders of the SCN or pineal gland. An identical pattern can occur in otherwise normal subjects with no detectable visual or neurological abnormality, probably because of a functional defect in the SCN or its connections which prevents the circadian sleep rhythm from being entrained by environmental factors.

Diagnosis

This requires a careful history and analysis of sleep diaries, supplemented by actigraphy to detect diurnal variations in movements which are an indirect marker of sleep and wakefulness.

Treatment

The symptoms of these partially or totally free running circadian rhythms are often difficult to eliminate, but treatment comprises sleep hygiene advice, chronotherapy, light therapy, melatonin or a combination of these. Melatonin is especially effective in blind people.

Irregular sleep–wake rhythm

The pattern of sleep may become irregular and fail to retain a constant relationship to the environmental time, or to light and darkness. The temperature and endocrine rhythmicity may also be lost or be dissociated from the sleep cycle. Insomnia, EDS or the need to nap during the day reflect the irregular sleep and wake patterns, but total sleep time is often normal.

Irregular sleep–wake rhythms may be due to rare endogenous disorders in which there is damage or dysfunction of the circadian rhythm generator or its connections (page 98). More commonly, it is the result of exogenous factors which not only influence the circadian rhythms but also affect the homeostatic and adaptive sleep drives. The most important examples are described below.

Social factors

There is a wide variety of personal and social factors which determine the regularity of each individual's sleep–wake habits. Variations in the time of going to sleep and waking up are usually insufficient to have much impact on the quality of sleep but can lead to severe daytime sleepiness. Even sleeping for longer in the mornings at weekends to catch up with the sleep debt that has accumulated during the week may be equivalent to a time zone change of 1–3 h and this will require subsequent adjustments of the circadian and sleep control mechanisms.

Time zone changes (jet lag)

CLINICAL FEATURES
Jet lag, which is the term used for the symptoms due to time zone changes, is due to a failure of the circadian rhythms to synchronize with the new environment after a sudden time zone shift. Jet lag does not occur with travel from north to south or south to north, but only with transmeridian journeys. It is not due to sleep deprivation, but this may contribute to the problems that develop. Sleep may be lost because of the timing of the departure and arrival, and the quality of sleep during the journey is often poor.

Jet lag is characterized by insomnia and EDS, usually with a reduction in total sleep time and sleep efficiency and with frequent naps during the day. The first night's sleep after the journey is least affected because of prior sleep deprivation. The circadian sleep rhythm adjusts more quickly to the new environment than the temperature rhythm and most endocrine rhythms, leading to internal desynchronization. Travellers who make frequent time zone changes may develop a persistent combination of insomnia and EDS.

Table 5.10 Jet lag prevention.

	Eastward travel	Westward travel
Before travel	Go to sleep and wake up early for 1–2 days Bright light exposure in morning for 1–2 days or melatonin on evening before journey	Go to sleep later for 1–2 days Bright light exposure in evening for 1–2 days Wear sun glasses in bright light in mornings for 1–2 days Melatonin early in morning before journey
During travel	Arrive between 5.00 AM and 9.00 PM Avoid hypnotics and alcohol except when travelling in the evening Avoid stimulants, e.g. caffeine, late in the journey	Arrive between 10.00 AM and 3.00 AM

After arrival	Adopt new time immediately
	Avoid naps on day of arrival
	Bright light exposure in morning for 1–2 days or
	   melatonin on evening after flight
		Adopt new time immediately
		Consider stimulants, e.g. caffeine, for 1–2 days
		Bright light exposure in the evening for 1–2 days or
		   melatonin in morning after flight

CAUSES

The severity of jet lag depends on the following factors.

1 Number of time zones crossed. Symptoms are usually significant if more than six time zones are crossed.
2 Individual susceptibility. This varies considerably and in general, jet lag is more severe in the elderly.
3 Direction of travel. Eastward travel is more disruptive than travelling westward. It leads to an earlier night and therefore requires a phase advance. This is more difficult to adapt to than a phase delay because the circadian sleep rhythm is longer than 24 h. The symptoms mimic the DSPS with a delay in sleep onset and difficulty in waking in the morning. In contrast, travelling westward mimics an ASPS and as the new environment is delayed relative to the old, sleep onset REM is common. Adaptation to the new time occurs at a rate of around 1 h per day travelling eastward and 1.5 h per day travelling westward.

TREATMENT

The treatment of jet lag depends on the duration and direction of travel. If transmeridian journeys are frequent, their need should be assessed and it may be preferable to travel less frequently, but stay abroad for longer to reduce the problems of jet lag. If the stay abroad is less than around three days it is usually best to remain on 'home time' to avoid any need for adjusting to the new clock time while abroad and again after the journey home. Day-time activities such as social contacts, exercise, meals and exposure to light should remain unchanged relative to home time.

The measures that should be taken for longer episodes depend largely on whether the journey is eastward or westward (Table 5.10). The new sleep onset time is ahead of 'home' bed time with eastward travel and occurs before the release of melatonin and often in the 'forbidden zone' when it is difficult to initiate sleep. Travelling westward, however, encourages sleep onset later than 'home time' so that sleep occurs readily on the first night. The sleep latency is short, sleep efficiency is high and there is a normal or increased duration of stages 3 and 4 NREM sleep. Awakening may occur early with loss of REM sleep which increases (rebounds) on the second night.

Short-acting hypnotics may be useful both during the flight and for a few nights after arrival if taken to establish sleep at the onset of night time at the destination. Resetting of the circadian rhythms can be accelerated by carefully timed exercise and exposure to light. Excessive light in the morning leads to a phase advance and in the evening to a phase delay (Chapter 2). Exposure to light in the early morning is useful with eastward travel since it advances the sleep phase, but it should be avoided in the evening by staying indoors or wearing sunglasses.

Arrival after 3.00 AM to 5.00 AM on eastward journeys, but before 9.00 PM, avoids any phase delay due to light exposure at the destination. Conversely, when travelling westward light should be avoided in the morning, but exposure obtained in the evening. An arrival time from 10.00 AM to 3.00 AM is best in order to avoid the phase advancing effect of light in the early morning. Whether travelling east or west, loss of sleep is minimized with daytime flights, but if sleep is lost it will enhance sleepiness and increase the duration of stages 3 and 4 NREM sleep on the first night after arrival. It is best to go to bed progressively more closely each night after arrival to the usual time of sleep at the destination.

The effects of melatonin are opposite to those of light. With eastward travel a fast release preparation should be taken 1–2 h before sleep onset at the new location, both for its hypnotic effect and to advance the sleep phase. It should be taken on waking in the morning, or even if waking occurs during the night with westward travel.

Shift work

In most westernized societies 20–30% of the adult workforce carry out some form of shift work. This was introduced early in the twentieth century following the development of the assembly line, interchangeable parts, mass production and the idea of continuous use of production equipment. Henry Ford first applied this to the development of his Model T car which was produced in 1908, and was thereby able to reduce its price and make it available to large sections of society. Public pressure in most westernized societies has subsequently prioritized short-term productivity and artificial working practices above the need for the individual worker to obtain adequate sleep. This and a lack of awareness of the importance of sleep, circadian rhythms and their disorders, has had wide ranging detrimental effects.

Shift work entails working outside conventional daylight hours on a regular or intermittent basis. Shifts may be either fixed, in which there is an unchanging pattern of work times, or rotating, in which they change regularly [5]. At these times there is often a 7–10 h change in the timing of sleep, equivalent to a time zone shift of this degree.

EFFECTS ON SLEEP

Complete adaptation to shift work is very rare even after many years of shift work, and as a result, it causes both insomnia and excessive sleepiness at times when wakefulness is desired. Subjects who have difficulty in coping with these problems often obtain alternative employment, but DIS and EMW insomnia may persist for months or years after shift work has ceased. The effects on sleep are due to the following factors.

1 A mismatch between the circadian sleep rhythms and the external environment. This is particularly important in rotating shifts in which the association between the circadian rhythms and external time frequently changes. An 8 h shift change may take the circadian sleep rhythms around a week to adjust to and this may be further slowed by exposure to light during the day. Internal desynchronization of the circadian

Table 5.11 Factors determining effects of shift work.

Shift work	Fixed or rotating shifts
	Duration of shifts
	Direction of shifts
	Frequency of shifts
	Interval between changes
Individual	Age
	Previous sleep habits and quality
	Motivation to alter sleep habits

rhythms is common, particularly since, for instance, the temperature cycle takes longer than the sleep cycle to adapt to any external change.

2 Poor quality of sleep, not only because attempts to sleep are out of phase with circadian rhythms, but also because of noise, light and other disturbances during the day [6].

3 Sleep restriction. This is a common but not inevitable consequence of shift work. Sleep has to compete with social and recreational activities and the sleep pattern often becomes irregular.

SHIFT WORK PATTERNS AND SLEEP

The degree of disruption to the sleep–wake cycle caused by shift work (Table 5.11) depends on the factors described below.

Whether the shift is fixed or rotating

The total sleep time of fixed-shift workers is less than that of regular daytime workers, but longer than that of rotating-shift workers.

Number of hours shifted

It is common for shifts to last from 6.00 AM to 2.00 PM, 2.00 to 10.00 PM and 10.00 PM to 6.00 AM. In the first of these the subject has to wake early and it is best to go to bed earlier, although because of both social and circadian rhythm factors this may be difficult. The sleeping time is therefore shortened and there may be difficulty in waking and sleepiness later in the day due to sleep restriction. A 30–60 min nap in the afternoon after the end of the shift may be help.

The 2.00 to 10.00 PM shift causes fewer problems, although many people find it difficult to mentally unwind after work and need time with their family and for social activities. This leads to a late onset of sleep with a reduction in time spent asleep unless the awakening time in the morning is also delayed.

Most workers feel tired during the 10.00 PM to 6.00 AM shift and it is common to nap during this time. After the shift many people sleep until around midday although this may be difficult because of external noise and light. It is important to avoid bright light in the morning after the shift since this can cause a sleep phase advance. After the morning sleep there is an interval of around 8–10 h of wakefulness before starting work. This is different to conventional daytime work which usually starts soon after waking. Tiredness during the next shift can be reduced by taking a 30–60 min nap in the evening with the duration determined by the degree of loss of sleep during the main sleep episode. An alternative is to remain awake during the morning until around 12.00 midday or 2.00 PM and then to obtain the main sleep episode. This has the advantage of utilizing the afternoon circadian tendency to fall asleep and also reduces the length of time awake before starting the next shift. Nevertheless, the total sleep time is often 2–4 h less than that of daytime workers because of the mismatch between the circadian rhythms and the opportunities for sleep.

Direction of shift

Adaptation is quicker and more complete if the shifts move forward rather than backwards. An early morning shift followed by a daytime shift and night-time shift is preferable to the opposite sequence.

Frequency of shift changes

More rapid shift changes cause the subject more difficulty in adapting to the environmental changes.

Interval between shift changes

A short interval between shifts, as with, for instance, working a 2.00–10.00 PM shift and then 6.00 AM–2.00 PM, leads to sleep restriction and hinders the adaptation that can take place to the new work pattern. An interval of 12–16 h, which usually in practice includes the main sleep period and one or more naps is of help, but whole rest days between shifts are preferable.

Individual adaptability

The factors that determine this are poorly established but include the following.

Age. Younger subjects adapt more quickly and more completely to shift changes. Over the age of around 45 years, increasingly troublesome symptoms appear.

Previous sleep habits. Workers often tend to select jobs which fit their natural sleep patterns. 'Owls', for instance, often work for some or all of the night, which fits their endogenous pattern of a late sleep-onset and wake-up time. Conversely, 'larks' would be better suited to work between 6.00 AM–2.00 PM. Mismatch between the natural sleep tendencies and the hours of shift work magnifies its adverse effects.

Personality and motivation. The achievement of good quality sleep of an adequate duration has to compete with the desirability of social, recreational and other activities outside work. The degree of motivation to modify these, in order to obtain a reasonably quiet and dark sleep environment, and to prioritize an adequate sleep time outside work above other activities varies considerably. The temptation to stay awake and keep socially active during the time when sleep is best entered often leads to sleep restriction and sleep being taken at the least appropriate time in the circadian rhythm. These and other aspects of sleep hygiene have a large impact on how successfully each individual copes with the potential disturbance of shift work on sleep–wake function.

GENERAL EFFECTS

Increase in accidents and reduction in work performance

Early morning shifts are often associated with subalertness because of the reduction in sleep quality and duration during the previous night, and because the shift is taking place at a time when the circadian drive to sleep is still strong. Work during the night shift takes place at the nadir of the circadian rhythm for alertness. Both these shifts are associated with an increase in the frequency of accidents at work and a reduction in productivity. The number of errors in repetitive activities increases, particularly in those who are unable to develop coping strategies to handle their sleepiness.

Increased use of hypnotics and alcohol

These are often used to help re-establish an acceptable sleep pattern, but may lead to dependency and chronic disturbance of the sleep pattern.

Shortened life expectancy

This has been shown in several studies, but the cause is uncertain. It may be related to repetitive cycles of internal desynchronization of circadian rhythms, but other factors including an increased alcohol consumption and tobacco smoking may be relevant.

Table 5.12 Coping with night shift work.

To promote sleep during the day	To stay alert at night
Avoid bright light in the morning	Take a nap before going to work
Delay going to bed, ideally until 12.00 midday	Take caffeine, but not after 5.00 AM
Develop pre-sleep routines, e.g. hot bath	Keep work area brightly lit
Avoid caffeinated drinks before sleep	Avoid excessive overtime working
Keep bedroom at 18°C and dark	Avoid heavy meals before night shift
	Avoid alcohol or hypnotics

MANAGEMENT

The management of sleep–wake problems due to shift work (Table 5.12) entails the following.

Minimization of impact of shift work
1 Optimization of shift schedules according to the principles described above.
2 Adaptation of activities outside work so that a reasonable total sleep time is obtained. This may be most easily achieved as a single sleep episode, but division into a main sleep with one or more naps before starting the night shift often improves alertness at work at night [7].

Hypnotics and stimulants

Hypnotics. These may be useful when taken intermittently, but only short-acting benzodiazepines, zaleplon, zopiclone and zolpidem should be considered. Their main value is in initiating sleep, and drugs with a prolonged action will accentuate sleepiness during the night shift.

Stimulants. Stimulants, especially caffeine, are useful before and during night shifts to relieve sleepiness, but should be avoided after around 5.00 AM because they may prevent sleep from being initiated after the shift.

Modification of circadian rhythms
This can be achieved by factors such as the timing of physical exercise but the most important factors are discussed below.

Light therapy. The timing of light exposure is determined by the details of the shifts that are being worked. Light exposure in the evening and at night will enhance alertness during the night shift. Early in the night it causes a phase delay so that sleepiness may not develop until the end of the shift on subsequent nights. Light exposure after 3.00–5.00 AM

may, however, cause a phase advance and light should be avoided in the morning, for instance by wearing sunglasses.

Melatonin. Melatonin may be used to alter the time of the main sleep episode in order to adapt to the changes in shift-working hours. It delays the next sleep phase if it is taken in the morning, but taken in the evening will advance this. Melatonin can also hasten readaptation of the circadian rhythms after a period of shift work.

References

1 Jensen E, Dehlin O, Hagberg B, Samuelsson G, Svensson T. Insomnia in an 80-year-old population: Relationship to medical, psychological and social factors. *J Sleep Res* 1998; 7: 183–9.
2 Bonnet MH, Arand DL. Hyperarousal and insomnia. *Sleep Med Rev* 1997; 1: 97–108.
3 Gambetti P. Fatal familial insomnia and familial Creutzfeldt–Jakob disease: a tale of two diseases with the same genetic mutation. *Curr Top Microbiol Immunol* 1996; 207: 19–25.
4 Reynolds CF, Hoch CC, Stack J, Campbell D. The nature and management of sleep/wake disturbance in Alzheimer's dementia. *Psychopharmacol Bull* 1988; 24: 43–8.
5 Akerstedt T. Shift work and disturbed sleep/wakefulness. *Sleep Med Rev* 1998; 2: 117–28.
6 Weibel L, Spiegel K, Follenius M, Ehrhart J, Brandenberger G. Internal dissociation of the circadian markers of the cortisol rhythm in night workers. *Am J Physiol* 1996; 170: E608–E613.
7 Sallinen M, Harma M, Akerstedt T, Rosa R, Lillqvist O. Promoting alertness with a short nap during a night shift. *J Sleep Res* 1998; 7: 240–7.
8 Nagtegaal JE, Kerkhof GA, Smits MG, Swart ACW, Van der Meer YG. Delayed sleep phase syndrome: a placebo-controlled cross-over study on the effects of melatonin administered five hours before the individual dim light melatonin onset. *J Sleep Res* 1998; 7: 135–43.

6 Excessive Daytime Sleepiness

Introduction

Sleepiness is a common and physiological event in certain circumstances such as while relaxing after a meal in the early afternoon, and it can be difficult to differentiate this from a pathological degree of, or tendency towards, sleepiness or falling asleep. The balance of the homeostatic, ultradian and adaptive drives and the circadian rhythms determines whether sleep occurs or wakefulness continues. Each of these forces may be accentuated, diminished or modified in sleep disorders. Many of the conditions causing excessive daytime sleepiness (EDS) influence more than one of these aspects of sleep–wake control, although there is often uncertainty about the exact mechanisms involved.

Excessive daytime sleepiness therefore is not a diagnosis, but only a symptom. The term is often used loosely to indicate different types of sleepiness.

Subalertness
Consciousness is the awareness of oneself and the environment but its level ranges from extreme vigilance and alertness to the state of barely perceiving any stimulation. Subalertness is a state of diminished arousal rather than true sleepiness. It varies according to the phase of the circadian rhythm and the duration and quality of the previous sleep episode.

Drowsiness
Drowsiness, or sleepiness, may be felt during the day but does not necessarily lead to sleep.

Excessive duration of sleep during the day
Frequent naps or a single main daytime sleep episode, usually in the afternoon, may be taken or patients may wake up late or go to sleep early in the evening. The sensation of sleepiness may not be prominent, but sleep is easily entered.

Micro sleeps
These are brief episodes of sleep, lasting only a few seconds. The subject may not have any recollection of falling asleep, but is usually aware of having been sleepy and of waking suddenly at the end of the micro sleep.

Hypersomnolence is usually taken to mean an excessive sensation of sleepiness or drowsiness during the day, but it differs from hypersomnia. The latter usually implies an increase in the duration of sleep during each 24-h cycle which may be taken either as a prolonged main nocturnal sleep episode without additional sleep during the day or by falling asleep during the day, or a combination of both of these.

Prevalence

Population surveys have indicated that EDS is associated with sleep deprivation, snoring and hypnotic use, and is commonest in young adults, shift workers and the elderly. Excessive daytime sleepiness has been documented to occur in around 5% of the adult population in westernized countries, but the prevalence varies according to its definition.

Excessive daytime sleepiness forms a spectrum which merges with normality on the one hand and an inability to remain awake at all during the day at the other extreme. The usual duration of sleep is longer in infants and young children than in adults, but even in adult life some otherwise normal people have normal sleep architecture, but require a long sleep duration to feel refreshed (long sleepers). They may fall into the conventional definition of hypersomnia because of the increase in their sleep requirements during each 24-h cycle. The degree of alertness or sleepiness also varies between individuals. Those who are habitually subalert may become significantly drowsy or fall asleep in response to minor stimuli or changes in lifestyle that would not affect other people.

The methods for assessing the severity of daytime sleepiness have been described in Chapter 4, but many of the tests do not assess the subjective component of the symptom. The complaint of sleepiness is related to the expectations and requirements of each individual.

In the elderly, who may be confined to their home, a degree of sleepiness during the day which does not elicit a complaint of sleepiness would be intolerable in, for instance, a professional vehicle driver. Patients also vary considerably in their ability to cope with a certain level of sleepiness. A complaint of EDS without any objective change in the quality or duration of sleep may be precipitated by stress either within the family, with friends or at work.

Behavioural and psychological effects of excessive daytime sleepiness

Pre-sleep behaviour

Severe sleepiness requires an increased mental effort to maintain wakefulness, keep alert, concentrate and maintain attention. Intermittent restlessness, which may be a mechanism of increasing alertness, alternates with a vacant expression with little eye movement, infrequent blinking, drooping of the eyelids, yawning and rubbing of the eyes. Simple motor tasks such as walking or driving may continue, but the response time to changes in environmental situations is prolonged with an increased risk of errors and accidents. The automatic behaviour of acute sleepiness is similar to that seen on waking from sleep (confusional arousals) and there is often poor or fragmented recollection with distorted perceptions of this pre-sleep phase. Micro sleeps lasting 1–10 s are common and identifiable by a fixed gaze, absence of blinking and a blank facial expression. Absence of recollection of the onset of a micro sleep is common, but the arousal from it is usually recalled.

Psychological effects

The psychological effects of chronic daytime sleepiness largely reflect dysfunction of the prefrontal cortex [1]. The level of alertness falls, concentration deteriorates, attention for prolonged monotonous tasks shortens, and mood changes, particularly irritability, are common. Stereotyped behaviours with a loss of innovative responses to stimuli, a more limited vocabulary, loss of creativity and flexibility of thought processes and easier distraction by irrelevant information develop. Hallucinations due to altered perceptions of reality, or to intrusion of rapid eye movement (REM) sleep into wakefulness, may appear and there is a deterioration in short-term memory.

Motor effects

Motor dysfunction includes a deterioration in physi-

Table 6.1 Consequences of EDS.

Motor	Automatic behaviour
	Impaired physical performance
Awareness	Reduced alertness and attention
	Mood swings, irritability
	Loss of mental flexibility
	Hallucinations
Social	Poor school and work performance
	Hyperactivity in children
	Impaired social interactions
	Accidents (travel, home, occupational)

cal performance, particularly for long or monotonous tasks, a sense of fatigue, lack of energy, weariness and episodes of automatic behaviour in which purposeful, but inappropriate actions are performed in association with diminished vigilance and with subsequent amnesia (Table 6.1). Automatic behaviour of this type includes inappropriate actions such as putting sugar into a kettle, writing nonsense and missing motorway exits while driving.

When EDS is severe, dysarthria, tremor, ptosis, nystagmus and epileptic seizures may develop. The respiratory drive and probably respiratory muscle strength and endurance are reduced.

Social effects of excessive daytime sleepiness

Excessive daytime sleepiness can have a serious impact on family and social life, particularly if the patient's relatives and friends do not understand about the sleep problem. Recreational activities may have to be curtailed or may become dangerous if the subject is excessively sleepy.

Children with EDS have difficulty in learning and often perform poorly at school and in examinations. They may develop secondary psychological responses such as hyperactivity or aggression which cause additional problems. Excessive daytime sleepiness may also cause difficulties with employment, since it may be interpreted as laziness, poor motivation or even drunkenness. The psychological and motor consequences of chronic EDS impair work performance, particularly at night or during shift work. Productivity may fall and decision making becomes slower with an increased number of errors. Long working hours may also contribute to sleep deprivation which worsens the EDS, and the ability to cope with work responsibilities.

Accidents due to excessive daytime sleepiness

Social and occupational accidents

An increased risk of accidents in the home, during recreational activities and at work is a recognized consequence of EDS. The reduction in life expectancy in chronic EDS is probably partly due to accidents and partly to the sustained increased state of physiological arousal needed to combat sleepiness. This may predispose to, for instance, myocardial infarction. The specific physiological consequences of the sleep disorder causing EDS, such as the hypertension and strokes associated with obstructive sleep apnoeas (OSA), may also contribute to premature death.

Accidents in the home may be as simple as falling off a chair because of sleepiness, but can be more wide ranging if, for instance, they involve cooking or electrical appliances. Working with heavy or moving machinery should be avoided. Accident rates have been recorded to increase by up to 25% during night shifts compared to early morning shifts and errors at work can have serious consequences.

Motor vehicle accidents

SIZE OF THE PROBLEM

The importance of motor vehicles has increased steadily during the last 100 years with the increasing emphasis on mobility both for work and social reasons. Comfort and speed of the vehicles have been the priorities and the safety of driving has been relatively neglected. In one survey, 25% of New York State drivers admitted to having fallen asleep at the wheel, particularly during long journeys at night after a lack of sleep. It is estimated that 1–3% of all road traffic accidents are due to driver drowsiness and perhaps 10% of serious accidents, and 20% of motorway accidents. These particularly involve males under the age of 30 who are driving alone and who are involved in single-vehicle accidents. The number of near misses is probably much greater.

TYPE OF ACCIDENT

It can be difficult to be certain whether an accident is due to drowsiness or not. This is, however, likely to be a least a contributory factor in single-vehicle accidents occurring at night, particularly between 2.00 and 6.00 AM, despite this being the time when there is least

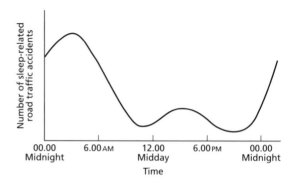

Fig. 6.1 Biphasic timing of accidents due to EDS.

traffic on the roads, and between 2.00 and 4.00 PM (Fig. 6.1). These accidents are often fatal and 40% occur on motorways or on dual carriageways.

CAUSES OF ACCIDENTS

Accidents are more common after working long hours or a night shift before driving, and in those who drive frequently when they are drowsy [2]. Sedative drugs and alcohol accentuate the sleepiness following sleep restriction and irregular sleeping patterns, particularly if these drugs are taken when the circadian rhythm facilitates sleep (2.00–6.00 AM or 2.00–4.00 PM). The effect of one drink of alcohol at these times may be equivalent to two or three taken at 10.00 AM. The risk of a sleep-related driving accident is three times greater in those taking hypnotics, such as benzodiazepines, and it is also increased with sedating tricyclic antidepressants. The effects of these drugs may exceed that of consumption of alcohol which is sufficient to raise the blood concentration above the legal limit of 0.8 g/l (80 mg/100 ml).

Medical causes of EDS are less frequent than social factors, but the presence of frequent OSAs increases the risk of motor vehicle accidents about 6-fold. The risk increases as sleep fragmentation worsens. The accident rate in those with narcolepsy appears to be less, probably because they are well aware of their limitations and of the possibility of sleepiness while driving.

Commercial drivers are particularly at risk of sleep-related accidents [3]. They often have to drive in order to meet deadlines or make emergency deliveries. This involves journeys at night, shift work and long driving times. The comfortable cabs and power steering of modern large goods and passenger carrying vehicles makes driving easier and less stimulating. Alertness falls after around 60 min driving and the mean duration of driving before a sleep-related accident is around 4 h.

Many commercial drivers are obese due to the ready availability of junk food between their journeys and the sedentary nature of their job. This obesity predisposes to OSAs and increases the risk of sleep-related accidents.

PRE-ACCIDENT BEHAVIOUR

The first observable sign of a sleepy driver is a change in speed due to intermittent loss of muscle activity in the leg controlling the accelerator. Shunting accidents at traffic lights or roundabouts are common, and it is common to weave or change lanes. If the driver veers off the road the vehicle may collide with an oncoming car or a static object. Articulated lorries may jack-knife if the driver suddenly regains alertness after a micro sleep and over reacts by making a sudden corrective steering action. This type of accident is most common on motorways early in the morning.

It is possible to drive for several miles while extremely drowsy or even lightly asleep. This type of automatic behaviour is characterized by a glazed expression, absence of blinking, reduced responsiveness to external stimuli and a loss of peripheral vision. Drivers are occasionally drawn towards lights or other features, for instance the rear of other vehicles, leading to fatal accidents. Micro sleeps are common and awakening may occur without any recollection of having fallen asleep or of changing lanes before the accident, although awareness of being sleepy before the incident is usually retained.

ACCIDENT PREVENTION

The risk of a motor vehicle accident due to sleepiness can be reduced by avoiding sleep deprivation and, if possible, shift work before driving, together with encouraging good sleep hygiene practice and a greater awareness of the problems of driving while sleepy. If driving after sleep deprivation is unavoidable it is best to sleep for around 30 min before starting driving and to take 50–100 mg caffeine. This has a stimulant effect within 30 min. Activities such as keeping the car windows open and playing music may have a slight stimulant action, but can encourage sleepiness in some people. It is essential to stop driving before sleepiness becomes marked and it is probably the drivers who ignore this warning symptom who are most likely to be involved in fatal accidents.

The design of roads also has a large influence on the frequency of sleep-related accidents. Accident blackspots on motorways are usually due to a combination of a previous monotonous stretch of driving, coupled with a complex junction or slip road system. Warning signs on motorways alerting drivers to be aware of sleepiness and the provision of laybys on major roads, so that drivers can stop to sleep should be encouraged. Ridged surfaces (rumble strips) are effective in alerting drivers to a lane change and have significantly reduced accident rates. Equipment to detect the driver's blink rate or eye closure and which then alerts the driver has been introduced, but is unlikely to be effective since accidents frequently occur before these signs develop. It is preferable to stop driving at the onset of sleepiness rather than to wait until this late stage before attempting to detect it.

These aspects of prevention of sleep-related motor vehicle accidents involve increasing the awareness of drivers and altering public policies regarding roads and driving. The doctor also has a role in advising patients about these aspects, in diagnosing any underlying sleep disorder, giving sleep hygiene advice, especially for shift workers, and in assessing whether or not the patient is fit to drive. This decision is influenced by the degree of sleepiness, the underlying sleep disorder and the distance and time of day that is usually driven. The doctor has a duty to inform the patient that he or she should notify the Driver and Vehicle Licensing Agency (DVLA) and the driver's insurance company of any sleep disorder that may impair the ability to drive. It is not the doctor's role to make these notifications except in exceptional circumstances when the duty to society as a whole may out-weigh the duty of confidentiality to the individual patient because of a substantial risk from an accident and the patient's unwillingness or inability to notify the authorities.

The DVLA do not require notification of EDS due to poor sleep hygiene, sleep deprivation, shift work or sedative medication, but the patient has a legal duty to report narcolepsy, irrespective of the extent of any perceived difficulty with driving. Medical disorders which affect the ability to drive may require a report from the doctor caring for the patient before a licence is issued, and if so, whether it is for a restricted period, such as 1–3 years, before being reviewed, or for a longer period. In general, the licence is usually retained in those with OSA if this is satisfactorily controlled with nasal continuous positive airway pressure (CPAP) for around three months and if there is satisfactory compliance with treatment. Large goods vehicle (LGV) and passenger carrying vehicle (PCV) licence holders with EDS due to OSA also require annual reassessment for at least 2 years to establish whether the improvement with CPAP has been maintained. Treatment of EDS and cataplexy in narcolepsy usually enables the licence to be retained for a limited period.

Assessment

The most important points to establish when assessing EDS are whether the sleepiness is physiological or pathological, its severity, its impact on the patient's lifestyle and its cause. These issues may be difficult to evaluate because of the normal changes in sleepiness with age and environmental factors that may promote sleep or wakefulness. The cause of EDS is often multifactorial and if it fails to improve with treatment the process of assessment should be reconsidered.

History

A careful history is essential in assessing EDS accurately (Table 6.2, Chapter 4). The following issues should be considered.

NATURE OF EXCESSIVE DAYTIME SLEEPINESS
Drowsiness and subalertness should be distinguished from similar symptoms such as fatigue. It should be established whether the subject is sleeping for more than the normal length of time during each 24-h cycle and the distribution of sleep during the day and night. Micro sleeps during the day are characteristic of sleep deprivation, whereas refreshing naps of 10–30 min are usual in narcolepsy, and longer, less refreshing naps are characteristic of idiopathic central nervous system hypersomnia (ICNSH).

SEVERITY OF EXCESSIVE DAYTIME SLEEPINESS
AND ITS IMPACT ON LIFESTYLE
This can be gauged by whether sleep occurs in situations in which a passive role is adopted or whether it extends into more active situations such as holding a conversation. Drowsiness, micro sleeps or prolonged sleeps while driving and deteriorating concentration and mood lability, usually with irritability, should be enquired of. Automatic behaviour is a feature of severe EDS.

The effects of EDS on the patient and his or her family, friends and colleagues at work, any accidents it has caused with moving machinery or while driving, and its influence on performance at school and work should be ascertained.

CAUSES OF EXCESSIVE DAYTIME SLEEPINESS
Questions should be asked regarding:
1 sleep hygiene, especially the duration and regularity of sleep times;
2 drugs, such as sedatives, analgesics or antidepressants;
3 causes of sleep fragmentation, such as OSA, periodic limb movements in sleep (PLMS), asthma, pain or discomfort at night;
4 REM sleep-related symptoms might indicate narcolepsy or a similar disorder;
5 neurological problems such as a previous head injury or encephalitis and current neurological symptoms that might indicate a focal lesion; and
6 systemic disorders, e.g. hypothyroidism.

Physical examination

Physical examination is often unrewarding, but an impression of the subject's mental state and level of alertness is important. Abnormalities of the upper airway and obesity which might be related to OSA should be sought. Examination of the nervous system is only indicated if a neurological cause is being considered.

Investigations

Further investigation is not required if the history and examination provide sufficient information for the cause and severity of the EDS to be established, and for treatment to be initiated. Disorders of sleep hygiene, including a suboptimal sleep environment, drug-related problems and systemic disorders such as hypothyroidism, can usually be managed without referral to a specialist centre, but in most other situations this is required for further investigations to be carried out (Table 6.3). Further investigations that may be performed are discussed below.

SLEEP STUDY
The complexity of the sleep study varies according to the suspected diagnosis. If OSA is most likely, an oximetry study may be sufficient, or combined with measurement of airflow and abdominal and ribcage movement. In most other situations polysomnography is needed to give information about sleep architecture, arousals, sleep-onset REM and the cause of arousals from sleep such as PLMS, central sleep apnoeas or gastro-oesophageal reflux. Serial sleep studies may be required to monitor progress with treatment.

ASSESSMENT OF SEVERITY OF EXCESSIVE
DAYTIME SLEEPINESS
This can be carried out with the tests described in Chapter 4, including the Epworth Sleepiness Scale and multiple sleep latency tests (MSLTs), which also demonstrate the sleep-onset REM characteristic of narcolepsy.

Table 6.2 Differential diagnosis of sleepiness.

	Characteristics	Causes
Physical tiredness	Sensation of fatigue or weariness	Organic illness and, less prominently with sleep deprivation, insomnia, and chronic fatigue syndrome or prolonged or intense exertion
Mental fatigue	Lack of attention Short concentration span Difficulty in assimilating information	Depression Chronic fatigue syndrome Sleep deprivation
Boredom	Loss of interest in immediate surroundings which lowers the threshold for sleep	Sleepiness predisposes but is not the cause
Automatic behaviour	Subalertness with poor motor control (ataxia) and complex but inappropriate actions	Any cause of sleepiness with entry into stages 1 and 2 NREM sleep
Confusional arousal (sleep drunkenness)	As for automatic behaviour, often with mental slowness and confusion	Partial arousal from sleep especially stages 3 and 4 NREM sleep
Hypnosis	A state of increased suggestibility	Occurs with EEG features of wakefulness not sleep
Meditation	A state of altered awareness	Dissociation of level of consciousness from reflex control
Fugue states	Amnesia with episodes of wandering	Psychogenic (hysterical), often precipitated by stress or depression Epilepsy, brief episodes often with other complex motor activities
Catalepsy	Prolonged maintenance of unusual postures	Hysteria: apparent unrousability but with EEG features of wakefulness Catatonia
Catatonia	Catalepsy with increased muscle tone and purposeless motor activity	Affective disorders, schizophrenia, metabolic disorders, drugs Organic brain damage
Confusion	Alertness with disorientation for time, place or person	Diffuse cerebral disorders, e.g. dementia Infection Metabolic disorders Drug effects and withdrawal

Continued on p. 116

Table 6.2 (cont'd)

	Characteristics	Causes
Delirium (toxic confusional state)	Confusion with restlessness and overactivity	As for confusion
Stupor	Unconsciousness and physical inactivity, but rousable to make brief verbal responses Merges into coma	As for coma
Coma	Unconsciousness, not readily reversible Responds reflexly but not with speech Regular EEG slow-wave activity, but not influenced by external stimuli	Diffuse bilateral cerebral cortical damage, e.g. encephalitis, head injury Upper brain-stem lesions Metabolic disorders Drugs
Persistent vegetative state (PVS)	Unresponsive and unaware of surroundings No communication A few simple movements	Extensive cerebral cortical damage
Akinetic mutism	Involuntary movements, except of eyes Some sleep–wake rhythms detectable	Extensive brain damage, especially to reticular activating system
Locked-in syndrome	Conscious and aware of surroundings Able to see and hear but paralysed except for vertical eye movements and blinking NREM and REM sleep alternate with wakefulness	Pontine lesions with intact midbrain and cerebral cortex
General anaesthesia	Reduced awareness and to a variable extent, memory, pain and movements Arousability brief and incomplete	Chemical agents with widespread CNS effects, in some cases affecting sleep control mechanisms

CNS, central nervous system; EEG, electroencephalogram; NREM, non-rapid eye movement; REM, rapid eye movement.

Table 6.3 Role of investigations in diagnosis of EDS.

Diagnosis	Investigation
Sleep deprivation	Sleep diary, PSG Actigraphy
Sleep fragmentation	Respiratory monitoring for OSA Arterial blood gases for ventilatory failure Polysomnography for PLMS or occasionally for other causes
Circadian rhythm disorders	Sleep diary Actigraphy 24 h temperature monitoring Diurnal cortisol secretion Melatonin profile
Neurological disorders	Narcolepsy: HLA type, PSG, MSLTs ICNSH: PSG to exclude other causes Focal lesions—head MRI or CT scan Prader–Willi syndrome: respiratory sleep study
Psychiatric disorders	Nil
Systemic disorders	Metabolic and endocrine investigations
Drugs	Blood and urine drug levels

CT, computerized tomography; HLA, human leucocyte antigen; ICNSH, idiopathic central nervous system hypersomnia; MSLTs, multiple sleep latency tests; MRI, magnetic resonance imaging; OSA, obstructive sleep apnoeas; PLMS, periodic limb movements in sleep; PSG, polysomnography.

INVESTIGATION OF THE CAUSE OF EXCESSIVE DAYTIME SLEEPINESS
1 Imaging techniques, e.g. computerized tomography (CT) and magnetic resonance imaging (MRI) scans of the brain to detect organic neurological disorders.
2 Human leucocyte antigen (HLA) typing, which is of use in narcolepsy.
3 Arterial blood gases, to assess ventilatory failure.

Principles of treatment

The aims of treatment (Fig. 6.2) are described below.

Assist adaptation

The nature of the disorder should be explained and advice should be given about lifestyle modifications to assist in managing any residual EDS despite optimal treatment. This may include coping strategies, advice about when to take naps and how to plan activities around episodes of sleepiness and driving. Explanation and reassurance about the nature of the condition to family, friends, school teachers, employers and colleagues at work may be helpful.

Optimize sleep hygiene

This is almost invariably an important aspect of the management of EDS. It entails:
1 altering the sleep environment so that the bed is comfortable and the bedroom warm, dark and quiet;
2 improving sleep–wake patterns, increasing physical activity, and light exposure during the day, regularizing sleep and wake times and avoiding daytime naps.

Treat the underlying cause

Disorders such as OSA, PLMS, hypothyroidism, gastro-oesophageal reflux and nocturnal asthma may all be amenable to treatment. Treatment of circadian rhythm disorders is described in Chapter 5.

Optimize drug treatment

HYPNOTICS
It is important to avoid sedatives and hypnotics such as alcohol, benzodiazepines and opiate analgesics.

CENTRAL NERVOUS SYSTEM STIMULANTS
These should be considered once all the above measures

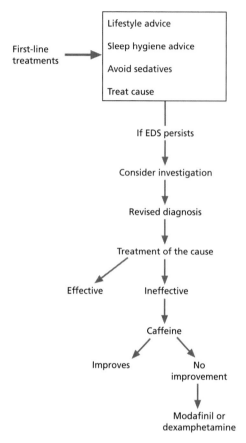

Fig. 6.2 Management of excessive daytime sleepiness (EDS).

have been implemented and if any residual EDS is sufficiently severe to have a significant impact on the subject's life, for instance by interfering with the ability to cope with interpersonal relationships, family responsibilities, driving or at work. The issues that should be addressed when choosing a stimulant preparation are as follows.

1 Effectiveness and duration of action. The ability to convert sleep to wakefulness and the level of alertness that can be achieved varies. Short-acting drugs are least likely to cause insomnia, unless they are taken late in the day, but are more likely to cause the level of alertness to fluctuate.

2 Specificity for sleep–wake actions. Stimulant preparations may affect mental function, changing the ability to perform complex mental tasks and causing emotional changes with euphoria, irritability or occasionally a psychosis. Motor hyperactivity, muscle tremor, autonomic effects such as sweating and

palpitations, and sensory changes including hallucinations, may appear.

3 Side-effects. These and the toxic : therapeutic ratio vary between individual stimulant drugs.

4 Drug interactions.

5 Potential for dependency.

6 Tolerance to therapeutic effects.

Caffeine is the usual first-line mild CNS stimulant for EDS, and is often taken in tea, coffee or cola drinks, or as caffeine tablets. Nicotine, which in low dose is a sedative, can be a stimulant in high doses and has a useful alerting effect. If EDS is more severe, modafinil should be considered before amphetamines and related drugs. It has a more specific sleep-promoting action with fewer other central or peripheral nervous system stimulant effects. Side-effects and drug interactions are uncommon and it has little potential for dependency. It has a more gradual onset and a longer duration of action than dexamphetamine, but lacks the 'lift' that amphetamines give. It is as effective as dexamphetamine as a wakefulness promoting drug, but should not be taken late in the day since its long duration of action may lead to insomnia.

Amphetamines should be reserved for those in whom modafinil is ineffective or for occasional patients who develop side-effects with this. Those who have been established on dexamphetamine or similar drugs, but who have side-effects or who have developed other management problems should be considered for transfer to modafinil, but this is not required for those who are both effectively treated with amphetamines and who do not have problems with them. A combination of modafinil and dexamphetamine is occasionally required and can provide the peaks of alertness due to the amphetamine on the background of wakefulness due to the modafinil.

Sleep deprivation

The duration of sleep required to feel refreshed on waking and alert during the day varies considerably, but is usually 6–9 h each night. Sleep deprivation is probably the commonest cause of EDS and is usually due to social or work pressures (Table 6.4, Fig. 6.3), arising from a conflict between the need to complete various activities and to obtain sufficient sleep. The increase in social and recreational activities, shopping outside normal daylight hours, the need to work shifts and to communicate across time zones for business purposes, has contributed to the development of a '24-hour society'. The possibility of carrying out these

Table 6.4 Age and excessive daytime sleepiness (EDS). ASPS, advanced sleep phase syndrome; CNS, central nervous system; DSPS, delayed sleep phase syndrome; ICNSH, idiopathic central nervous system hypersomnia; OSA, obstructive sleep apnoeas; PLMS, periodic limb movements in sleep.

Childhood	Adolescence	Young and middle-aged adults	Old age
		Sleep deprivation	
		Drugs	
			ASPS
	DSPS		
		Shift work	
		OSA	
			PLMS
			Pain and discomfort
		Narcolepsy	
		ICNSH	
		Focal CNS lesions	
	Kleine–Levin syndrome		
	Prader–Willi syndrome		
	Myotonic dystrophy		
Cerebral palsy			
		Head injury	
	Encephalitis		
		Cerebral irradiation	
	Psychiatric disorders		
	Metabolic and endocrine disorders		

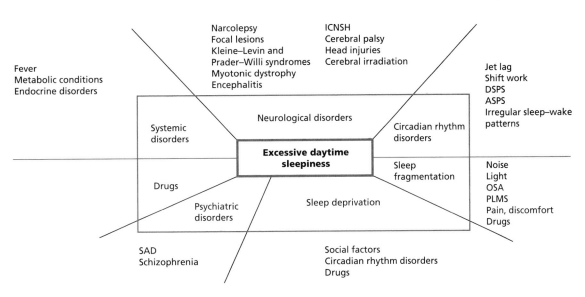

Fig. 6.3 Causes of excessive daytime sleepiness (EDS). ASPS, advanced sleep phase syndrome; DSPS, delayed sleep phase syndrome; ICNSH, idiopathic central nervous system hypersomnia; OSA, obstructive sleep apnoeas; PLMS, periodic limb movements in sleep; SAD, seasonal affective disorder.

activities at any time has enabled them to take priority over obtaining sufficient sleep and regular sleeping times.

Sleep deprivation can be caused by circadian rhythm disorders, such as the delayed sleep phase syndrome (DSPS) and advanced sleep phase syndrome (ASPS). Either the end or start of the sleep period becomes truncated in order to comply with social or cultural norms. A more complex pattern of sleep restriction may be due to irregular sleep–wake rhythms or to stimulant drugs such as caffeine and amphetamines which prevent sleep from being entered and thereby reduce the total sleep time.

Acute loss of sleep increases the degree of sleepiness during the next day and EDS gradually worsens if this is perpetuated. It is probably worse if non-rapid eye movement (NREM) sleep, which occurs particularly during the first third of the night, is preferentially lost, as in voluntary sleep restriction with a late onset of sleep. Shift work may affect either sleep onset or involve an early wake-up time with preferential loss of REM sleep. Polysomnography during sleep deprivation shows a reduced sleep latency, sleep-onset REM and a slightly increased duration of NREM sleep but with less stage 1 sleep. During the first one or two nights after sleep deprivation has been relieved, the duration of NREM sleep increases, but on subsequent nights there is an increase (rebound) in REM sleep. If this loss of sleep is not compensated for by these changes and an increase in sleep duration, a 'sleep debt' builds up with a tendency to EDS, a short sleep latency and an ability to prolong the nocturnal sleep episode.

Sleep deprivation reduces the ability to maintain attention. This can be partially offset by mental effort and by drugs such as caffeine, amphetamines and probably modafinil. Motor performance deteriorates and the time to respond to stimuli lengthens. There is a linear decline in performance of tasks requiring attention over the first 72 h of sleep deprivation, but this can be significantly improved by naps of as short as 30 min. Sensory changes such as a reduction of the visual field and visual illusions, but not hallucinations, may develop and speech becomes flat with little intonation. Decision making is impaired and memory worsens. Frontal lobe functions involving flexibility and originality of thought, foresight and word fluency all deteriorate. There is less control of mood, and uninhibited behaviour may appear together with paranoia and a failure to recognize or admit to errors. These mental changes cannot be compensated for by

an increase in effort or motivation and neither caffeine nor amphetamines are effective. The efficacy of modafinil has not been established. These frontal lobe functional changes are similar to those seen in the elderly, but are completely reversed once adequate sleep is obtained.

Short term sleep deprivation has an immunosuppressant effect. It reduces production of interferons, natural killer (NK) cell activity and phagocytic activity. It leads to changes in carbohydrate metabolism and endocrine function similar to those that are often seen in the elderly. Glucose intolerance develops, possibly due to reduced cerebral glucose utilization and changes in autonomic control of pancreatic function so that less insulin is released. The afternoon and evening plasma cortisol levels rise and the normal increase in thyrotrophin (TSH) at night is reversed. Increased sympathetic activity during the day leads to hypertension and changes in renal function.

Long-term NREM sleep deprivation may cause short stature in children, possibly due to under secretion of growth hormone. Chronic REM deprivation probably impairs neuropsychiatric development in children.

A careful history should elicit the nature and extent of sleep deprivation and the reasons for this. It is important to explain the effects of loss of sleep to the patient and to discuss methods of altering the balance between daytime activities and sleep in favour of the latter. Constraints such as fixed working hours may be difficult to change, but advice about regularity of sleep times, an earlier onset of sleep, planning of naps during the day to compensate for sleep restriction at night, improving the sleep environment in order to maximize the quality of sleep, avoiding stimulant drugs such as caffeine in the evening, and other aspects of sleep hygiene such as taking exercise during the day to increase alertness may all be of value. The management of circadian rhythm disorders, including shift work problems, is described in Chapter 5. Excessive daytime sleepiness due to sleep restriction improves with increasing the duration of sleep, in contrast to idiopathic CNS hypersomnia with which it can easily be confused.

Sleep fragmentation

This is the failure to sustain sleep or a stage of sleep because of frequent transitions to a lighter stage of sleep or to wakefulness. The time spent in bed and the duration from the start to the end of sleep may be normal, but continuity of sleep is broken. This fragmentation of sleep, particularly stages 2–4 NREM sleep, is thought to be a separate factor from sleep deprivation in causing EDS, although the evidence is not conclusive. It is not certain how much the severity of EDS is influenced by the duration of each arousal or whether there is a minimum length of sleep between arousals which is required to retain the refreshing function of sleep.

Sleep fragmentation may be due to one or more of the following factors.

1 External factors. These may be a noisy, light, hot or cold sleep environment, or an uncomfortable bed. These problems should be corrected.

2 Conditions which only appear during sleep. This important group of disorders includes OSA and central sleep apnoeas (Chapters 9 and 10), PLMS (Chapter 7) and occasionally other behavioural disorders during sleep if they occur frequently. Sleep apnoeas may also lead to drowsiness or coma due to hypercapnia. The history and examination may need to be supplemented by blood gas analysis and a sleep study, usually polysomnography, to confirm the diagnosis and assess the severity of these disorders.

3 Medical disorders which are exacerbated by sleep. These include gastro-oesophageal reflux, nocturnal angina and asthma (Chapter 8). They often present with the primary symptom of the disorder, but EDS can be significant. A history should be supplemented by relevant investigations.

4 Symptoms that are largely unrelated to sleep. These include pain and discomfort due to rheumatoid arthritis or other types of arthritis and neurological diseases, such as Parkinsonism and multiple sclerosis.

These symptoms require appropriate investigation and treatment of their cause, together with analgesic and other symptomatic treatment and modification of the sleep environment and sleeping position.

5 Drugs. These may fragment sleep through different mechanisms. Firstly, stimulant drugs such as caffeine and amphetamines cause frequent sleep-stage shifts and arousals. Tricyclic antidepressants may increase the frequency of PLMS and drugs such as dopamine agonists may cause awakening due to vivid dreams. Alcohol and short-acting hypnotics cause rebound insomnia at the end of the night and other drugs cause side-effects which may develop during sleep leading to frequent arousals and awakenings. A careful drug history and assessment of the need for each drug and the possible substitution by alternative treatments is required.

Circadian rhythm disorders

These may cause either EDS or insomnia or both (Chapter 5).

Rapid eye movement sleep-related disorders

Rapid eye movement sleep-related disorders share several important characteristics (Table 6.5). Excessive daytime sleepiness often occurs as a 'sleep attack' which may be hard to resist. Fragments of REM also intrude into wakefulness. The two manifestations of the loss of muscle tone, which is a feature of REM sleep, are cataplexy, which occurs while awake,

Table 6.5 Features of REM-related causes of EDS.

Feature of sleep		Abnormality
Changes in sleep	*Night*	Short sleep latency
		Insomnia
	Day	Sleep attacks
		Subalertness
Dreams		Vivid
		Occur while going to sleep, asleep, waking up and occasionally while awake
Motor control		Sleep paralysis
		Cataplexy
		Other behavioural disorders, e.g. PLMS, REM behaviour disorder

PLMS, periodic limb movements in sleep; REM, rapid eye movement.

usually in response to a sudden emotional stimulus such as laughter, and sleep paralysis in which the ability to move is lost either while falling asleep or at the point of waking up. Rapid eye movement sleep fragments may also be represented by vivid dreams during sleep, or similar impressions such as visual or auditory hallucinations either during drowsiness, while falling asleep, or waking up and occasionally while fully awake.

Pontine and midbrain lesions

These are usually considered to be distinct from narcolepsy but cause very similar symptoms with intense daytime sleepiness with 'sleep attacks' and often sleep paralysis, cataplexy and hallucinations. These lesions isolate the pedunculopontine and laterodorsal tegmental (PPN/LDT) nuclei from rostral brainstem inhibition so that motor inhibition can develop during wakefulness. The REM sleep behaviour disorder, in which muscle tone is intermittently retained during sleep, may also occur, especially with central or bilateral lesions that damage the tegmento-reticular tract which helps to maintain atonia. Intense colourful visual hallucinations (peduncular hallucinosis) are characteristic. Lesions affecting the reticular activating system (RAS) in the rostrocentral midbrain tegmentum cause a combination of EDS, hallucinations and a vertical gaze palsy. Lesions confined to the pontine tegmentum may reduce or alter the nature of both NREM sleep and REM sleep and there may be no recognizable NREM or REM sleep if they are severe enough to cause the locked-in syndrome.

Narcolepsy (narcoleptic syndrome)

OVERVIEW

The term narcolepsy was for many years used almost synonymously with the symptom of EDS, but it now usually implies a specific disorder of REM sleep which has various manifestations both during sleep and wakefulness.

OCCURRENCE

Narcolepsy affects around one in 2000–3000 people in most societies, although it is much less frequent in Israeli Jews. In the UK there are an estimated 20 000 people with narcolepsy of whom 80% are currently untreated and most of these are undiagnosed. Narcolepsy is equally common in males and females. It occasionally appears before the age of 5 years, develops before the age of 10 years in around 10%,

and in one-third the first symptom is present before the age of 15 years. The most frequent age of onset is 20–40 years and it is unusual for it to appear after the age of 55.

Patients with narcolepsy often give a family history of EDS, but in only around 10% is there a relative with narcolepsy and this is a first-degree relative in only 1–2%. The risk of a child of a narcoleptic having the disease is around 1%. Twin studies have been inconclusive, but the familial tendency to narcolepsy probably does have a genetic basis.

PATHOGENESIS

Narcolepsy is primarily a disorder of the control and structure of REM sleep, but NREM sleep and wakefulness may also be abnormal. It can be regarded as a tendency to a mixed sleep–wake state or as a sleep state boundary control disorder in which REM sleep intrudes into NREM and wakefulness. A characteristic feature is, however, that only fragments of REM sleep may appear. The reduced awareness of external stimuli which is characteristic of sleep may become separated from dreams and from the motor inhibition of REM sleep and any one or a combination of these three components may be present at any one time. Each component is also less stable than normal. It is uncertain whether REM sleep in narcolepsy is as effective in promoting mental associations as in normal subjects. The deeper stages of NREM sleep are shortened and, perhaps because the lighter stages are more prevalent, there are more arousals to wakefulness during sleep.

The neurochemical basis of narcolepsy is uncertain, but it probably involves an increase in cholinergic activity relative to activity mediated by noradrenaline and dopamine. The abnormalities are probably mainly located in the pons and midbrain, but higher centres such as the hypothalamus and basal forebrain may also be involved, for instance in the triggering of cataplexy by emotion.

AETIOLOGY

There is usually no obvious trigger for narcolepsy but a number of factors may contribute to its appearance. These are detailed below.

Genetic factors

There is an abnormality in the short arm of chromosome 6 which is closely associated with the HLA type DR2 and subtype DR15 and more particularly with the subtype DQB1*O602 (Table 6.6). Human leuco-

Table 6.6 Human leucocyte antigen type and narcolepsy.

HLA type Population (% positive)	African-American		Caucasian		Japanese	
	Narcolepsy	Normal	Narcolepsy	Normal	Narcolepsy	Normal
DQ1	95–100	75	90–100	67	100	75
DQB1*0602	90–95	35	95–100	25	100	12
DR2						
DR15	65–75	30	90–100	25	100	35
DRB1*1501	10–20	7	95–100	25	100	12

cyte antigen is a protein which is present in cell membranes and is linked to a susceptibility to autoimmune diseases. Narcolepsy could be due to an immune process localized to the brain, but there is no direct evidence for this and no histopathological abnormalities have been found in the brains of those with narcolepsy. The link with the immune processes may be through a genetic tendency to release a particular pattern of inflammatory mediators, such as cytokines, which lead to the sleep abnormalities.

The association of narcolepsy with this HLA type is the strongest of any disease. Its presence does not, however, invariably lead to narcolepsy since its HLA type is present in around 25% of Caucasian populations. The expression of the genetic tendency requires other factors which may act through altering the immune state.

Experimental evidence in dogs and mice suggests that a genetically determined change in the receptors on the surface of neurones for small transmitter molecules (hypocretins or orexins), or a lack of hypocretins, can induce a syndrome similar to narcolepsy. The relevance of these findings to narcolepsy in humans is uncertain.

Acquired states
Narcolepsy is associated with several conditions which can both alter the immune response and the balance of cholinergic, adrenergic and dopaminergic transmitters in the brain. The causes of a clinical picture similar to narcolepsy have been described on page 122, but the following conditions can lead to the appearance of narcolepsy.

Pregnancy. Narcolepsy may appear during pregnancy at which time the immune state is altered so that the fetus can be tolerated by the mother, but it persists after the birth of the child.

Infection. This has been postulated as a trigger factor for narcolepsy but is poorly documented, except for encephalitis lethargica in which it was probably due to pontine or midbrain inflammation.

Lymphomas. Non-Hodgkin B-cell lymphomas have been associated with narcolepsy even in the absence of the typical HLA type. The narcolepsy may be due to focal infiltration with lymphoma cells into the pons and the midbrain, and improves with treatment by radiotherapy.

Head injuries. Head injuries may trigger narcolepsy which usually appears immediately afterwards or within a few weeks or months of the injury. Direct damage to the structures controlling REM sleep may be responsible, but more probably the injury initiates changes in neurotransmitters or an inflammatory response, the type of which is dictated by the HLA type, and which leads to symptoms of narcolepsy.

CLINICAL FEATURES
The most common symptoms of narcolepsy in children are prolongation of the main sleep episode with EDS, but the tiredness that is experienced can lead to paradoxical hyperactivity. This may be incorrectly diagnosed as the attention deficit hyperactivity disorder (ADHD).

In adults the onset is sudden in around 15%, particularly in older subjects in whom the various manifestations tend to arise almost simultaneously and often in a severe form. In younger adults EDS usually appears before cataplexy. This is often seen within the next two years, but may be delayed for up to 30 years, and other symptoms subsequently develop. Complete remissions are uncommon, although the symptoms may fluctuate in severity, probably either due to a change in the intrinsic severity of the disorder, to external factors, or to the patient's lifestyle and ability to cope with the problems that arise [4]. Sleep paralysis, cataplexy and vivid dreams are more likely to spontaneously improve than EDS.

The specific effects of narcolepsy are as follows.

Disorders of sleep

Insomnia. It is usual for those with narcolepsy to fall asleep within 5 min of going to bed, but the sleep pattern is then unstable. Awakenings from sleep or shifts from deeper to lighter stages of NREM sleep are frequent. During awakenings there is often a craving to eat sweet food and this, together with a reduction in physical activity during the day time, may cause obesity. The total duration of sleep during the night is only slightly reduced, and episodes of REM sleep are shorter than in normal subjects. Most narcoleptics feel unrefreshed when they wake in the morning.

Excessive daytime sleepiness. The total sleep time during each 24 h is normal or only slightly increased because the loss of sleep time at night is only just outweighed by the time spent asleep during the day. There are two components to daytime sleepiness.
1 Daytime naps. These are usually of 10–30 min duration and rarely last for more than 1 h. They are temporarily refreshing and there is usually a refractory period of over an hour before the next nap is taken, often at a time corresponding to the 90 min ultradian REM sleep cycle. Sleep-onset REM is common during the naps. The naps may occur in situations where sleep might be anticipated, such as while sitting as a car passenger, but sleep 'attacks' may be sudden and irresistible and occur in such situations as while talking, walking or during sexual intercourse.
2 Subalertness. This is probably due to a disorder of wakefulness rather than of sleep, although sleep fragmentation and poor quality of NREM sleep may contribute. Cognitive function is normal, but attention and concentration span are reduced. Poor memory is often reported, but this is probably due to low self esteem, subalertness and the anterograde amnesia of micro sleeps rather than a true memory defect.

Automatic behaviour is closely related to subalertness during the day. Semi-purposeful behaviour in which familiar and often complex tasks are carried out without any subsequent recollection may include inappropriate actions such as stacking dishes in a refrigerator and may lead to accidents. Automatic behaviour should be distinguished from the stereo-typed behaviour of epilepsy and fugue states.

Disorders of dream control

Dreams during sleep. These are vivid and there is usually good recall. The dream theme may continue even after interruption by a period of wakefulness. Dreams occur at sleep onset and the perception of dreaming all night is common. Dreams may be in colour with vivid sounds as well as taste, smell and pain. A sensation of levitation such as flying or swooping, or being pushed up or pressed down is common, probably representing fluctuations in the inhibition of muscle spindle activity. The dreams are often sufficiently unpleasant and realistic to become nightmares.

Dreams during wakefulness. Dreams often occur shortly before sleep (hypnagogic hallucinations) or shortly after waking (hypnopompic hallucinations), but can occur during wakefulness. They represent partial REM sleep intrusion into wakefulness or the intrusion of consciousness into partially formed REM sleep at the end of a sleep episode. These dreams merges into wakefulness and are usually vivid and sufficiently realistic for the subject to be unsure whether they represent reality or not. Awareness of semi-formed images, the presence of people, or animals such as insects is common and a feeling of levitation (and even 'out of body' experiences) with a visual and auditory content usually comprising voices, is usual. The subject is sufficiently awake to be able to think and talk during the dream. This temporary loss of contact with reality can be embarrassing and the dream images may lead to vague but intense emotions, particularly fear.

Migraines are common in narcolepsy and may cause sensory disturbances, but they can usually be readily distinguished from dream disorders.

Disorders of motor control

Motor disorders during sleep. Narcolepsy is associated with a variety of parasomnias due to fluctuations in the degree of motor inhibition in REM sleep. Sleep terrors, sleep talking and walking are common, and irregular jerking movements and periodic limb movements may be seen during REM sleep because of a failure of motor inhibition. This also underlies the appearance of REM sleep behaviour disorder. Obstructive sleep apnoeas are more common than in normal subjects, probably because of an alteration in the inhibition of the activity of the dilator muscles of the upper airway and also because of obesity.

Sleep paralysis is a motor disorder which has been particularly associated with narcolepsy. It is the inability to move while consciousness is retained, either at the onset of sleep or less commonly when waking up. The respiratory muscles, or more probably only the diaphragm, retain activity but speech is impossible. The episodes usually last for less than 2 min but can occasionally persist for up to 30 min. The intense relaxation may be pleasurable, but much more commonly it is perceived as frightening because of the inability to move, the loss of control, and the occasional association with vivid dreams. Sleep paralysis episodes are less common in the upright position and can be terminated by an intense effort to move or by a touch from the partner, who may be alerted to the situation by a change in the pattern of breathing or faint sounds that may be uttered.

Cataplexy. This is the sudden onset of muscle weakness during wakefulness. It usually appears within two years of the development of EDS, although it precedes this in around 10% of narcoleptics.

It may follow an abnormal sensation around the mouth or face, which is succeeded by twitching of the lower face, and occasionally the upper limbs, and rapid eye movements due to an intermittent loss of muscle tone. This usually leads to symmetrical muscle weakness which may remain localized or become generalized. Mild episodes may simply cause drooping of the face, double vision, dysarthria or nodding of the head. The weakness may spread to cause loss of strength in the arms, trunk muscles and legs, causing the knees to buckle and the subject to fall to the ground, occasionally with persisting twitching of the limbs. Consciousness and memory of the episode are retained, although paralysis may be complete apart from the respiratory and extra-ocular muscles. Incontinence and tongue biting are not features of cataplexy.

Recovery from an episode of cataplexy is usually sudden and complete. Cataplexy attacks usually last for a few seconds or up to two minutes, but can occur repetitively for up to 20–60 min (status cataplecticus) and are then usually followed by REM sleep.

Cataplexy in narcolepsy is almost invariably triggered by a sudden intense emotion. There is no disorder of emotional control, but laughter or anger, or the anticipation of these emotions, or surprise are usually the triggers. It may also occur during or after sexual intercourse. It varies considerably in frequency and severity, but is more common and more severe if the subject is tired. It is similar but more intense than the transient loss of muscle 'tone' which is common with emotion including laughter and exercise in normal subjects. This is not accompanied by twitching of the face or jerking of the limbs and there is usually weakness of the limbs rather than the head and neck which are most commonly involved with cataplexy.

Situations in which sudden or intense emotions may be felt tend to be avoided and techniques of controlling the emotions, and a flattened affect are often developed to avoid cataplexy. The attacks can sometimes be prevented by tensing the muscles at the onset of an attack, for instance by clenching the fists. Injuries and accidents including drowning may occur because of cataplexy.

INVESTIGATIONS

Human leucocyte antigen typing
This is useful in excluding narcolepsy if the characteristic subtype is absent. It is of little value in confirming the diagnosis since the subtype is present in a significant percentage of normal subjects in most populations (see Table 6.6).

Polysomnography
This may help to establish the diagnosis of narcolepsy, exclude other diagnoses and assess the presence of complications, such as insomnia, PLMS, OSA or REM sleep behaviour disorder. It characteristically shows a short sleep latency, usually less than 5 min, without an increase in the total sleep time at night, although the total sleep time during each 24-h cycle is slightly greater than normal because of the daytime naps (Fig. 4.5). Sleep-onset REM (defined as the appearance of REM sleep within 20 min of onset of sleep) is present in around 50% and REM episodes are often shorter in duration and have more variable

Table 6.7 Differential diagnosis of vivid dreams in narcolepsy.

Schizophrenia
Epilepsy
Alcohol and benzodiazepine withdrawal
Hallucinogenic drugs
Parkinsonism
Occipital lobe lesions

muscle tone than normal. The duration of stage 1 NREM sleep is increased, and stages 3 and 4 are shortened. Sleep efficiency is increased and parasomnias, particularly PLMS, REM behaviour disorder and OSA may be detected.

Multiple sleep latency tests
These show a short sleep latency with a mean of less than 5 min in 80% of narcoleptics. Sleep-onset REM in two or more of the four or five MSLTs is present in most narcoleptics, but may also be seen in depression, REM sleep deprivation due to sleep restriction or fragmentation due to OSA and in drug and alcohol withdrawal.

Maintenance of wakefulness test
This is usually reduced to around 10 min, but this finding is not specific to narcolepsy and 15% of those with narcolepsy remain awake for 20 min.

DIFFERENTIAL DIAGNOSIS
Before the widespread use of polysomnography and HLA typing, narcolepsy was often confused with or misdiagnosed as schizophrenia. The combination of an unusual affect and auditory and visual hallucinations led to this error, and the overlap of the symptoms of these two conditions led to the theory that schizophrenia was a REM sleep disorder. The two conditions are, however, unrelated.

The diagnosis of narcolepsy is highly likely if there is a combination of EDS and well documented or observed cataplexy. The probability of this being present is only slightly increased by positive polysomnography or MSLT findings. The likelihood is increased if other clinical features are present, including a short sleep latency, nocturnal insomnia, vivid dreams, both during wakefulness and sleep, sleep paralysis and parasomnias. Each of the last four of these only occur in around 50% of those with narcolepsy.

Some of these features are often absent which leaves the diagnosis in doubt. Some examples of situations that arise are as follows.
1 *Cataplexy without EDS.* This is unusual since EDS usually precedes rather than follows cataplexy. One view is that narcolepsy cannot be diagnosed in this situation since EDS is considered to be a prerequisite, but if the HLA type is appropriate and polysomnography and MSLT findings are typical of narcolepsy, this is likely to be the correct diagnosis.
2 *The only symptom is EDS.* If the HLA type is appropriate, the diagnosis remains uncertain unless

Table 6.8 Differential diagnosis of cataplexy.

Familial cataplexy
Norrie disease
Niemann–Pick disease type C
Prader–Willi syndrome
Epilepsy, especially gelastic and atonic
Vertebro-basilar insufficiency
Drop attacks
Myasthenia gravis
Periodic paralysis
Faints
Hysteria

polysomnography and MSLT findings are typical of narcolepsy.
3 *Excessive daytime sleepiness without cataplexy,* but with dreams during wakefulness or parasomnias, such as sleep paralysis. This may represent an early or mild form of narcolepsy which can be diagnosed if the polysomnography and MSLT findings are typical. If they are not, the diagnosis may only become clear at a later stage when cataplexy develops.

The absence of the appropriate HLA subtype in any of these clinical situations makes it unlikely that narcolepsy is the correct diagnosis. It should be suspected in the REM behaviour disorder and in those with PLMS in REM sleep, and the HLA type tested for.

The differential diagnosis of narcolepsy is wide because of its multiple symptoms (Tables 6.7 and 6.8). The hallucinations of epilepsy are more stereotyped than in narcolepsy. Sleep paralysis occurs in normal subjects, usually in adolescents and the elderly, especially with REM sleep rebound following sleep deprivation. There is also a familial tendency to sleep paralysis which should be distinguished from the generalized fatigue on waking which is common in the chronic fatigue syndrome and depression. This is due to a lack of motivation rather than true paralysis. It lasts longer than sleep paralysis and small movements, for instance of the fingers, are possible.

Cataplexy may arise as an isolated familial disorder, but needs to be distinguished from epilepsy, especially if this is triggered by laughter (gelastic epilepsy), or is associated with loss of muscle tone (atonic seizure) or if cataplectic twitches are present (although depression of the level of consciousness is usual in each of these types of epilepsy), and other disorders listed in Table 6.8. Similar episodes of cataplexy which are not always triggered by emotion occur in Norrie disease, Niemann–Pick disease type C, the Moebius syndrome, and the Prader–Willi syndrome.

SOCIAL EFFECTS

The impact of narcolepsy on the quality of life varies according to its severity, the combination of symptoms, age of onset and the patient's understanding and ability to cope with the symptoms, as well as the availability of support from those around the patient. The impact is, in general, comparable to that of epilepsy or multiple sclerosis.

Narcolepsy particularly affects interpersonal relationships. Social activities are avoided because of the risk of falling asleep or of cataplexy during any excitement, and alcohol may precipitate an irresistible sleep attack. Problems may arise during marriage, particularly if the partner does not have a full understanding of the difficulties arising from the condition. Failure to adapt to this often causes confusion and anger, and separation or divorce is frequently attributed to the disorder by those with narcolepsy.

The children of those with narcolepsy may be exposed to danger if the parent falls asleep or during a cataplexy episode. Accidents to children may occur, for instance, if the narcoleptic parent is carrying the child and has a cataplectic episode or if the children are alone with the parent who has an irresistible sleep attack which leaves the children unsupervised. Parental anxiety about whether the children may also develop narcolepsy, and guilt about the restrictions that this condition imposes on how they care for their children, may be intense.

Intelligence is normal in narcolepsy, but the poor concentration and attention span reduces educational achievements. Falling asleep in class and during examinations is common. An inability to take part in many sports often leads to a feeling of being different from other children and after leaving school there may be difficulties in employment. Monotonous work may precipitate sleep and computer and desk jobs and those involving frequent meetings are particularly difficult to cope with. Working at heights or with moving machinery may be unsafe, and frequent job changes are common, as well as limitations on which types of employment are suitable.

Recreational opportunities are also restricted, both because of the risk of accidents, and because any emotional response may cause cataplexy which is usually embarrassing. Accidents occur at home or at work, but particularly during driving, although the exact risk of this is uncertain. There is usually sufficient warning of sleepiness to be able to pull over to the side of the road and cataplexy is infrequent while driving.

As a result of these difficulties secondary psychological problems are common. Emotional development may be retarded if narcolepsy appears in childhood, and a low self esteem, little confidence and anxiety are common. Awareness of being under-achievers, depression, embarrassment about their symptoms and weight gain, both due to a craving for carbohydrates and a lack of physical activity, are common. These aspects are especially important in adolescence when the individual's pattern of interpersonal relationships is becoming established.

The only influence of narcolepsy on lifespan is through increasing the risk of accidents, such as road traffic accidents, and those related to drowning and fire.

TREATMENT

Treatment of narcolepsy is often delayed for many years because of a failure to make the diagnosis early in its natural history. The diagnosis is delayed by a mean of 14 years after the onset of EDS and 7 years after cataplexy appears. During this time important psychological responses to the problems of narcolepsy develop and these may be only partially reversible once they have become established. The most important aspects of treatment are discussed below.

Advice

Understanding of narcolepsy. Explanation and reassurance about the nature of the symptoms and the outcomes of narcolepsy is important, not only for the patient but also for the parent, partner, school teachers and employers, where appropriate. Those with narcolepsy are often thought to be depressed, lazy, or have a mental disorder and their sleep and cataplexy attacks often generate resentment, anger or occasionally guilt, all of which can harm interpersonal relationships.

Sleep hygiene. The nocturnal sleep episode should not be shortened, and regular sleep–wake routines should be adopted. These may be difficult to achieve, particularly in adolescence. Other aspects of sleep hygiene which are detailed in Chapter 5 are also important.

Modification of daytime activities. Alertness can be increased by exercise and exposure to bright light, but exercise should be avoided in situations where falling asleep or cataplexy might be dangerous, e.g. boxing, mountaineering, or while swimming alone. Alcohol and large meals, particularly those containing carbohydrates, are likely to induce sleep and should be avoided.

Naps during the day should be planned to coincide either with the circadian rhythms so that they are taken between 2.00 and 4.00 PM, or around essential activities. Naps should be taken before events for which it is important to be particularly alert, but equally, the timing of these events should be coordinated with the optimal time for naps.

Coping strategies. It is important to accept that narcolepsy is a life-long condition which has to be managed and integrated into the everyday lifestyle. Coping strategies including cognitive techniques, may help.

School activities. An understanding of narcolepsy by teachers and others at school is important. Narcolepsy does not affect the intelligence or memory, but concentration and attention span are often reduced. Careful planning of study schedules should be adopted. Examinations should be arranged for the mornings or at whatever time of day alertness is greatest. The length of the examination may need to be extended in order to take into account the periods of sleep that are needed. Individualized careers advice should be offered.

Employment. An awareness and understanding of narcolepsy by the employer is important so that planned short naps, and regular breaks from tasks involving immobility or prolonged concentration can be taken. The work area should be well lit.

The most suitable work for those with narcolepsy involves exercise and contact with other people together with a stimulating environment, e.g. shop assistant, hairdresser, porter. Shift work, particularly rotating shifts, should be avoided, and part-time work should be timed for when alertness is greatest, which is usually in the morning. Occupations where continuous concentration is required, e.g. air traffic controller, and those involving confrontation or situations which might induce cataplexy, such as a policeman or traffic warden, should be avoided. Work involving moving or heavy machinery could be dangerous because of cataplexy, and jobs involving water, such as a swim-

ming pool attendant are unsuitable because of the risk of drowning due to cataplexy or a sudden sleep attack. Work with computers may be satisfactory if there is a particular interest in this, but if not, episodes of sleep are likely and these may increase the chance of dismissal.

Driving. Narcoleptics need to be aware that driving while drowsy is dangerous since the reaction time is increased, peripheral vision is reduced and judgement is impaired. Once narcolepsy has been diagnosed, the individual has a duty to notify the DVLA and their own insurance company. The DVLA usually seeks a medical report regarding the fitness to drive, and a licence is granted for one to three years if this is satisfactory, before the situation is reviewed.

Awareness of the times of day when sleepiness is most likely enables these to be avoided for driving. Taking a nap before driving, and timing stimulant medication so that alertness is optimized at the time of driving may help, and driving for any longer than has previously been found leads to drowsiness should be avoided. Cataplexy is rarely a problem during driving. Situations which could lead to sudden or intense emotions, such as anger or laughter and which might trigger this should be avoided, but there remains a risk of sudden unexpected events involving other cars or pedestrians which might cause cataplexy.

Drugs
These may be indicated for the following conditions.

Excessive daytime sleepiness. Both subalertness during wakefulness, and episodes of sleep, respond to CNS stimulants. The timing of the dose of stimulant treatment needs careful consideration so that the level of alertness can be raised to cope with planned activity, and so that the effect wears off before the desired nocturnal sleep time in order to minimize the risk of insomnia. Large quantities of caffeinated drinks are often taken, but stronger stimulant medication is usually needed. The amphetamines and related drugs have been the mainstay of stimulant treatment for many years, together with drugs such as mazindol which are chemically unrelated, but which have similar effects. Dexamphetamine is the most commonly prescribed drug in this group [5], but has important drawbacks (Chapter 3). These usually limit the dose that can be prescribed so that EDS is often undertreated. The residual sleepiness commonly causes secondary effects such as loss of self esteem, depression and unemployment which are potentially avoidable.

Modafinil is as effective as amphetamines and improves alertness in around 75% of patients [6]. It has been shown to improve the quality of life and reduce the number of daytime naps. It has fewer unwanted CNS actions and side-effects [7]. It is preferable to dexamphetamine as initial treatment for EDS in narcolepsy. Patients who have developed side-effects with amphetamines and those at risk of side effects of amphetamines because of, for instance, ischaemic heart disease should be considered for a trial of modaflnil instead. Dexamphetamine is indicated for patients who have already been established on it with improvement in EDS and without side-effects, and in those who either fail to improve with modafinil or fall into the small group who develop troublesome side-effects. Modafinil can be combined with dexamphetamine so that it provides the background improvement in EDS with dexamphetamine taken shortly before activities for which alertness is particularly important.

Cataplexy. Amphetamines, and to a lesser extent mazindol, have an anticataplectic action which may be partly due to increasing the level of alertness. Modafinil, which has the same effect on alertness, does not have this action but may increase the blood level of anticataplectic drugs such as clomipramine. The most effective anticataplectic drugs are the tricyclic antidepressants and the selective serotonin re-uptake inhibitors (SSRIs). Their mechanism of action is probably different from their antidepressant action since the anticataplectic effect is apparent within one day, whereas relief of depression often takes around two weeks. The 5HT and probable noradrenergic promoting actions of these drugs may be responsible for their efficacy. Their anticholinergic effects may also contribute.

Tricyclic antidepressants such as clomipramine 10–150 mg nocte, imipramine 25–150 mg nocte, protriptyline 5–20 mg nocte, and desipramine 75–200 mg nocte, have been extensively used. Selective serotonin re-uptake inhibitors such as fluoxetine 20–60 mg daily and paroxetine 20–60 mg daily are effective, and selective noradrenaline re-uptake inhibitors, e.g. viloxazine 300 mg daily may also be useful. In general, the tricyclic drugs are more effective than the SSRIs, but have more side-effects, particularly weight gain, and may exacerbate EDS. MAOI antidepressants are also effective but are rarely used because of their drug interactions. Second-line drugs include venlafaxine 37.5–375 mg daily which also improves daytime alertness, clonazepam 1–4 mg nocte, and clonidine 150–300 µg daily.

Dreams and nightmares. Antidepressants reduce the frequency and duration of dreams and nightmares through their action in reducing the duration of REM sleep.

Insomnia. This usually responds to hypnotics such as zopiclone or a benzodiazepine, e.g. temazepam 10 mg nocte, which consolidates sleep, or to sedating tricyclic antidepressants such as imipramine. Sleep hygiene advice may also be needed.

Motor disorders during sleep. These may require specific treatment (Chapter 7). Care should be taken to ensure that any drug treatment does not exacerbate other symptoms of narcolepsy, particularly EDS.

Depression. This is a frequent response to the problems of narcolepsy and may require a tricyclic or SSRI antidepressant.

Non-rapid eye movement sleep neurological disorders

Narcolepsy and other REM sleep-related conditions have already been described, but all the remainder of the neurological disorders causing EDS significantly increase the total time asleep. This is not a feature of narcolepsy, in which insomnia commonly occurs at night and the extra sleep during the day leads to a normal or only slightly increased total sleep duration. In these disorders, however, either the nocturnal sleep episode is extended or there are frequent or prolonged naps during the day. In some of these conditions, the evidence for a CNS abnormality is strong, but in others it remains doubtful. Excessive daytime sleepiness may be due to sleep fragmentation resulting from OSA, as in multiple system atrophy and central sleep apnoeas due to disorders of the medulla (Chapter 9), PLMS or the distruption of the circadian sleep rhythm with, for instance, hypothalamic lesions. In most conditions, however, the exact mechanisms underlying the need to sleep for prolonged periods is uncertain, but these may involve primarily the homeostatic drive which may lead to secondary changes in the adaptive drive.

Characteristic	ICNSH	Narcolepsy
Age of onset (years)	15–30	15–30
Gender	M = F	M = F
Family history	Occasional	Occasional
EDS	Yes	Yes
Insomnia	No	Yes
REM sleep features		
Cataplexy	Nil	Prominent
Sleep paralysis	Nil	Common
Dreams	No	Prominent
Naps		
Duration	30–120 min	10–30 min
Refreshing	No	Yes
Night time sleep episode	Prolonged	Slightly shortened
Arousability on waking	Difficult	Variable
Natural history	Lifelong	Lifelong
Polysomnography		
Sleep latency	↓	↓↓
SOREM	No	Common
NREM sleep	Consolidated	Fragmented
MSLT	Short	Very short
HLA	No association	DQB1*0602 almost invariable

Table 6.9 Narcolepsy and idiopathic CNS hypersomnia.

EDS, excessive day-time sleepiness; F, female; HLA, human leucocyte antigen; M, male; MSLT, multiple sleep latency test; NREM, non-REM; SOREM, sleep-onset REM.

Idiopathic central nervous system hypersomnia

OCCURRENCE

This is an uncommon condition, but its true incidence is uncertain because of the variable criteria which have been used to make the diagnosis. The term is often used when no definite diagnosis for EDS has been established. Patients diagnosed as ICNSH will therefore form a heterogeneous group unless a comprehensive clinical and investigative evaluation has been undertaken.

Idiopathic central nervous system hypersomnia (ICNSH) is equally common in males and females and it usually appears between the ages of 15 and 30 years. It is usually sporadic, but is occasionally familial, and is then associated with autonomic disorders e.g. migraines, postural hypotension and cold hands and feet.

PATHOGENESIS

Idiopathic central nervous system hypersomnia is thought to be due to an increase in the intensity or amplitude of the homeostatic drive to sleep. This overcomes the circadian and adaptive drives more readily during the day leading to EDS, and at night causes prolonged sleep. No abnormality of neurotransmitters has been identified, but this may be responsible for the sleep abnormalities.

CLINICAL FEATURES

Excessive daytime sleepiness is the sole symptom of ICNSH (Table 6.9). Frequent naps during the day with a sensation of subalertness are characteristic and there is often a long nocturnal sleep. In contrast to narcolepsy the nocturnal sleep episode is undisturbed, but it is unrefreshing despite the normal or greater than normal duration of stages 3 and 4 NREM sleep. Daytime naps are also unrefreshing and often last for 30–120 min. They are not associated with dreams. It is difficult to arouse the subject from sleep, either during the night, during naps, or in the morning, even with alarms, and confusional arousals, occasionally associated with aggression, are common if the subject is awoken.

Idiopathic central nervous system hypersomnia may

merge into the category of 'long sleepers', although they are not sleepy during the day as long as their main sleep episode at night is not curtailed. The condition tends to progress steadily over the weeks or months after its appearance and then persists throughout life with little change although occasionally it improves spontaneously. It may cause secondary psychological reactions, particularly depression, loss of educational opportunities or employment and an inability to take part in recreational activities.

INVESTIGATIONS

Polysomnography reveals a short sleep latency with a long total sleep time, high sleep efficiency and few arousals (Fig. 4.5). Sleep architecture is normal, except that the NREM sleep episodes may not shorten in duration during the night as in normal subjects and the duration of stages 3 and 4 NREM sleep may be increased. There is no sleep-onset REM, but there is often high spindle activity at the start and end of sleep.

Multiple sleep latency tests confirm a short sleep latency, usually 5–10 min, but with no sleep-onset REM.

DIFFERENTIAL DIAGNOSIS

Clinical evaluation is insufficient to exclude other causes of EDS and polysomnography is required, often with MSLTs. An MRI head scan may be needed to exclude an organic disorder. Idiopathic central nervous system hypersomnia can be distinguished from narcolepsy as shown in Table 6.9, although secondary depression may shorten REM sleep latency. Hypersomnia following head injuries, neurosurgery and viral infections should be identifiable from the history. Sleep restriction may cause EDS with similar polysomnography findings but EDS improves with an increase in the time spent asleep, unlike ICNSH.

TREATMENT

The principles of treatment are similar to those for narcolepsy. Counselling, lifestyle and sleep hygiene advice are important and the response to CNS stimulants is at least as good as in narcolepsy. Modafinil is effective and has fewer side-effects than dexamphetamine and related drugs which are best reserved for patients who fail to improve with modafinil.

Focal neurological lesions

PONS AND MIDBRAIN

These often cause abnormalities of REM sleep, but lesions affecting the ascending RAS, which promotes wakefulness, will induce sleep without necessarily specifically altering REM sleep. There are usually focal neurological signs which help to identify these lesions.

HYPOTHALAMIC AND THALAMIC LESIONS

Diffuse lesions in the hypothalamus are probably responsible for the sleep abnormalities in the Kleine–Levin and Prader–Willi syndromes, some types of encephalitis, and following head injuries, but the most common focal lesions are hypothalamic tumours, surgical trauma, radiotherapy and, occasionally, multiple sclerosis. Lesions of the posterior hypothalamus damage its reticular activating system leading to a disturbance of the homeostatic sleep drive and circadian rhythms. They are often associated with endocrine and autonomic abnormalities.

Thalamic lesions more frequently cause insomnia than EDS, but this is occasionally seen with, for instance, thalamic infarcts or trauma.

Kleine–Levin syndrome (recurrent hypersomnia)

OCCURRENCE

This rare syndrome is three times more common in males than females. The onset is usually in early adolescence and, while it may gradually improve later in life, it rarely resolves completely.

PATHOGENESIS

It occasionally follows a head injury, or more frequently a febrile illness, suggesting that it can be a post-encephalitic syndrome which runs a relapsing and remitting course. It is thought to result from an instability of hypothalamic control of sleep, feeding, mood and sexual activity [8]. There is little direct evidence for any neurotransmitter abnormality, but a reduction in dopamine availability during exacerbations and an increase in 5HT have been proposed.

CLINICAL FEATURES

The clinical features are an alternation of apparent complete normality with episodes lasting between two days and three weeks (usually less than one week) occurring 2–12 times per year. Secondary psychiatric problems and social isolation are common consequences of these episodes. There are three specific features of these.

Excessive daytime sleepiness

This may appear suddenly or develop over a few days and up to 20 h sleep per day may be obtained. The subject is difficult to wake and between the sleep episodes may be confused, depressed and agitated, but able to eat, micturate and defaecate. Euphoria may appear as the attack resolves, but there is often amnesia for the episode.

Overeating

A voracious appetite ('megaphagia'), equivalent to compulsive eating without satiety, is characteristic. There is no preference for any particular type of food, such as carbohydrates, and considerable weight may be gained during the attacks.

Sexual disinhibition

About 25% of patients make inappropriate sexual advances or repeatedly masturbate, and behaviour may be aggressive.

INVESTIGATIONS

The main value of polysomnography is to exclude other causes of EDS since it is normal between attacks, and even during them only shows an increased total sleep time.

DIFFERENTIAL DIAGNOSIS

The Kleine–Levin syndrome may be difficult to distinguish from the early stages of narcolepsy or from depression with EDS in adolescence, bipolar mood disorder and psychogenic hypersomnia (page 134).

TREATMENT

The frequency and severity of attacks may be reduced by lithium and CNS stimulants.

Prader–Willi syndrome

PATHOGENESIS

This multisystem disorder is associated with absence of part of chromosome 15. This impairs the development of the hypothalamus which leads to a loss of the sensation of satiety, leading to continual overeating and gross obesity.

CLINICAL FEATURES

Subalertness during the day is common and day time naps are frequent. These are usually due to sleep fragmentation caused by OSA, but there may also be a hypothalamic abnormality causing EDS. The obesity and narrow upper airway contribute to the OSA. The reduced respiratory drive and generalized respiratory muscle weakness also predispose to central sleep apnoeas. There may be an atypical form of cataplexy, but narcolepsy does not appear to be related to this syndrome.

INVESTIGATIONS

Polysomnography shows an increase in the total sleep time with an increase in the duration of stages 3 and 4 NREM sleep, reduction in REM sleep latency, increase in the number of REM sleep episodes, with reduction of the inter-REM sleep interval.

TREATMENT

Treatment of OSA with nasal CPAP is effective, although compliance may be difficult to achieve and sustained weight loss is uncommon.

Cerebral palsy

This is usually due to birth trauma and the extent of the brain damage correlates with the degree of sleep disturbance. Excessive daytime sleepiness is common and is partly due to an abnormality of sleep control, but also to drugs, especially anticonvulsants, and to poor sleep hygiene. Polysomnography is hard to interpret because of the poor definition of NREM and REM sleep, particularly in those who are severely affected. The number of arousals is increased, there are few spindles or K-complexes and the duration of stages 3 and 4 NREM and REM sleep appear to be reduced.

Myotonic dystrophy (dystrophia myotonica)

Excessive daytime sleepiness is occasionally due to sleep fragmentation due to OSA or PLMS, or to hypercapnia due to nocturnal hypoventilation associated with a disorder of the respiratory drive and weak respiratory muscles. It may also be due to a disturbance of the sleep-controlling mechanisms, perhaps associated with damage to the dorso-medial thalamic nuclei. There is some evidence that the circadian rhythms are disorganized, or that time givers, such as light exposure, are less effective than in normal subjects. Most patients who have EDS are also HLA DQB1*0602-positive, raising the possibility that there may be an overlap with narcolepsy.

Head injuries

Sleep disorders commonly follow closed head injuries, especially if these are severe enough to initially cause loss of consciousness. Injury may cause direct brain damage, or complications such as intracerebral haemorrhage, subdural haematoma or epilepsy which can damage the sleep controlling mechanisms and circadian rhythms. The sleep disorder may also be due to sedative drug therapy, e.g. anticonvulsants, related to loss of vision (page 105) or to secondary psychological responses to the injury and its effects.

The initial coma is usually due to either diffuse cerebral cortical damage due to intracerebral haemorrhage or cerebral oedema, or to malfunction of the brainstem. It is often followed by a phase of continuous sleepiness, usually with a reduction in REM sleep, which is punctuated by increasingly frequent awakenings. A gradual increase in the duration of REM sleep has been correlated with an improvement in cognitive function after the injury, but there is often poor dream recall. In the recovery phase the poor differentiation of NREM and REM sleep may prevent accurate sleep staging. Excessive daytime sleepiness may improve for up to around a year, but recovery is often incomplete, so that there is a prolonged nocturnal sleep episode with frequent and prolonged naps during the day, and subalertness between these. The clinical features are similar to ICNSH.

Head injuries may be the trigger for the development of narcolepsy and occasionally for the Kleine–Levin syndrome. They may also cause a delayed sleep phase syndrome, probably due to damage to the pathways between the pineal gland and the SCN, as is seen with whiplash injuries to the neck. These causes of EDS should be distinguished from the insomnia that often accompanies the post-concussion sydrome, and the effects on sleep of the post-traumatic stress disorder.

Encephalitis

The acute phase of encephalitis characteristically causes a deterioration in the level of consciousness and even coma. There may be a full recovery of consciousness, but EDS may be a permanent result. This is usually due to inflammation in the midbrain and posterior hypothalamus which alters both the homeostatic sleep drive and circadian rhythms. Persistent EDS may also be due to central or OSAs which cause sleep fragmentation and occasionally to carbon dioxide narcosis when hypoventilation due to damage to the medullary respiratory centres is severe.

The most important examples of EDS due to encephalitis are as follows.

INFECTIOUS MONONUCLEOSIS
This infection with the Epstein–Barr virus (EBV) may be followed by EDS which can persist for several years. This may be difficult to distinguish from the chronic fatigue syndrome that is often caused by an EBV infection.

HUMAN IMMUNODEFICIENCY VIRUS INFECTION
A variety of sleep disorders occur with human immunodeficiency virus (HIV) infection. Patients who are HIV positive without features of the acquired immunodeficiency syndrome (AIDS) have an increased duration of stages 3 and 4 NREM sleep with reduction in REM sleep in the second half of the night so that REM sleep is more evenly distributed. As it advances, there is a decrease in sleep efficiency, increase in the number of arousals, and a reduction in stages 3 and 4 NREM sleep which correlates with the fall in the CD4 lymphocyte count. Complaints of insomnia, daytime fatigue, drowsiness, poor concentration and memory are common.

These changes in sleep structure may be due to cytokines and other mediators of the immune response and changes in growth hormone secretion which initially promote NREM sleep. The later changes occur when the immune response is failing and may be partly due to neuronal death or dysfunction caused by direct effects of the HIV or to changes in production or release of neurotransmitters.

AFRICAN SLEEPING SICKNESS (AFRICAN TRYPANOSOMIASIS)
This is due to a protozoan, *Trypanosoma brucei*, which is transmitted to humans by the tsetse fly from wild animals. It occurs in a wide belt of Africa between latitudes 22° north and south. The initial febrile illness is followed by a meningoencephalitis with demyelination, especially in the periaqueductal region of the midbrain but also in the pons, medulla, hypothalamus and frontal lobes. The mechanisms controlling sleep become severely disorganized due both to the destructive nature of the inflammation and the release of cytokines. Sleepiness usually appears weeks or even years after the acute infection, is linked to the severity of the illness, and is often associated with fits, ataxia and tremor. Excessive daytime sleepiness is progressive and death usually occurs within around a year without antitrypanosomal drug treatment.

The total sleep time remains approximately normal, but the circadian rhythms of sleep, temperature and hormone secretion are lost, and a polyphasic sleep pattern appears. Nocturnal insomnia with severe sleep fragmentation is associated with EDS (sleep reversal) and the concentration of PGD2 is raised in the cerebrospinal fluid. Sleep episodes during the day often last 3–4 h, but become shorter as the disease progresses. Polysomnography shows loss of definition of NREM sleep, with absence of spindles and K-complexes, but the proportions of NREM and REM sleep are unaffected. The normal features of REM sleep are retained and sleep-onset REM is common [9].

Treatment with trypanosomicidal drugs such as melarsoprol can reverse the loss of circadian function and lead to longer sleep episodes with more cycles of stages 3 and 4 NREM sleep and less sleep-onset REM.

ENCEPHALITIS LETHARGICA

This has caused several large epidemics of which the last was between around 1915 and 1927. Cocksackie and Echo viruses have been isolated from some subsequent sporadic cases. Cerebral damage is extensive, but sleep disorders are most prominent when the inflammation involves the midbrain and hypothalamus.

The manifestations include EDS, which appears to have had similar features to narcolepsy and sleep 'inversion' which probably represents a delayed sleep phase syndrome with an onset of sleep at around 3.00 AM. Occasionally patients remain awake all night, especially shortly after the acute phase of the illness and the encephalitis also causes central alveolar hypoventilation due to damage to medullary respiratory centres.

POLIOMYELITIS

This can cause both central and OSAs associated with EDS due to damage to the medullary respiratory centres and weakness of the upper airway and chest wall muscles. Nocturnal hypoventilation may be severe enough to lead to carbon dioxide narcosis (Chapters 9 and 10).

WESTERN EQUINE ENCEPHALITIS

This can damage the medullary respiratory centres and cause central alveolar hypoventilation. This may present with EDS due to respiratory-induced arousals from sleep and carbon dioxide narcosis.

GENERAL PARESIS

This form of neurosyphilis can cause EDS.

Multiple sclerosis

Physical fatigue related to muscle weakness is common in multiple sclerosis but this should be distinguished from mental fatigue and from EDS. The latter is usually due to sleep fragmentation caused by discomfort, muscle spasms, nocturia and occasionally central or obstructive sleep apnoeas. Periodic limb movements in sleep have also been reported as being common in multiple sclerosis and depression may

have an important impact on sleep. The HLA DR2 type is present in 50–60% of those with multiple sclerosis, but there is little evidence that narcolepsy, which shares this HLA type, is any commoner in multiple sclerosis than in the general population.

Cerebral irradiation

Excessive daytime sleepiness often occurs within 6 weeks of radiotherapy to the brain. It may be due to a direct effect of the radiotherapy, possibly acting through cytokines and other inflammatory mediators, but occasionally the symptoms may be due to a raised intracranial pressure due to worsening of the tumour for which the radiotherapy was given. Excessive daytime sleepiness is common when a large volume of brain is irradiated, for instance with prophylactic treatment for leukaemia or small cell carcinomas of the bronchus, whereas localized radiotherapy even close to the hypothalamus for pituitary tumours causes less EDS. Excessive daytime sleepiness following cranial irradiation should be distinguished from the physical fatigue that follows radiotherapy to areas outside the brain.

Psychiatric disorders

Excessive daytime sleepiness is much less frequently caused by psychiatric problems than is insomnia. It may develop as a protective psychological reaction to circumstances which are difficult to cope with. If it persists it may be difficult to distinguish from ICNSH but MSLTs are usually normal. Excessive daytime sleepiness occasionally arises in depression, particularly the seasonal affective disorder (SAD), and is often associated with weight gain, whereas depression and weight loss often leads to insomnia. The daytime sleepiness seen in schizophrenia is occasionally due to the disorder itself, but more commonly to sedative medication.

Systemic disorders

Like the neurological disorders other than those related to REM sleep, the systemic disorders causing EDS increase the duration of sleep during each 24 h, often with a long nocturnal sleep episode. The sleep abnormalities are due to a wide range of mechanisms, most of which involve alterations in sleep factors such as cytokines.

Fever and infection

Fever in response to an infection is due to pyrogens,

such as IL-1, some of which are also sleep factors. Both Gram positive and negative bacteria and, to a lesser extent, viral infections cause an initial increase in sleepiness and in the duration of NREM sleep with inhibition of REM sleep and later an inhibition of stages 3 and 4 NREM sleep. The induction of the fever and of NREM sleep are independent effects of cytokines. Prolongation of sleep is associated with a better survival in severe infections. The altered sleep pattern modifies the profile of melatonin secretion and this also affects the immune response to the infection.

Metabolic disorders

These rarely cause EDS, but may alter the state of consciousness as in, for instance, hypoglycaemia, carbon monoxide poisoning and lead encephalopathy. Hepatic encephalopathy causes EDS with difficulty in initiating sleep and a delay in the onset of melatonin secretion, similar to the delayed sleep phase syndrome.

Hypothyroidism

Excessive daytime sleepiness, apathy, stupor and coma may develop, either due to the metabolic abnormality or to OSA caused by obesity. The duration of stages 3 and 4 NREM sleep is reduced but this and the EDS return to normal with thyroxine treatment.

Premenstrual sleepiness

This usually occurs in adolescence for a few days before the onset of each menstrual period. A long sleep at night is associated with naps during the day and occasionally with an increased appetite. Polysomnography may be required to exclude other possible causes, including premenstrual exacerbation of the periodic limb movements in sleep, but is normal in this condition. Multiple sleep latency tests are shortened.

Pregnancy sleepiness

This usually occurs during the first trimester with an increase in total sleep time and in the number of daytime naps.

Drugs

Drugs may cause EDS by fragmenting sleep through a variety of mechanisms as described on page 121, or by causing sedation during wakefulness (Table 6.10). These effects may occur either while the drug is being taken or during the withdrawal phase.

Drugs are a common cause of EDS and a careful drug history should always be taken. Blood and urine

Table 6.10 Sedative drugs which cause EDS.

Hypnotics
Antipsychotics
Antidepressants, especially MAOIs and tricyclics
Anticonvulsants
Alpha-agonists, e.g. clonidine, methyldopa
Alpha-blockers, e.g. prazosin, indoramim
Antihistamines (older drugs, e.g. chlorpheniramine)
Melatonin (slight effect)
Nicotine (slight effect in low dose)
Withdrawal of amphetamines and related drugs

MAOIs, monoamine oxidase inhibitors.

testing is indicated if there is doubt about whether the drug has been taken or if a combination of drugs may be contributing to the symptoms.

References

1 Harrison Y, Horne JA. Sleep loss impairs short and novel language tasks having a prefrontal focus. *J Sleep Res* 1998; 7: 95–100.

2 Suratt PM, Findley LJ. Driving with sleep apnea. *N Engl J Med* 1999; 340: 881–3.

3 Mitler MM, Miller JC, Lipsitz JJ, Walsh JK, Wylie CD. The sleep of long-haul truck drivers. *N Engl J Med* 1997; 337: 755–61.

4 Parkes JD, Chen SY, Clift SJ, Dahlitz MJ, Dunn G. The clinical diagnosis of the narcoleptic syndrome. *J Sleep Res* 1998; 7: 41–52.

5 Mitler MM, Aldrich MS, Koob GF, Zarcone VP. Narcolepsy and its treatment with stimulants. *Sleep* 1994; 17: 352–71.

6 Schwartz JRL, Schwartz ER, Veit CA, Blakely EA. Modafinil for the treatment of excessive day-time sleepiness associated with narcolepsy. *Today's Therapeutic Trends* 1998; 16: 287–308.

7 Pigeua R, Naithoh P, Buguet A *et al*. Modafinil, d-amphetamine and placebo during 64 hours of sustained mental work. I. Effects on mood, fatigue, cognitive performance and body temperature. *J Sleep Res* 1995; 4: 212–28.

8 Merriam AE. Kleine–Levin syndrome following acute viral encephalitis. *Biol Psychiatry* 1986; 21: 1301–4.

9 Buguet A, Gati R, Sevre JP, Develoux M, Bogui P, Lonsdorfer J. 24 hour polysomnographic evaluation in a patient with sleeping sickness. *Electroencephalogr Clin Neurophysiology* 1989; 72: 471–8.

7 Behavioural Abnormalities in Sleep

Introduction

The organization of motor activity during sleep is very different from during wakefulness. The higher centres are active, particularly in rapid eye movement (REM) sleep, but there is greater inhibition of lower motor neurone activity, especially in the postural muscles, in REM sleep. As a result there is less movement during sleep with a reduction in muscle tone and in reflex responses, despite the activity of the higher centres. Motor activity can, however, break through either if the central activity increases, or if its inhibition fails, even transiently. The central activity may be intense and pathological as in an epileptic seizure, or more subtle and normal, or near normal. Motor inhibition may be lost in young children in whom the sleep regulation systems are immature, in the elderly and in patients with degenerative neurological disorders (in whom sleep control degenerates). There are fewer motor disorders in REM sleep than in non-rapid eye movement (NREM) sleep because of the intense motor inhibition, but an exception is the REM sleep behaviour disorder in which release of motor inhibition allows complex movements, usually reflecting the content of vivid dreams, to be enacted. An abnormality of motor control which is present in both NREM and REM sleep probably underlies the occasional assoication of abnormal behaviour during both these sleep states (parasomnia overlap syndrome). An example is the combination of sleep walking and REM sleep behaviour disorder.

The term 'parasomnia' is commonly used to describe most of these type of events during sleep. They are usually defined as unusual, undesirable and episodic events which are not due to disorders of the sleep or wake mechanisms themselves. This definition is unsatisfactory for several reasons. Firstly, inclusion of an undesirable element leads to a subjective assessment of what is, or is not a parasomnia. Secondly, the sleep–wake mechanisms interact in a complex manner with the abnormal events during sleep, and

cannot be clearly differentiated from them. Thirdly, the range of unusual events occurring during sleep is so diverse that the concept of a parasomnia has little value in understanding their nature or in guiding their management in clinical practice. A complex, and often inconsistent, classification of descriptive syndromes has been built up around the concept of parasomnias without sufficient regard for the underlying pathophysiological processes.

The distinction between sleep and wakefulness is not always clear cut. Features of both these states may coexist, for instance during sleep paralysis and in automatic behaviour when NREM sleep intrudes into wakefulness. The transitions between sleep stages are also associated with various mixtures of the features of sleep and wakefulness. At these times awareness of the environment and of activities may be suppressed, while movements take place which are often complex. The common mechanism of transition from a deeper to a lighter stage of NREM sleep or to wakefulness which underlies these different types of motor activity probably accounts for their familial association.

There are numerous classifications of the motor disorders during sleep, but in this chapter they will be regarded primarily according to which stage of sleep they arise in and whether they are associated with a transition into or out of this sleep stage (Tables 7.1, 7.2). The movement disorders which are present during wakefulness but which are affected by sleep will be discussed last.

The presenting feature is usually the report of the abnormal behaviour by the patient or more usually the partner, other members of the family, friend or carer. Occasionally, the patient or bystander may be injured during the episode, but excessive daytime sleepiness (EDS) and insomnia are unusual, except in periodic limb movements in sleep (PLMS). Excessive daytime sleepiness with snoring is a feature of motor abnormalities of the upper airway which are discussed in Chapter 10. Excessive daytime sleepiness and medical complications of respiratory failure, including

Table 7.1 Sleep-state transition behavioural disorders.

Wake–REM	*Wake–NREM*
Cataplexy	Hypnic jerks
Sleep paralysis	Benign neonatal and fragmentary myoclonus
	Rhythmic movement disorder
REM–wake	*NREM–wake*
Sleep paralysis	Confusional arousal
Post-traumatic stress disorder	Sleep terror
	Sleep walking
	Sleep talking
	Sleep eating and drinking
	Panic attack
	Nocturnal cramp

NREM, non-rapid eye movement; REM, rapid eye movement.

Table 7.2 Sleep-state specific behavioural disorders.

NREM sleep	*REM sleep*
Epilepsy	REM sleep behaviour disorder
Sleep bruxism	Status dissociatus
PLMS	

NREM, non-rapid eye movement; PLMS, periodic limb movements in sleep; REM, rapid eye movement.

conditions affecting the chest wall muscles and other components of the respiratory pump, are considered in Chapter 9.

Assessment

History

A careful history is essential to accurately assess motor disorders during sleep (see Chapter 4). The issues that should be considered are as follows.

1 What is the nature of the movements? Do these affect the whole body or are they localized to one part, such as the limbs in periodic limb movements in sleep, or jaw movements as in sleep bruxism? Is there a sequence of movements as in Jacksonian epilepsy? Is the type of movement repetitive and what is its frequency and amplitude? Are the movements simple or complex and is violence a feature, either spontaneously or if restraint is attempted?

2 Are there any associated features such as sensory symptoms, dreams, autonomic activation or incontinence?

3 What is the mental state during the episode? Is the patient responsive to questions or commands? Is there any recall of the events and do any of the activities appear to be premeditated? Are there signs of anxiety? What happens after the event? Can the patient fall asleep readily or are there any abnormal behaviours?

4 How does the event relate to sleep, wakefulness or the transition between the two? Do similar episodes occur during wakefulness during the day time? The age of the subject, the time during the night of the events and the presence of a family or previous history of similar types of sleep disorder may suggest a relationship of the episodes to sleep, wakefulness or the transition between the two.

5 What is the cause of the events? Are they precipitated by sleep deprivation, poor sleep hygiene, drug intake, including alcohol or its withdrawal, or caffeine? Is there any underlying neurological disorder such as dementia or Parkinsonism?

Physical examination

Physical examination may reveal signs of injury or effects of the abnormal movements such as ground-down teeth as a result of sleep bruxism. Neurological examination may be required, but is usually of limited value, except in REM behaviour disorder, epilepsy and movement disorders that are present during wakefulness.

Investigations

The history may suggest a diagnosis with a sufficient degree of certainty for management to be planned without the need for further investigation. This is usually the situation with sleep walking, sleep talking, rhythmic movement disorder and sleep bruxism. In most other situations, particularly when the movements are complex, potentially dangerous to the patient or to others, troublesome to the partner or carer, or if their nature is uncertain, referral to a specialist centre for more detailed assessment and investigation is needed. Investigations are directed to ascertaining the following.

NATURE OF THE ATTACKS

Polysomnography with video and audio recording is important in establishing the nature of the events, their relationship to the stage of sleep or to wakefulness, and the presence of other factors which may contribute to the clinical picture.

CAUSE OF THE ATTACKS

This may be established by the following methods.
1 Blood tests, e.g. ferritin, urea and electrolyte estimation in PLMS.
2 Electro-encephalogram (EEG) in wakefulness to assist the diagnosis of epilepsy.
3 Brain imaging techniques, e.g. computerized tomography (CT) and magnetic resonance imaging (MRI) scans of the head, particularly to investigate REM behaviour disorder, frontal lobe epilepsy and involuntary movement disorders which are worse during wakefulness than sleep.

Principles of treatment

The aims of treatment are as follows.
1 Explain the nature of the disorder to the subject and reassure when appropriate.
2 Sleep hygiene advice. This minimizes the risk of sleep deprivation which may precipitate motor disorders during sleep, and can also be directed to reduce the risk of arousal which is important in preventing sleep–wake transition disorders. Changes in the use of any drugs that may be adversely affecting the sleep–wake patterns should be considered.
3 Treat the underlying disorder, e.g. by treating the cause of iron loss and replacing iron in PLMS, use of anticonvulsants for epilepsy, dopamine agonists for PLMS and Parkinsonism, and benzodiazepines in REM behaviour disorder.
4 Modification of sleep–wake patterns by drugs, e.g. use of benzodiazepines to consolidate stage 2 NREM sleep and thereby reduce the risk of sleep–wake transition disorders, the use of tricyclic antidepressants to reduce the duration of REM sleep to minimize, for instance, sleep paralysis; or avoiding stimulants such as caffeine in order to reduce the risk of arousal and of sleep–wake transition disorders.

5 Protection. This may be required for the patient in the form of a helmet, locking the bedroom door, or constructing a stair gate. Localized movement disorders need specific equipment, such as a gum shield for sleep bruxism. Protection for the partner usually takes the form of sleeping in a separate bedroom, if necessary with the door locked.
6 Lifestyle advice. This may be required to cope with any stress which may be contributing to the movement disorders and also in order to cope with the impact of the movement disorder. Psychotherapy is occasionally needed.

Wakefulness–non-rapid eye movement transition movements

Propriospinal myoclonus

These irregular jerking movements occur during relaxed wakefulness before sleep and are inhibited by sleep. They last 150–300 ms and involve large muscles, including those of the neck, chest and abdomen. They appear to be generated by a spreading wave of activity in the propriospinal system in the spinal cord due to loss of brain stem or higher centre inhibition. They have no clinical significance, but can be confused with hypnic jerks, which only occur during sleep, and PLMS.

Hypnic jerks (sleep starts, hypnic myoclonus)

OVERVIEW

Hypnic jerks are brief twitching movements that occur only at the onset of sleep. They may be associated with vivid sensations, particularly a feeling of falling.

OCCURRENCE

They are very common, occurring occasionally in 60–70% of normal adults. They are equally frequent in males and females.

PATHOGENESIS

They are probably due to momentary failure of inhibition of lower motor neurone activity during the unstable phase of sleep onset. Sensory symptoms reflect a transient lowering of the threshold for muscle spindle, vestibular and auditory impulses to excite the cerebral cortex (page 164). Hypnic jerks may be provoked by central nervous system (CNS) stimulants such as caffeine, sleep deprivation and stress.

CLINICAL FEATURES

Hypnic jerks are usually single, although occasionally

a few jerks may follow in quick succession. They involve especially the legs, are usually bilateral, but can occasionally be asymmetrical. The jerks last less than 1 s and occur at or soon after the onset of sleep. They arise from stages 1 or 2 NREM sleep. They may be evoked by external stimuli, and are followed by a brief arousal to wakefulness or EEG features of arousal, including K-complexes. Occasionally there is a brief cry or autonomic changes, including an increase in heart or respiratory rate, and sweating. They fluctuate in their severity and frequency, but can lead to a fear of falling asleep.

INVESTIGATIONS
None are usually needed.

DIFFERENTIAL DIAGNOSIS
1 Periodic limb movements in sleep. These are repetitive, of longer duration and affect predominantly the legs.
2 Fragmentary myoclonus. These are of small amplitude.
3 Myoclonic epilepsy.
4 Startle disease (Hyperekplexia). This is a rare, and often familial disorder of motor control causing an exaggerated response to stimuli, often with loss of balance and falls. There is no loss of consciousness, but injuries are common since the arms are held stiffly during the fall. Repetitive jerky movements of the limbs occur at night and hyper-reflexia is present. Clonazepam and sodium valproate may be effective.

PROBLEMS
Occasional sleep-onset insomnia due to either fear of falling asleep or repeated awakenings, or to anxiety regarding the nature of the symptoms.

TREATMENT
1 Reassurance.
2 Sleep hygiene advice, especially with regard to avoiding sleep deprivation.
3 Avoid stimulants such as caffeine.
4 Benzodiazepines, such as clonazepam or temazepam, are occasionally required.

Benign neonatal myoclonus and fragmentary myoclonus (partial myoclonus)

Benign neonatal myoclonus is often familial and is seen soon after birth. It may last for a few months and is characterized by twitching of the fingers, toes and face during the lighter stages of NREM sleep.

Similar, but often asymmetrical, focal jerks of the limbs and occasionally the face are a feature of fragmentary myoclonus. They last for less than 150 ms, are associated with K-complexes and occur only during NREM sleep. Like benign neonatal myoclonus, they either represent an increase in higher centre activation which overcomes a normal level of motor inhibition or, more probably, a transient recurrent failure of the latter.

Rhythmic movement disorder (head banging, jactatio capitis nocturna)

OVERVIEW
This disorder is characterized by repetitive movements of large muscle groups before and soon after the onset of sleep. Head banging is the best recognized pattern.

OCCURRENCE AND AETIOLOGY
This is three to four times more common in males than females. Body rocking usually appears at around 6 months and head banging and head rolling at around 9 months. These movements often disappear by around 18 months old and are uncommon after the age of 4 years. They can occasionally persist into early adult life, particularly if there are abnormalities such as mental retardation, autism or following a head injury. Daytime head banging is a separate entity which is usually suppressed during sleep. It is a transient phase in young children, but in adults is associated with learning disabilities, autism and psychotic states.

PATHOGENESIS
Little is known about the cause of this disorder. It is not usually associated with any other abnormality in children. The movements may assist development of vestibular function.

CLINICAL FEATURES
The repetitive stereotyped movements usually begin during drowsiness and persist into light NREM sleep, often for 10–15 min. They often appear to be pleasurable, possibly because of the vestibular stimulation that they provide and they may promote the onset of sleep. The usual frequency of the movements is 0.5–2/s. Head banging against a pillow, the framework of the bed or a wall is the most common pattern, but head rolling from side to side and rocking or rolling of the entire body with flexion and extension or lateral movements may be seen. The child often squats on his hands and knees or rocks in a sitting position, and

there may be repetitive vocalizations or humming. Scalp lacerations and even subdural haemotomas can occur, but other injuries are uncommon.

INVESTIGATIONS
Polysomnography is rarely required but shows rhythmic movement artefacts during drowsiness and in stages 1 and 2 NREM sleep. There are no EEG features of arousal from sleep by the rocking movements. Video recordings confirm the nature of the movements.

DIFFERENTIAL DIAGNOSIS
1 Epilepsy, e.g. infantile spasms.
2 Periodic limb movements in sleep.
3 Bruxism.

PROBLEMS
1 Parental anxiety and insomnia.
2 Occasional injury such as subdural haematoma.

TREATMENT
1 Explanation to, and reassurance of, family and treatment of any psychological cause.
2 Protection of the child, e.g. by padding the bed-head or provision of a protective helmet.
3 Benzodiazepines or tricyclic antidepressants may occasionally be required.

Non-rapid eye movement sleep–wakefulness transition movements

There are three types of normal movements associated with arousals from NREM sleep towards wakefulness.
1 Benign neonatal myoclonus. This is often familial and is seen in the first weeks or months after birth. It is characterized by twitching of the fingers, toes, other limb muscles and face during the lighter stages of NREM sleep.
2 Fragmentary myoclonus (partial myoclonus). This causes asymmetrical focal jerks of the limbs, and occasionally the face, which last for less than 150 ms. They are associated with K-complexes and occur only during NREM sleep. Like benign neonatal myoclonus, they either represent an increase in high centre activation which overcomes a normal level of motor inhibition or more probably a transient recurrent failure of the latter.
3 Gross body movements. Arousals commonly cause minor postural movements or shifts in position which are associated with a slight elevation of heart rate and blood pressure. The eyes may open briefly but sleep is soon re-entered and there is no recall of the microarousal. These usually occur either at sleep onset, during stages 1 and 2 NREM sleep or at the start or end of a REM sleep episode. They are most common in the second half of the night and often occur 3–4 times per hour.

Disorders of the transition from a deeper to a lighter NREM sleep stage or to wakefulness ('disorders of arousal') are due to incomplete adaptation to this sleep stage change. Loss of muscle inhibition allows the higher-centre activity to be expressed. This usually reflects the stage of sleep after the transition, although the level of alertness remains at the stage of sleep before the transition or somewhere between this and full alertness.

This group of disorders has several features in common (Fig. 7.1).
1 There is a failure to attain the level of alertness of normal wakefulness. Awareness of the surroundings is reduced or absent and the subject is uncontactable or virtually uncontactable by other people. This loss of awareness is greater than with sleep inertia.

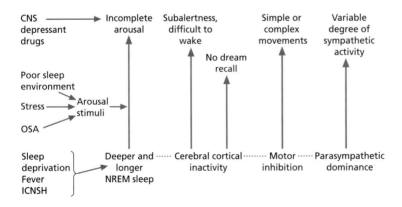

Fig. 7.1 Non-rapid eye movement sleep–wakefulness transition movements.

2 There is no dream content and little or no recall of the event. There may be a vague recollection of a frightening image or of an imminent catastrophe.

3 Inhibition of motor activity is released. The movements may be simple and repetitive, or complex.

4 There is a variable degree of autonomic activation. The parasympathetic usually predominates over the sympathetic activity during sleep, but at the time of these arousals sympathetic activity may be marked, especially in sleep terrors and panic attacks.

5 It is difficult to wake the subject from the attacks, but if challenged he or she may become angry, startled and violent.

6 They tend to occur during the first third of the night when NREM sleep, especially stages 3 and 4, is most prolonged.

7 These episodes do not cause insomnia or EDS.

8 There is often a family history, probably reflecting a similarity in neurodevelopmental problems responsible for the manifestation of the disorder, and more than one of these disorders often occurs either in the same individual or in the same family.

The origin of the disorders from stages 3 and 4 NREM sleep makes them particularly frequent in any situation in which these stages are increased or in which there is a tendency to arouse.

1 Causes of increase in stages 3 and 4 NREM sleep and incomplete arousal. In childhood the duration and intensity of stages 3 and 4 NREM sleep are increased and the immaturity of the sleep regulating mechanisms predisposes to incomplete arousals. The latter is common with CNS depressant drugs, such as hypnotics, antipsychotics, tricyclic antidepressants and alcohol. The duration of stages 3 and 4 NREM is increased by sleep deprivation, due to, for instance, shift work, and in fevers and occasionally in idiopathic central nervous system hypersomnia (ICNSH).

2 Causes of frequent arousals (sleep fragmentation). These include a noisy external environment, pain, stress causing anxiety, obstructive sleep apnoeas or forced awakenings by a parent or carer.

The most important individual disorders are described below.

Confusional arousal (sleep drunkenness)

OVERVIEW

Confusional arousals occur at the transition from stages 3 and 4 NREM sleep to wakefulness when the attainment of full alertness is delayed. The subject appears confused and carries out inappropriate actions.

Table 7.3 Differential diagnosis of complex activities in sleep and on arousal.

Confusional arousal
Frontal lobe epilepsy
Temporal lobe epilepsy
REM sleep behaviour disorder
Sleep walking
Panic attack
Sundown syndrome

REM, rapid eye movement.

OCCURRENCE

Confusional arousals are equally common in males and females, and are almost universal in children under the age of 5 years if they are woken from stages 3 and 4 NREM sleep. They occur in around 1% of susceptible adults, particularly, for instance, when they are sleep deprived, and are less common in the elderly because of the reduction in duration of stages 3 and 4 NREM sleep.

PATHOGENESIS

Confusional arousals are the manifestation of a delayed and partial reorganization of cortical activity at the transition from stages 3 and 4 NREM sleep to wakefulness. They are more common when these sleep stages are enhanced, as in, for instance, ICNSH, and following sleep deprivation, shift work, alcohol and obstructive sleep apnoeas (OSA) which may all lead to rebound NREM sleep. They are also more common with hypnotics and in disorders that reduce the normal level of alertness, such as hepatic and renal encephalopathy and narcolepsy.

CLINICAL FEATURES

Confusional arousals occur most frequently during the first third of the night when stages 3 and 4 NREM sleep are most prolonged. They may arise spontaneously or in response to external stimuli or forced awakening. Sleep is not re-entered after arousal but a period of subalertness manifested by confusion follows. Disorientation in time and space with slow and inappropriate responses to questions and commands are common.

Confusional arousals are an exaggerated form of sleep inertia but the state of subalertness and confusion is combined with abnormal and often complex motor activity (Table 7.3). Children may cry, call out, roll around the bed, or move around the room. Adults may carry out activities such as walking or climbing stairs, and may carry out inappropriate activities such as picking up a glass instead of the telephone or putting sugar into the kettle. Restraint is resisted, often aggressively, but violence is never premeditated.

Confusional arousals may last for several minutes and afterwards full alertness is regained, but there is little recall of the event, except for brief flashbacks of what has happened. There is no dream content, anxiety or autonomic activation. The features of confusional arousals may merge into the end of a sleep terror or episode of sleep walking, and the subject then falls asleep readily. If there is more than one confusional arousal per night the earlier episodes are usually the more intense.

INVESTIGATIONS

Polysomnography is only occasionally required in children to distinguish confusional arousals from other conditions, but is more often needed in adults or if there are atypical features. It shows frequent arousals from stages 3 and 4 NREM sleep even when confusional arousals do not develop. The arousals occur both during daytime naps and night-time sleeps, and there may be some residual delta waves combined with alpha and theta during the arousal suggesting that electrophysiological aspects of both wakefulness and sleep are present simultaneously. Video recordings may clarify the nature of the activities carried out during these episodes.

DIFFERENTIAL DIAGNOSIS

1 Sleep terrors.
2 Sleep walking.
3 Sleep talking.
4 Epilepsy.
5 Episodic nocturnal wanderings.
6 REM sleep behaviour disorder.
7 Nightmares.
8 Fugue states.

PROBLEMS

There is danger both to the subject and to witnesses.

TREATMENT

1 Reduce any tendency to excessive stages 3 and 4 NREM sleep, e.g. sleep hygiene advice.
2 Minimize the risk of arousals during the first third of the night, especially in children.
3 Promotion of attainment of full alertness, e.g. discontinue hypnotics.

4 Treat the cause of subalertness, e.g. narcolepsy, hepatic failure and obstructive sleep apnoeas.

Sleep terrors (night terrors, pavor nocturnus, pavor incubus)

OVERVIEW

Sleep terrors are sudden and brief episodes which occur especially in children and which are characterized by panic and confusion with intense autonomic activation.

OCCURRENCE

They are more common in males than females, are often familial, and there is an association with confusional arousals and sleep walking. They occur from the age of around 1 year, are most common between 5 and 7 years and arise in around 3% of children aged 4–12 years, but they then become increasingly uncommon. If they persist after the age of 20 there is often associated psychopathology such as anxiety, depression or phobias. They are very uncommon in old age in which stages 3 and 4 NREM sleep are much reduced. They are common in those who sleep walk or sleep talk and also in Gilles de la Tourette syndrome.

PATHOGENESIS AND AETIOLOGY

Sleep terrors are due to incomplete arousal from stages 3 and 4 NREM sleep and the same factors that predispose to confusional arousals can provoke them. Fever is an additional risk factor, possibly through predisposing to arousal from stages 3 and 4 NREM sleep, or by impairing the arousal process itself. Some episodes are precipitated by stress.

CLINICAL FEATURES

Sleep terrors appear especially during the first half of the night, mainly in the first NREM sleep cycle, and may occur more than once per night. The child suddenly appears to waken with a gasp, loud scream or cry and with the appearance of extreme fear, agitation and panic (Table 7.4). Sweating, dilated pupils, rapid respiratory and heart rates and an increase in muscle tone are characteristic and enuresis occasionally occurs. The child may sit up or leap out of bed, utter meaningless speech, and occasionally run wildly around the room. This is more common in adolescence than in younger children, but there may be injuries through, for instance, running out of doors or jumping through windows. The child is unresponsive to questions or commands and resists restraint, often causing harm to both the patient and others.

Table 7.4 Differential diagnosis of autonomic activation in sleep and on arousal.

Sleep terror
Nightmare
REM sleep behaviour disorder
Panic attack
Post-traumatic stress disorder

REM, rapid eye movement.

These episodes may last for only a few seconds, or for up to 10–20 min. They may be followed by an awakening with confusion and incoherent speech, and behaviour which is identical to a confusional arousal. Sleep is then re-entered promptly. There is little recall of the event but there may be an awareness that something frightening has happened or of vague images, particularly if alertness is attained before the subsidence of autonomic activation. No detailed recall of the event or of any dream content is given.

INVESTIGATIONS
Polysomnography is only occasionally needed but shows abrupt arousal from stages 3 or 4 NREM sleep usually within 1–4 h of sleep onset at the onset of a sleep terror. There are also frequent transitions to lighter stages of NREM sleep at other times which are not associated with sleep terrors. Video recordings show the details of the episode.

DIFFERENTIAL DIAGNOSIS
1 Confusional arousals.
2 Sleep walking.
3 Sleep talking.
4 Epilepsy.
5 Episodic nocturnal wanderings.
6 REM sleep behaviour disorder.
7 Nightmares.
8 Nocturnal panic attacks.
9 Post-traumatic stress disorder.

PROBLEMS
1 Sleep disruption and anxiety for the parents.
2 Embarrassment for the child.
3 Occasional injury to the child or others.

TREATMENT
1 Reassurance and explanation. This may be sufficient if the attacks are infrequent.

2 Sleep hygiene advice and in particular avoidance of sleep deprivation and caffeine.
3 Scheduled awakenings 15–30 min before the usual time of the sleep terror.
4 Benzodiazepines.
5 Beta blockers such as propranolol which may reduce the autonomic effects.
6 Measures to prevent injury to the child, e.g. remove any breakable objects and if necessary lock doors and windows of the bedroom.
7 Explore any psychological causes of anxiety or stress which might precipitate the attacks.

Sleep walking (somnambulism)

OVERVIEW
Sleep walking is a common manifestation of incomplete arousal from stages 3 and 4 NREM sleep in children and young adults.

OCCURRENCE
This is equally common in males and females and is often familial. It only occurs after the ability to walk has been attained, but similar episodes occur in infancy in which the child may simply crawl around. Its onset is usually after around 18 months and it is most common between the ages of 4–8 years. It becomes less common after adolescence, and if it begins in adult life there is usually significant psychopathology. It may be associated with other arousal disorders, such as confusional arousals and sleep terrors but is rare in the elderly.

PATHOGENESIS AND AETIOLOGY
Any factor which promotes stages 3 and 4 NREM sleep or arousal from sleep will increase the likelihood of sleep walking in a susceptible subject. Factors such as a noisy sleep environment, a distended bladder, pain, stress, fever or obstructive sleep apnoeas may all precipitate sleep walking in a susceptible subject. It is common in Gilles de la Tourette syndrome.

Sleep walking is said to be more common in those with migraines suggesting that an abnormality of 5HT transmission may be linked to both these conditions.

CLINICAL FEATURES
Sleep walking usually occurs during the first third of the night. The subject may sit up in bed, open the eyes, pick at the bedclothes, move around semi-purposefully and then usually attempt to leave the bed (Table 7.5). Children may walk into their parents'

Table 7.5 Differential diagnosis of walking during sleep.

Sleep walking
Sleep terror
Frontal lobe epilepsy
Temporal lobe epilepsy
REM sleep behaviour disorder
Confusional arousal
Sundown syndrome
Psychogenic fugue
Malingering

REM, rapid eye movement.

bedroom and enter their bed and make simple responses to questions and commands. Micturition occasionally occurs. He or she may try to dress and then walk around the bedroom indecisively, but often avoiding obstacles. A few words may be spoken and the subject may climb stairs, handle kitchen utensils and attempt to prepare a meal, open the front door of the home, walk considerable distances and even drive a motor vehicle. Injuries may result from falling down stairs or through windows, or after walking outside the home.

He or she usually allows themselves to be put back to bed without resistance, but attempts to restrain or waken the sleep walker should be avoided. They can cause a confusional arousal with disorientation, anxiety and a desire to escape which may evoke violence [1]. There is no autonomic activation or dream content during sleep walking and no recall of the event. Sleep is readily entered afterwards.

INVESTIGATIONS
Polysomnography may be required to differentiate sleep walking from other behavioural abnormalities in sleep. It often shows hypersynchrony of high voltage delta waves for a few seconds on a background of stages 1 and 2 NREM sleep without any epileptic features before the episode of sleep walking, as well as frequent arousals directly from stages 3 and 4 NREM sleep to wakefulness which may be unassociated with episodes of sleep walking. Video recording will show the pattern of activities.

DIFFERENTIAL DIAGNOSIS
1 Confusional arousals.
2 Sleep terrors.
3 Epilepsy.
4 Episodic nocturnal wanderings.

5 REM sleep behaviour disorder.
6 Psychogenic fugues.
7 Malingering.

PROBLEMS
1 Embarrassment.
2 Risk of injury such as falling down stairs or out of a window, and occasionally to others through resisting restraint.

TREATMENT
Treatment is usually not required, but if the attacks are frequent or if the subject is at risk of injury the following measures should be considered.
1 Attention to sleep hygiene.
2 Reduction of stress and sleep deprivation.
3 Scheduled awakenings 15–30 min before the usual time of the sleep walking.
4 Benzodiazepines, such as clonazepam or diazepam, prevent arousals and consolidate stages 1 and 2 NREM sleep, although they are usually used only intermittently.
5 Environmental protection. This includes closing and locking windows, locking stairs with a stairgate, putting bells on the bedroom door to alert the parents, sleeping in a low bed, and avoiding an upper bunk, moving sharp or breakable objects from the bedroom and staying in ground floor accommodation, for instance in hotels.
6 Psychotherapy may be of help in adults.

Sleep talking (somniloquy)

OVERVIEW
This common disorder is characterized by speech which may be incoherent and which does not significantly contribute to communication to others.

OCCURRENCE
It is equally common in males and females in childhood, but is more frequent in males in adult life. It is occasionally familial and becomes less common during adolescence. Most adults who sleep talk have done so since childhood but in those whom the age of onset is over around 25 years there is usually significant psychopathology.

PATHOGENESIS
Sleep talking is associated with brief arousals from stages 1 and 2 NREM sleep, and while it may occur

Table 7.6 Differential diagnosis of sleep vocalization.

Sleep talking
Sleep terror
Frontal lobe epilepsy
REM sleep behaviour disorder
Confusional arousal

REM, rapid eye movement.

without any external stimulation, it may be triggered by factors that cause arousal from sleep.

CLINICAL FEATURES
Sleep talking usually occurs during the first third of the night and only lasts for a few minutes. Speech is usually incoherent or unintelligible, and often has little meaning (Table 7.6). Words are spoken in short sentences and usually without emotion, although occasionally long tirades are delivered which are related to a preoccupation of the sleep talker. The speech may be in any language that the subject is capable of speaking. There is no autonomic activation or recall of the events. Sleep talking may be followed by a confusional arousal and can be associated with sleep walking.

INVESTIGATIONS
Polysomnography may be required, especially in adults, to distinguish sleep talking from other disorders that lead to vocalization. It shows brief arousals from stages 1 and 2 NREM sleep in most subjects. If arousals from sleep talking occur in REM sleep and there is dream content, the probable diagnosis is REM sleep behaviour disorder.

DIFFERENTIAL DIAGNOSIS
1 REM sleep behaviour disorder.
2 Confusional arousals.
3 Sleep terrors.
4 Talking during brief spells of wakefulness which occur between sleep episodes.
5 Epilepsy.
6 Fugue states.

PROBLEMS
Annoyance to bed partner, especially if the sleep talking occurs frequently.

TREATMENT
1 Reassurance and explanation.

2 Advice on sleep hygiene, especially avoidance of sleep deprivation, and of any factors that may cause arousal from sleep.
3 Benzodiazepines, such as clonazepam, used intermittently or in short courses may help to consolidate stage 2 NREM sleep.

Sleep eating and drinking (sleep-related eating disorder)

CLINICAL FEATURES
There are several patterns of eating and drinking during sleep [2]. The most frequent is probably an arousal disorder related to confusional arousals and sleep walking and which is most common between the ages of 20 and 40 years, particularly in females. It is characterized by recurrent, often nightly, episodes of eating, drinking and preparing food during sleep. These episodes usually occur in the first 2–3 h of sleep and may occur with partial arousals from stages 3 and 4 NREM sleep. They are not prevented by eating a large meal before going to sleep. There is little awareness or recall of the activities. No food preference has been observed, but alcohol is rarely taken. Subjects occasionally choke while eating and there is also risk of fire from the cooker being left on after the episode of eating or preparing food. There is no evidence of any eating disorder during wakefulness, but considerable weight may be gained.

DIFFERENTIAL DIAGNOSIS
This disorder should be distinguished from the following.

Night eating
This occurs in adults during wakefulness before the initiation of sleep and during awakenings from sleep. It is commonest in insomnia of the DIS (difficulty in initiating sleep) type and is associated with anxiety states and stress. Night eating in children often follows going to sleep while still hungry. Carbohydrate-containing food is often preferred. The serum melatonin levels are low during sleep, predisposing to wakefulness, and the level of leptin, which suppresses appetite, is also reduced.

Bulimia nervosa
Binge eating at night is uncommon but is usually associated with similar episodes during the day, self-induced vomiting and often DIS. Nocturnal eating

tends to occur when daytime symptoms are most marked and there is often a history of an arousal disorder such as sleep walking.

Narcolepsy
Awakenings during sleep are often associated with eating, particularly carbohydrates.

Kleine–Levin syndrome
Intermittent episodes of EDS occur in conjunction with a voracious appetite (megaphagia).

Awakenings from other sleep disorders
Eating at night often occurs during awakenings from, for instance, PLMS and, less frequently, obstructive sleep apnoeas. There is no food preference.

TREATMENT
Treatment of sleep eating and drinking due to partial arousals from NREM sleep is unsatisfactory, but clonazepam, L-dopa and dopamine agonists have been recommended. Food which the subject might be allergic to should be locked away or removed from the accommodation.

Sexual activity in sleep
This is a rarely reported disorder which is more common in males and usually appears in early adult life. Sexual intercourse is usually attempted and often achieved, but with no recollection of the event. Sexual activity with children may lead to the allegation of sexual abuse or assault. There is usually a history of other behavioural disorders in sleep, especially sleep walking, and often a family history of these conditions as well. The events may be triggered by sleep deprivation, sleep fragmentation due to, for instance, obstructive sleep apnoeas, alcohol and stress. Benzodiazepines such as clonazepam are effective, but treatment of the precipitating factors may be sufficient.

This disorder should be distinguished from sexual approaches during wakefulness but with no recall admitted subsequently, and dissociative states in which complex movements take place during wakefulness as demonstrated electrophysiologically. These states are associated with severe psychopathology and there is amnesia for the activity. The REM behaviour disorder is not generally recognized to lead to sexual activity in sleep, but may sometimes be the cause.

Nocturnal cramps

OVERVIEW
These are painful episodes due to sudden muscle tension which usually cause arousal from sleep.

OCCURRENCE
They are most common in elderly subjects, in pregnancy and in those on diuretics, glucocorticoids, in Parkinson's disease and in peripheral neuropathies due to, for example, diabetes mellitus.

PATHOGENESIS
The cramps are due to sudden contraction of skeletal muscles. Their cause is obscure, but they represent a sudden localized loss of motor inhibition. They occur during NREM sleep and usually cause arousal to wakefulness. They are not a feature of REM sleep, probably because of the more intense motor inhibition.

CLINICAL FEATURES
The cramps cause intermittent episodes of tightness and pain in the muscles, particularly of the calves and feet, and there may be soreness of the muscles afterwards. The frequency of the cramps fluctuates. They often occur on most nights for several days or weeks and then go into remission. There is no dream recall on arousal at the time of the cramp.

INVESTIGATIONS
None is necessary.

DIFFERENTIAL DIAGNOSIS
Periodic limb movements in sleep.

PROBLEMS
1 Leg pain.
2 Early morning wakening (EMW).

TREATMENT
1 Stretch muscles, e.g. by dorsiflexion of foot.
2 Quinine sulphate 200–300 mg nocte is usually effective but clonazepam, carbamazepine, verapamil and vitamin E have been used.

Panic attacks
Panic attacks occur during wakefulness, usually in the morning but also in sleep, particularly during the first third of the night and usually at the time of NREM sleep transition from stage 2–3 or 3–4. They are not

associated with dreams and the patient awakens fully, often with a sensation of intense fear, choking, breathlessness, palpitations, tremor and hyperarousal which prevents subsequent sleep. There is no tendency towards aggression or violence, but recall of the fear experienced during the event is retained.

DIFFERENTIAL DIAGNOSIS
The differential diagnosis includes hyperventilation, gastro-oesophageal reflux, OSA, vocal cord adduction and left ventricular failure.

TREATMENT
Treatment of the cause, or reassurance, psychotherapy or anxiolytics may be indicated.

Wakefulness–rapid eye movement sleep transition movements

The most important movement disorder of this type is cataplexy which is the sudden loss of muscle strength in response to emotional stimuli, usually laughter or anger. It is characteristic of narcolepsy and is discussed in Chapter 6. Sleep paralysis at the transition from wakefulness to sleep also falls into this category but is discussed in the next section.

Rapid eye movement sleep–wakefulness transition movements

The body movements described on page 140 are normally seen at the moment of arousal from REM sleep to wakefulness, but disorders of this transition phase are as follows.

Sleep paralysis

OVERVIEW
Sleep paralysis is the inability to move at the onset or end of sleep while the subject is alert. It is the converse of the REM sleep behaviour disorder in which muscle tone is preserved, but sleep persists.

OCCURRENCE
The onset of sleep paralysis is usually between the ages of 15 and 35 years. It occurs in three situations.

Sporadic
This is the most common type and males and females are equally frequently affected. Of normal subjects

25–50% have one or more episodes of sleep paralysis, usually if they are sleep deprived due to, for instance, shift work. It is more common on awakening than before falling asleep.

Familial
This is rare, but the tendency can be inherited as a dominant X chromosome-linked condition. It usually affects women and recurrent episodes, usually at sleep onset, are characteristic.

Narcolepsy
Sleep paralysis, usually at sleep onset, occurs in 20–40% of narcoleptics. Narcolepsy is the most likely diagnosis if sleep paralysis is frequent, particularly if other features of this condition are present.

PATHOGENESIS
Sleep paralysis occurs when the motor inhibition of REM sleep persists despite alertness being regained. Dissociation of these two major aspects of REM sleep is a feature of narcolepsy in which the function within the pons is disturbed.

CLINICAL FEATURES
Sleep paralysis is often triggered by sleep deprivation, irregular sleep–wake schedules or psychological stress. There is an inability to move, although respiration, usually due to diaphragmatic activity, continues. Some eye movements may still be possible as in REM sleep. The episode usually lasts from a few seconds to several minutes. There is awareness of the situation which is usually frightening, although occasionally it is felt to be enjoyably relaxing. Hypnagogic and hypnopompic hallucinations (page 164) occur in 75% of subjects and often contribute to the sensation of fear. The episode either terminates spontaneously through intense efforts to move, a noise or more commonly by a sudden touch by the bed partner.

INVESTIGATIONS
Polysomnography is rarely needed but may confirm that these episodes occur at the transition into and out of REM sleep.

DIFFERENTIAL DIAGNOSIS
1 Periodic hypokalaemic paralysis, although this occurs at rest while awake as well as on awakening, especially in adolescent males after alcohol or a large carbohydrate meal. A low serum potassium is detectable during the attacks.

2 Epilepsy (atonic seizures).
3 Hysteria.
4 Drop attacks.
5 Faints.

PROBLEMS
Anxiety for the subject.

TREATMENT
1 Sleep hygiene advice.
2 Tricyclic antidepressants, e.g. clomipramine if the episodes are a recurrent problem.

Movement disorders in non-rapid eye movement sleep

Epilepsy

OVERVIEW
The wide variety of clinical manifestations of epilepsy are all due to a synchronized and excessive electrical discharge in different regions of the brain. Sleep and the transition to wakefulness affect the threshold for these discharges to occur or propagate.

PATHOGENESIS
Intermittent synchronized excessive generalized or focal electrical discharges within the brain are responsible for epilepsy. They may arise either in a central core of malfunctioning neurones which lead directly to the epileptic seizure, or in afferent neurones which provide an abnormal influence on healthy neurones and predispose them to initiate the seizure. The site and spread of the electrical discharge determines the clinical features, which, particularly with temporal and frontal lobe epilepsy, may include complex motor activities.

The influences of NREM and REM sleep on epilepsy are very different. The diffuse cortical synchronization in NREM sleep, due to the thalamocortical projections, predisposes towards the discharge of epileptic foci or propagation of the discharge. Any factor which increases NREM sleep will tend to precipitate epilepsy. This includes sleep deprivation and after alcohol ingestion. In contrast, the desynchronization of cortical activity in REM sleep acts as an anticonvulsant, protecting against epilepsy, and the intense motor inhibition, characteristic of REM sleep, may also play a part.

CLINICAL FEATURES
There is a bimodal time distribution of nocturnal

Table 7.7 Differential diagnosis of limb jerking.

Hypnic jerks
Fragmentary myoclonus
Startle disease
PLMS
REM sleep behaviour disorder
Epilepsy, e.g. frontal lobe epilepsy
Arousals due to, for example, OSA

OSA, obstructive sleep apnoeas; PLMS, periodic limb movements in sleep; REM, rapid eye movement.

epilepsy. Seizures tend to occur either early in the night, particularly in stages 1 and 2 NREM sleep, or 1–2 h before or after the transition from sleep to wakefulness in the morning.

Epileptic seizures rarely lead to a complaint of insomnia despite the events interrupting sleep. They only cause EDS if seizures are frequent during the day and are followed by episodes of sleep or through the sedative effects of anticonvulsants. The usual complaint by the partner, parent or carer is of frightening or disturbing movements during sleep (Table 7.7).

Sudden, unexpected death in epileptics usually occurs during sleep. Its cause is uncertain but it is more frequent in males aged around 30 years, particularly if their epilepsy is poorly controlled. Death may result from cardiac dysrhythmias due to a sleep related pattern of excessive sympathetic activation or to metabolic changes, such as transient increase in serum potassium after the seizure. It may also be caused by central apnoeas caused by a failure of the respiratory centres to generate any respiratory movements or alternatively to persistent tonic activity of the chest wall muscles preventing inspiration and leading to hypoxia.

The most important types of epilepsy that are related to sleep are as follows.

Infantile spasms (West's syndrome)
These occur particularly between the ages of 3–9 months. The child briefly flexes the neck, lumbar spine and often the knees and elbows ('salaam spasms'). These occur particularly when the child is drowsy or soon after waking, but rarely during sleep although the EEG pattern of hypsarrhythmia (irregular high voltage slow waves with spikes or sharp waves) may only be seen during sleep.

Lennox–Gastaut syndrome
This appears between the ages of 3 and 6 years and

one-third of children present with the features of infantile spasms. A variety of types of seizure appear, but during NREM sleep these are usually of the tonic type. Mental retardation is characteristic and the prognosis is poor.

Febrile convulsions
These occur in 3% of children, especially between the ages of 6 months and 5 years, and are usually associated with a temperature of greater than 38°C. Fifty per cent of febrile convulsions occur either close to the start or end of sleep, and a further 25% soon after wakening.

Landau–Kleffner syndrome
This usually appears before the age of 7 years and is characterized by multifocal spikes detectable on the EEG. Seventy per cent of children have generalized or partial seizures and there is an acquired dysphasia and auditory inattention.

Electrical status epilepticus of sleep
This condition is defined by the EEG appearances of continuous 2–2.5 Hz spike and wave activity occupying more than 85% of NREM sleep. It is only rarely seen in REM sleep. The condition is equally common in males and females and arises between the ages of 5 and 15 years. Nocturnal seizures may be present, but the EEG abnormality often improves after a few years although learning difficulties and behavioural abnormalities usually persist.

Absence seizures (petit mal epilepsy)
These sudden episodes of loss of muscle tone usually cause brief episodes of blinking or staring and occur most frequently soon after waking and during drowsiness. Spike and wave discharges of 3 Hz are common, especially in stages 2–4 NREM sleep.

Benign Rolandic epilepsy (benign epilepsy with centro-temporal spikes, Sylvian seizures)
These seizures occur more frequently in males than females and usually between the ages of 2–12 years. They are the most common simple partial seizures in childhood and represent 25% of childhood epilepsy. Twitching of the face, lips and tongue associated with dysarthria and drooling are characteristic. Seventy-five per cent of subjects only have these seizures during sleep and in a further 15% they are seen both during sleep and wakefulness. They occur particularly in stages 1 and 2 NREM sleep.

Janz syndrome (juvenile myoclonic epilepsy)
This is equally frequent in males and females and usually occurs between the ages of 10 and 25 years. The synchronized bilateral myoclonic jerks of the limbs, particularly the arms, usually occurs soon after wakening, especially if the subject is sleep deprived or waking from NREM sleep. There may be confusion but no loss of consciousness. The EEG shows synchronized frontal bilateral spike and wave or polyspike and wave discharges at a frequency of 4–6 Hz during the episode, at sleep onset, or on awakening.

Generalized seizures
Generalized tonic–clonic seizures usually occur soon after falling asleep or on awakening. They occur during sleep in up to 25% of subjects and daytime seizures are unlikely to develop if they have not appeared within 2 years of the onset of the nocturnal episodes.

Myoclonic seizures in adults also occur, especially at sleep onset and on wakening, and are associated with a brief loss of consciousness.

Temporal lobe epilepsy (complex partial seizures, psychomotor epilepsy, limbic epilepsy)
These seizures are associated with inappropriate complex behaviour patterns (automatisms) such as picking at clothing, smacking the lips or wandering around the room. There may be hallucinations, particularly of smells and taste, illusions of familiarity with strange environments and intense feelings of anxiety and fear. The seizures are mainly diurnal and it is rare for them to be exclusively nocturnal. They are, however, associated with a low sleep efficiency due to either frequent or prolonged awakenings unrelated to nocturnal seizures. They have been thought to be related to the start or end of REM sleep episodes but are much more common in NREM sleep. Longer lasting epileptic fugues with less change in the level of consciousness, complex behaviour patterns and with a tendency to wander should be distinguished from the more protracted hysterical fugues and from postictal sleepiness and automatic behaviour.

Frontal lobe seizures
These may be focal motor seizures with unilateral movements of the limbs, head and neck or complex partial seizures. They probably equate to paroxysmal arousals, nocturnal paroxysmal dystonias and episodic nocturnal wanderings [3] and are described below.

INVESTIGATIONS

Electroencephalogram
High-amplitude abnormal electrical activity, particularly spikes (less than 70 ms) or waves (70–120 ms) may be detected between or during seizures, especially in NREM sleep. They are due to synchronized depolarization causing the spikes and hyperpolarization causing the waves. A standard full montage EEG during wakefulness may be sufficient to detect electrical epileptic activity, especially with hyperventilation or photic stimulation.

A sleep EEG is indicated if epilepsy is suspected and the EEG while awake is non-diagnostic, especially if seizures are mainly nocturnal or infrequent. Sleep may be entered during the day following sleep deprivation, on the previous night or if sedation is given, although this will not induce a physiological sleep state. Sleep deprivation is usually induced by asking the subject to go to bed 2 h later and to wake up 2 h earlier than usual on the night before the EEG. Epileptic features may be detected even if only stages 1 and 2 NREM sleep occur, as is common with daytime sleep EEGs. The alternative is to carry out an EEG examination during overnight sleep. A full montage EEG is preferable to the standard polysomnograpy EEG montage since more of the cerebral cortex is sampled. A 24 h or even longer 'ambulatory' recording may be required, but the signals are often of poor quality, artefacts are common and fewer electrodes can be used than with a standard EEG. Absence of abnormalities between seizures with any of these techniques does not exclude epilepsy.

Polysomnography
This is insensitive at detecting epileptic discharges, but if they do occur they make any further sleep staging during the seizure impossible. Video recordings show the nature of the movement disorder which in epilepsy is more repetitive and stereotyped than in most other motor disorders. Polysomnography may demonstrate frontal lobe epilepsy, rarely confirms a diagnosis of temporal lobe epilepsy, but is of most value in demonstrating non-epileptic behavioural abnormalities during sleep.

Computerized tomography and magnetic resonance imaging scans
Computerized tomography and MRI scans may show the presence of the cause for the epilepsy, such as a space occupying lesion or cerebrovascular disease.

DIFFERENTIAL DIAGNOSIS
This includes faints, panic attacks, hyperventilation, hypoglycaemia, transient cerebral ischaemic attacks, drop attacks, PLMS, REM sleep behaviour disorder and rhythmic movement disorders. These can usually be distinguished since epileptic seizures are repetitive, often complex and the subject is uncontactable during the episode, and often sleepy afterwards with little recall of the event.

Obstructive sleep apnoeas may lower the threshold for epilepsy by inducing sleep deprivation through fragmentation of sleep. Commonly, however, the twitching movements associated with an arousal at the end of an apnoea are mistaken for epileptic seizures. Treatment of OSA may improve epileptic control, but conversely, treatment for presumed epilepsy usually worsens OSA and makes the nocturnal arousal movements more frequent. Any of the sedative anticonvulsants can have this effect and phenytoin also leads to hypertrophy of the tissue of the upper airway which predisposes to OSA.

TREATMENT
Treatment of any condition causing sleep deprivation or fragmentation may improve the control of nocturnal epilepsy.

The actions of anticonvulsant drugs on seizures during sleep may differ from their effects during wakefulness, according to their differing tendencies to promote or abolish NREM sleep.

Paroxysmal arousal, nocturnal paroxysmal dystonia and episodic nocturnal wandering

OVERVIEW
These three similar disorders differ in their duration and the complexity of the episodes that they cause. They probably all represent forms of frontal lobe epilepsy.

OCCURRENCE
They are slightly more common in males and usually arise before the age of 50 years. They are occasionally familial, probably inherited in an autosomal dominant manner, and there is an increased prevalence of other types of epileptic seizures in these patients.

PATHOGENESIS
Most of these episodes represent the effects of epileptic discharges in the anterior and medial parts of the frontal lobes.

CLINICAL FEATURES

Paroxysmal arousals are brief and only last for a few seconds or occasionally up to a few minutes [4]. They occur up to 20 times per night and on most nights. They usually continue for many years unless they are treated. Nocturnal paroxysmal dystonias are more prolonged and episodic nocturnal wanderings may last for several minutes. Unlike temporal lobe seizures, these attacks usually occur only during sleep.

In all three disorders there is a sudden arousal from NREM sleep, usually stage 2, but also stages 3 and 4. The episodes are stereotyped for each individual. The first manifestation is usually a brief scream, moan or howl associated with opening of the eyes and an expression of fright or surprise. In paroxysmal arousals there may also be brief dystonic or athetoid semipurposeful limb movements with signs of autonomic activation such as a tachycardia. In nocturnal paroxysmal dystonias the dystonic posturing of the head, trunk and limbs and choreoathetoid movements are more marked and may even lead to opisthotonus. The episode may terminate with repetitive limb movements such as grasping, punching, flailing, shaking, running, jumping, cycling or kicking. Occasionally pelvic thrusting, genital manipulation or tonic posturing is seen. In episodic nocturnal wanderings the patient may leave the bed and resist restraint with violence. There is no dream content, a rapid resumption of consciousness, and little or no recall of the episode with no tongue biting or incontinence. In all three of these disorders the episode terminates with a return to sleep.

INVESTIGATIONS

1 Polysomnography. This shows movement artefact at the onset of the episode and no detectable epileptic discharges, probably because the focus is deep in the frontal lobe. Video recording reveals the types of movements.
2 Interictal EEG. This may show abnormalities indicative of epilepsy, but is often normal.

DIFFERENTIAL DIAGNOSIS

1 Other epileptic episodes, especially temporal lobe epilepsy.
2 Fugue states in which global amnesia is associated with wandering, although the subjects are awake and in touch with the environment.
3 Periodic limb movements in sleep.
4 Sleep terrors.
5 REM sleep behaviour disorder.

PROBLEMS

1 Insomnia, which may occur if the episodes are frequent.
2 Physical injuries.
3 Disruptive sleep for the bed partner.

TREATMENT

All three types of episodes respond to anticonvulsant treatment such as carbamazepine, phenytoin and sodium valproate and possibly to gabapentin and lamotrigine.

Sleep bruxism (tooth grinding or crunching)

OVERVIEW

The repetitive movements of sleep bruxism are confined to the muscles moving the lower jaw and they cause a range of dental and jaw disorders.

OCCURRENCE

Sleep bruxism is equally common in males and females and occurs occasionally in up to 50% of children and frequently in 5–20%. It is often familial and the prevalence decreases linearly with age. It is most frequent between the ages of 3 and 12 years but occurs in only 2–5% of young adults and around 1% of the elderly.

PATHOGENESIS

Sleep bruxism is due to contraction of the masseter, temporalis and pterygoid muscles, but more frequently, repetitively and with more force than is normal. It may represent a disorder of dopaminergic movement control. In adults it may be precipitated by oral problems and dental conditions such as malocclusion, mandibular or maxillary disorders, and anxiety, sleep deprivation, L-dopa, SSRI antidepressants and alcohol. If it occurs during wakefulness as well as sleep it usually has a different aetiology and is associated with diffuse brain damage, mental retardation or cerebral palsy.

CLINICAL FEATURES

Sleep bruxism is manifested by repetitive rhythmic chewing movements leading to grinding or crunching of the teeth. It varies in severity, but there are often hundreds of episodes each night. They usually occur at around one each second and in runs of 5–10. The noise is usually felt to be unpleasant and the movements cause grinding down of the teeth, dental decay, periodontal damage, increased tooth mobility and temporo-mandibular joint dysfunction with pain which is usually worse on waking.

INVESTIGATIONS

Polysomnography is rarely needed to establish the diagnosis but may be required to establish whether any other sleep disorder is present and exacerbating bruxism. It shows masseter and temporalis muscle activity as an artefact, especially during stage 2 NREM sleep and occasionally stage 1 NREM or REM sleep. It can also occur during stages 3 and 4 NREM sleep, and the bruxism often leads to brief arousals.

DIFFERENTIAL DIAGNOSIS

Epilepsy with rhythmic jaw movements.

PROBLEM

Dental and jaw disorders.
Insomnia for the partner.

TREATMENT

1 Sleep hygiene, especially with regard to avoiding sleep deprivation and relevant drugs.
2 Correction of any dental malocclusion or other oral disorders.
3 Dental moulds and mouth guards which protect the teeth from damage from friction.
4 Relief of anxiety.

PLMS in sleep (PLM syndrome, nocturnal myoclonus) and restless legs syndrome (Ekbom's syndrome)

OVERVIEW

These two conditions are often regarded as distinct, but there is a continuum of clinical features and similarities in their aetiology, pathogenesis and treatment which makes it likely that they have the same basic causes (Tables 7.8 and 7.9).

Neonatal	Childhood	Adolescence	Young and middle-aged adults	Old age
Benign neonatal myoclonus				
		Confusional arousal		
	Sleep terror			
		Sleep walking		
		Sleep talking		
		Sleep eating		
		Panic attacks		
				Nocturnal cramps
		Hypnic jerks		
	Rhythmic movement disorder			
		Cataplexy		
		Sleep paralysis		
		Post-traumatic stress disorder		
		PLMS		
		Epilepsy		
	Sleep bruxism			
			REM behaviour disorder	
			Status dissociatus	

Table 7.8 Age and behavioural abnormalities in sleep. PLMS, periodic limb movements in sleep; REM, rapid eye movement.

Table 7.9 Restless legs and periodic limb movement syndromes.

	RLS	PLMS
Cause	Metabolic disorders Drugs	Metabolic disorders Drugs CNS disease
Wake–sleep	Awake	Asleep
Sensory symptoms	Limb 'ache', etc.	Nil
Motor effects	Voluntary movements Involuntary jerks	Limb movements
Sleep symptoms	Nil	EDS Insomnia Restlessness

CNS, central nervous system; EDS, excessive daytime sleepiness; PLMS, periodic limb movements in sleep; RLS, restless legs syndrome.

OCCURRENCE

Periodic limb movements in sleep (PLMS) and the restless legs syndrome (RLS) are both equally common in males and females. A family history is obtained in over one-third of subjects and they are probably autosomally dominantly inherited. Both conditions may arise at any age, including childhood, but their prevalence increases rapidly after the age of 50 years (Table 7.9). The prevalence of PLMS is uncertain, but may be around 5% between the ages of 30 and 50 years, 30% between 50 and 65 years and 45% in the population over the age of 65. These figures include mild forms of PLMS which may not require any treatment. Restless legs syndrome is thought to occur in 5–15% of the adult population. Around 35% of PLMS subjects have RLS and 80% of RLS patients have PLMS but the severity of both PLMS and RLS fluctuates throughout life.

PATHOGENESIS

The regular periodicity of PLMS suggests that there is a CNS oscillator which is able to overcome the motor inhibition of stages 1 and 2 NREM sleep. Periodic limb movements in sleep are less common in stages 3 and 4 NREM and REM sleep, probably because motor inhibition is more intense [5]. The movements occur at intervals of 15–40 s which is a similar periodicity to the cyclic alternating pattern (CAP) cycle of 40 s and the oscillations in the heart rate and blood pressure (Mayer waves) which represent fluctuations in sympathetic nervous system activity. If PLMS has a similar origin this would imply that its appearance is due to a failure to inhibit the movements due to an oscillator which is universally present.

The location of the oscillator is uncertain, but it probably has functional connections with the basal ganglia, particularly the caudate and putamen which are closely connected with the substantia nigra in the midbrain. The red nucleus may also be involved in the motor aspects of PLMS and subcortical sensory processing disorders may involve the thalamus. Dopamine is a neurotransmitter at most of these nuclei, but mu-opioid receptor function in the cerebellum may also be impaired in PLMS.

Periodic limb movements in sleep can also be present even with a complete spinal cord transection or during spinal cord anaesthesia, suggesting that loss of inhibition from higher motor centres may be an important factor. The limb movements may be generated by the propiospinal system in the spinal cord which spreads activity to adjacent spinal segments. Dysfunction of the pyramidal tract and reticulospinal tract probably contributes to the motor features and the latter may be responsible for the sensory aspects of RLS through influencing the dorsal horns in the spinal cord.

The oscillator may also be under the control of the circadian rhythms or a sleep related mechanism. This could be related to the reduction in serum ferritin or the increase in dopamine production during sleep or to changes in blood-borne chemical stimuli which influence the stability of the oscillator and which reach the brain from other sites in the body.

Restless legs syndrome occurs during wakefulness,

in contrast to PLMS, and its pathogenesis probably involves cortical mechanisms and sensory processing as well as the generation of limb movements. The increasing frequency of PLMS and RLS in the elderly is probably due to degenerative processes within the CNS which facilitate the expression of the movements or sensations, or fail to suppress or control the oscillator.

AETIOLOGY

Both PLMS and RLS are usually idiopathic, especially in females, but in one-third of subjects there is a family history of one or other of these conditions. Inheritance appears to be through an autosomal dominant mechanism. They have also been associated with a wide variety of chronic and some acute disorders. Most of these links are poorly substantiated, but both conditions are probably associated with the following.

Iron deficiency
Periodic limb movements in sleep and RLS are common in iron deficiency, for instance during pregnancy and in rheumatoid arthritis, but may also be due to abnormalities in iron metabolism without any iron deficiency. Tyrosine hydroxylase is an enzyme which requires ferrous ions to function, and converts L-tyrosine to L-dopa. This can be the rate-limiting step in the synthesis of dopamine. There is no evidence for iron deficiency altering the function of the D2 receptors. Iron is mobilized as transferrin in which form it crosses the blood–brain barrier, but it is stored as ferritin.

The serum ferritin level is inversely proportional to the severity of RLS symptoms and to sleep efficiency as shown by polysomnography. The serum ferritin levels drop by 30–50% at night and an increased iron availability is required to cope with the increased dopamine production at night. Periodic limb movements in sleep might appear if iron is not available, either because of total body deficiency or because of a failure to transfer iron across the blood–brain barrier or into the dopamine synthesizing areas of the brain. Iron occurs particularly in the substantia nigra, striatum, deep cerebellar nuclei and the red nucleus. Correction of iron deficiency leads to improvement in the symptoms of both PLMS and RLS.

Magnesium deficiency
This may contribute to PLMS and RLS. Magnesium shares with iron the same protein for assisting transfer of the ion into cells.

Renal failure
This causes anaemia, but PLMS and RLS in renal failure appear to be independent of this. They occur in 20–40% of those with renal failure and are not relieved by haemodialysis, suggesting that this does not remove whatever chemical is responsible for initiating these syndromes. Renal transplantation does, however, relieve both PLMS and RLS.

Peripheral neuropathies
Periodic limb movements in sleep and RLS are associated with some types of peripheral neuropathy, especially that due to vitamin B12 deficiency, which presumably modify the sensory input to the spinal cord and brainstem.

Pregnancy and menstruation
Restless legs syndrome occurs in at least 15% of pregnancies, usually in the 2nd and 3rd trimester, and RLS and PLMS are often worse premenstrually.

Sleep deprivation or sleep fragmentation
These can be due to any cause, including OSAs.

Drugs
In general, CNS stimulants and dopamine antagonists worsen PLMS and RLS. The most important drugs are caffeine, glucocorticoids, monoamine oxidase inhibitors (MAOI) and tricyclic antidepressants, lithium, antipsychotics such as phenothiazines, antihistamines, calcium channel blockers, and metoclopramide. Withdrawal from anticonvulsants and hypnotics such as benzodiazepines and barbiturates and chronic alcohol consumption also worsen PLMS and RLS.

PLMS, but not RLS, is associated with the following.

Narcolepsy. Periodic limb movements in sleep often occur in REM as well as NREM sleep. Restless leg syndrome is not associated with narcolepsy.

Movement disorders. Periodic limb movements in sleep are common in both idiopathic and secondary Parkinsonism, possibly because of abnormalities in dopamine availability, but RLS is much less common. They are also a feature of Huntington's disease and Gilles de la Tourette syndrome.

CLINICAL FEATURES

Periodic limb movements in sleep

Periodic limb movements in sleep lead to complaints of insomnia and EDS from the patient and of restlessness during sleep from the partner whose sleep is often disturbed. The limb movements cause frequent awakenings during the night and the patient may then be distressed about the need to move the legs and to keep them cool. This awareness and these movements take place during wakefulness so, strictly speaking, they are distinct from the limb movements during sleep, and fall into the RLS category.

Limb movements. The periodic limb movements in sleep are characterized by sudden movements of the limbs, usually the legs, although they are not as brief as myoclonic jerks and the muscles may take longer to relax than to contract [6]. The movements last from 0.5–5 s, but usually 1.5–2.5 s. They are usually bilateral and symmetrical, but can be unilateral or asynchronous. There may be more than one type of movement in any individual, but each type occurs repetitively. The most common is extension of the big toe with ankle dorsiflexion and knee and hip flexion. This pattern is similar to a Babinski response which probably, like PLMS, reflects loss of supra-spinal inhibition of the lower motor neurone by pyramidal tract influences. If the arms are affected, the movements are often more writhing, flailing or flinging, and other muscles such as the abdominal and paraspinal muscles may be involved. Occasionally PLMS is so severe that the whole body moves relentlessly for hours on end and unusual positions are adopted to obtain temporary relief.

There is considerable variation from night to night in the frequency of PLMS, but the movements occur in clusters at intervals of 5–120 s, usually 15–40 s. The intervals are often constant in any one sleep stage during a single night in an individual patient. They are most frequent in stages 1 and 2 NREM sleep, less frequent in stages 3 and 4 and almost absent in REM sleep in which motor inhibition is maximal. They also occur in quiet wakefulness before sleep and during episodes of wakefulness during the night, even if there are no symptoms of RLS.

Effects on sleep. Periodic limb movements are most frequent shortly after sleep onset when stages 1 and 2 NREM sleep are developing, and they frequently cause brief arousals or prolonged awakenings. The subject is aware of difficulty in initiating sleep, and it may be impossible to fall asleep for several hours. Later in the night, when stages 1 and 2 NREM sleep recur, the PLMS tend to fragment sleep and there may be long periods of sleeplessness since movements occur even during wakefulness and prevent a return to sleep. Protruding the feet from the bed clothes to cool them or leaving the bed to walk about is often needed.

The insomnia caused by PLMS may therefore be DIS, difficulty in maintaining sleep (DMS) or EMW and is often associated with EDS which can be severe. Excessive daytime sleepiness is probably due both to the prolonged episodes of wakefulness which lead to sleep restriction, as well as to micro arousals from the PLMS. However, EDS is very variable and it is unknown which properties of the limb movements lead to micro arousals. The frequency of the movements, a change in their frequency, the amplitude of movement or the termination of a cluster of PLMS have all been proposed as arousal stimuli. Arousal may, however, occur before the limb movement is detectable which suggests that it is not the movement, but the neurological activity that it represents which causes arousal. It is likely that it is the ability of the output from the oscillator generating the movements to break into the brainstem and thalamic mechanisms promoting NREM sleep which is significant.

If PLMS are very severe they may cause immediate arousals from sleep even if sleep deprivation is marked. In this situation the subject feels excessively sleepy throughout the day, but is unable to establish sleep. The intense sleepiness may cause accidents and injuries through falling during micro sleeps and episodes of automatic behaviour.

Restless legs syndrome

This is characterized by both sensory and motor symptoms while the subject is awake.

Sensory. The characteristic sensation is an unpleasant, uncomfortable, creeping, crawling, irritating, pulling, stretching, heavy, tired and occasionally tingling, pins and needles, burning, aching, itching or painful sensation which is sometimes described as being like insects or worms inside the legs. The sensation is felt deep within the legs, particularly around the knees, but also in the thighs, calves, and even the buttocks and lower back, but rarely in the feet or arms, and not in the hands, and is usually bilateral.

The sensations only occur at rest, for instance while sitting in a seat, as a car or train passenger, in an aeroplane, cinema, theatre or lecture. They are relieved by movements such as walking or stretching the limb and the patient often feels an irresistible need to move. Massage of the muscle, but not isometric contraction, may relieve the unpleasant sensation. Cooling the legs or occasionally warming them may give relief. It is possible to distract the subject from the unpleasant sensations if they are mild, but not once they become severe. They are relieved by sleep, even if this is a brief nap, but are not helped simply by lying down.

These sensations are almost invariably worse in the evening and early in the night, but in more severe cases they spread back into the day. They may prevent sleep onset and the maintenance of sleep and can occur even if the limb has been amputated (phantom RLS).

Motor. Two types of movements are characteristic of this condition. Firstly, voluntary 'fidgety' movements to relieve the unpleasant limb sensations and, secondly, involuntary jerks which cannot be consciously suppressed. These have similarities to PLMS in that they involve extension of the big toe and flexion of the ankle, knee and hip. They can be partially suppressed by adopting a flexed position and are less regular in their periodicity than PLMS. They tend to coincide with most intense moments of the unpleasant limb sensations. These movements also occur during awakenings from sleep due to PLMS.

INVESTIGATIONS

Blood tests
Blood tests can be used to test, for example, for haemoglobin, ferritin, urea and electrolytes. These may indicate the cause of PLMS and RLS.

Polysomnography
Polysomnography is useful in distinguishing PLMS from other behavioural abnormalities during sleep, showing the severity of the PLMS and their relationship to EEG arousals (Figs 4.5 and 5.7). The PLMS can be detected using anterior tibial electro-myogram (EMG) electrodes. Video recordings reveal the type and frequency of the movements. The sleep stage during which the movements occur, the effects on sleep architecture, frequency of arousals and the presence of other factors contributing to sleep disruption can all be demonstrated. Polysomnography usually shows that the movements are most common in stages 1 and 2 NREM sleep, but, particularly in the REM sleep

behaviour disorder and narcolepsy, they may appear in REM sleep.

The current methods of quantifying PLMS on polysomnography are unsatisfactory. They are conventionally recorded as the number of clusters of movements per hour of sleep, but this does not represent the total number of movements. The frequency of arousals per hour associated with the PLMS can also be calculated. Frequent or prolonged awakenings are not recognized by either of these scoring systems, which also ignore the limb movements occurring during wakefulness at night.

Actigraphy
Detection of PLMS by acceleration monitors can be performed without polysomnography. These are suitable for out-patient and serial use, for instance to monitor the effects of treatment. The frequency and type of limb movements can be quantified.

DIFFERENTIAL DIAGNOSIS

Periodic limb movements in sleep
The movements may be confused with hypnic jerks which are usually single and occur at the onset of sleep, epilepsy, leg movements due to arousals from, e.g. OSA, and other causes of limb movements (Table 7.7). Obstructive sleep apnoeas and PLMS often coexist, although they do not appear to share the same central oscillator. PLMS may increase in frequency after OSA are treated with nasal continuous positive airway pressure (CPAP) possibly because the duration of stages 1 and 2 NREM sleep is increased.

Restless legs syndrome
This may be confused with the following.

Paraesthesia due to peripheral neuropathies. The sensations tend to be more constant and, unlike the RLS, there are often neurological abnormalities on examination.

Akathisia. This is usually due to antipsychotic drugs or idiopathic Parkinsonism. There is an urge to move the limbs, especially the legs, in response to a general inner feeling of restlessness. Akathisia is not related to any particular time of the day or night. It is not worsened by immobility and may involve persistent repetitive movements of large muscle groups leading to body rocking and walking. It often responds to withdrawal of the antipsychotic drug, or administration of benzodiazepines or propranolol.

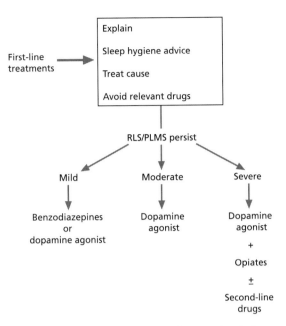

Fig. 7.2 Treatment of restless legs syndrome and periodic limb movements in sleep.

PROBLEMS

Periodic limb movements in sleep
1 Insomnia or EDS for the patient.
2 Sleep disturbance and minor injuries for the bed partner.

Restless legs syndrome
Unpleasant sensations and difficulty in initiating and maintaining sleep.
   Social difficulties such as inability to travel as a car passenger or sit in a cinema.

TREATMENT
The treatment of PLMS and RLS is similar, but in the RLS advice should be given about keeping the legs moving during the day and the feet cold, through for instance wearing loose footwear. If PLMS are asymptomatic they do not require treatment, but if the movements are troublesome or if the sensations of RLS are severe the following steps should be followed (Fig. 7.2).
1 Explanation and reassurance.
2 Give sleep hygiene advice, especially if sleep deprivation is a factor.
3 Treat the cause, e.g. iron deficiency.
4 Avoid relevant drugs, e.g. discontinue tricyclic antidepressants or reduce caffeine intake.

5 Drug treatment. This is often effective, but rotation of drugs or even a 'drug holiday' so that therapy is intermittent rather than continuous may be required to reduce tolerance and the risk of dependency. Drug treatment in children should be avoided wherever possible because of the unknown long-term toxicity of the treatment. Drugs should also be avoided if possible during pregnancy, in which iron replacement may be of help. Most of the effective treatments cross the placenta, enter breast milk, and can cause sedation of the infant. Dopamine agonists also reduce prolactin release and inhibit lactation.

First-line drugs

Benzodiazepines. Long-acting drugs such as diazepam should be avoided because of the risk of sedative effects, but clonazepam, temazepam and nitrazepam are often useful. They tend to consolidate stage 2 NREM sleep and reduce sleep-stage transitions and arousals from sleep but only partially relieve the movements through their muscle relaxant effect. The patient therefore obtains more benefit than the partner. They are best if the condition is mild, and especially when insomnia is a problem, but may worsen other associated disorders, e.g. OSA. They should be used intermittently, usually in short courses.

L-dopa and dopamine agonists. L-dopa is usually given with a dopa decarboxylase inhibitor such as carbidopa or benserazide which prevents peripheral metabolism to dopamine, but does not itself cross the blood–brain barrier. This combination increases the dopamine level in the CNS and reduces peripheral side-effects. To treat PLMS 50–400 mg L-dopa can be given 30–60 min before sleep and a second similar dose repeated during the night if the patient wakes, unless a slow release preparation is used before sleep.
   In 75% of subjects with PLMS, L-dopa exacerbates RLS symptoms before sleep even if it improves the PLMS. This augmentation worsens when the dose is increased or L-dopa is taken before the onset of the RLS symptoms. A change to a dopamine receptor agonist such as: ropinirole 0.25–0.75 mg nocte, pergolide initially 0.05 mg nocte, or bromocriptine initially 1 mg nocte, is usually effective since these drugs only cause 'augmentation' of RLS symptoms in 10–15% of patients. Ropinirole has been implicated as a cause of sudden 'sleep attacks' and in the UK it is not recommended if the patient drives a motor vehicle.

Opiates. These may be useful in severe PLMS. Codeine 30–60 mg nocte, dextropropoxyphene 65 mg nocte, tramadol 50–150 mg nocte, or even methadone 5–10 mg nocte or morphine 5–15 mg nocte are effective. Tolerance and dependency on these drugs occasionally occurs and there is a risk of respiratory depression.

Second-line drugs
Second-line drugs which may be required in severe or resistant cases, either alone or in addition to one or more of the first-line drugs include the following.

Anticonvulsants. Carbamazepine, gabapentin and sodium valproate are probably the most effective.

Baclofen. This is occasionally helpful in severe PLMS and reduces the amplitude of the movements and the number of arousals, but not the frequency of the movements.

Beta blockers. Propranolol, for example.

Clonidine.

Melatonin. This may reduce the frequency of PLMS by modifying any underlying circadian rhythm disorder.

Movement disorders in rapid eye movement sleep

Only a few movements normally prevail over the intense motor inhibition of REM sleep. The saccadic rapid eye movements and movements of the middle ear muscles, posterior crico-artenoid, diaphragm and parasternal intercostal muscles are well recognized. Jerky movements of the facial and distal limb muscles lasting less than 1 s also occur irregularly, at times when REMs are present.

The most important abnormalities of movement in REM sleep are as follows.

Rapid eye movement sleep behaviour disorder

OVERVIEW
The essential features are the vivid, often unpleasant, dreams and abnormal movements in REM sleep ranging from twitches to complex and often aggressive actions.

OCCURRENCE
This is occasionally seen in children and young adults, but is much more common over the age of 50 years. It affects males four times more frequently than females and is occasionally familial.

PATHOGENESIS AND AETIOLOGY
The characteristic feature of REM sleep behaviour disorder is the failure of motor inhibition during REM so that muscle tone returns and movements related to cortical activities and dream mentation take place. The abnormality is probably located in the pons or medulla in the areas that are responsible for inhibition of muscle activity during REM sleep. The exact location and extent of the lesions probably determines the type and degree of the REM sleep behaviour disorder.

This condition may be seen with narcolepsy or transiently due to drug toxicity or during REM sleep rebound during withdrawal, from, for instance, tricyclic antidepressants, amphetamines or alcohol. No cause is found in around 60% of patients, but in the remainder organic brain disease is detectable. This is usually degenerative, e.g. dementia, fatal familial insomnia, multiple system atrophy, idiopathic and secondary Parkinsonism, following strokes and in multiple sclerosis. The features of REM sleep behaviour disorder may precede other features of these disorders by up to five years [7].

CLINICAL FEATURES
Dreams are often, but not invariably, recalled, but there is no recollection of the movements during sleep. The vivid dreams and abnormal movements can occur during any REM sleep cycle but are most common during the first. This is usually around 90 min after sleep onset and symptoms tend to recur at around 90-min intervals during the night (Table 7.10). In mild cases the limb and trunk movements may represent an exaggeration of the normal irregular muscle twitches or jerks that can be seen in REM sleep, and periodic limb movements may appear.

When the condition becomes more severe, complex, organized actions, including flailing of the arms, hand waving, finger pointing, punching, laughing, talking, screaming, swearing, sitting up, kicking, getting out or diving out of bed, walking, running and jumping may be seen. The movements appear to represent exploratory or aggressive behaviour. These actions may injure either the subject or the bed partner. The subject resists restraint and can be violent

Table 7.10 Confusional arousal, frontal-lobe epilepsy and REM sleep behaviour disorder.

Characteristic	Confusional arousal	Frontal-lobe epilepsy	REM sleep behaviour disorder
Age	Especially children	Adults	> 50 years
Gender	M = F	M > F	M > F
Family history	Common	Occasional	Occasional
Time during night	First third	Any	Last third
Sleep stage	3 and 4 NREM	2, 3 and 4 NREM	REM
Dream content	Nil	Nil	Vivid
Recall	Nil	Nil	Intense
Behaviour	Slow complex activity, aggressive if restrained	Screams with repetitive movements	Simple and complex movements
Autonomic activation	Nil	Nil	Variable

F, female; M, male; NREM, non-rapid eye movement; REM, rapid eye movement.

and appears to feel intense emotion, but there are no sexual or feeding activities.

If awakened during the episode a vivid dream, often with an unpleasant or aggressive and violent content, is reported and similar dreams may be recalled even between the episodes of movements. Ordinary dreams are not enacted physically. Dreams are often repetitive, and involve being threatened, persecuted or confronted, leading the subject to react by fleeing or fighting back. The arousals from sleep may occasionally cause EDS if they lead to sufficiently severe sleep fragmentation.

INVESTIGATIONS

Polysomnography
This is important in establishing the diagnosis and excluding other disorders. It shows normal sleep architecture, except for an occasional increase in REM sleep duration and density, and slightly prolonged stages 3 and 4 NREM sleep. Muscle tone is maintained during some or all of REM sleep and there is an increase in phasic motor activity and generalized restlessness in REM sleep. Periodic limb movements may be seen in both REM and NREM sleep. There are no epileptic features. Video recordings show the pattern of activity.

Magnetic resonance imaging or computerized tomography head scans
These may be required to diagnose the cause of REM sleep behaviour disorder.

DIFFERENTIAL DIAGNOSIS
1 Nightmares.
2 Confusional arousals.
3 Sleep terrors.
4 Sleep walking.
5 Post-traumatic stress disorder.
6 Epilepsy.
7 Episodic nocturnal wanderings.
8 Sudden arousals from OSAs.
9 Panic attacks.

PROBLEMS
Danger to patient and partner.

TREATMENT
1 Benzodiazepines, e.g. clonazepam. These reduce muscle tone and are usually promptly effective and suppress phasic REM sleep.
2 Second-line drugs include L-dopa, tricyclic antidepressants, such as desipramine and imipramine, carbamazepine, clonidine and possibly gabapentin and L-tryptophan.
3 Protection of the patient and partner if violence appears likely. Implements that can be used aggressively should be removed from the sleeping area.

Status dissociatus
This rare disorder may represent a severe form of the REM sleep behaviour disorder, but EEG recording during sleep does not show any distinction between REM and NREM sleep, and features of wakefulness may also be seen [8]. Sleep is characterized by

frequent muscle twitches, vocalizations, and vivid dreams. Sleep is refreshing and patients do not complain of EDS.

Status dissociatus may be caused by degenerative disorders such as multiple system atrophy, and fatal familial insomnia, but may also be due to narcolepsy and withdrawal from alcohol after protracted abuse. Clonazepam is often effective.

Sleep and movement disorders of wakefulness

Effects of sleep on movement disorders

Movement disorders which are most prominent during wakefulness persist to a variable extent during sleep. The extent of the influence of sleep on these movements depends on their origin.

PSYCHOGENIC MOVEMENT DISORDERS

These disappear during sleep, except perhaps in stage 1 NREM sleep, but may reappear during arousals from sleep.

UPPER MOTOR NEURONE MOVEMENT DISORDERS

These movement disorders, such as Parkinsonism and Huntington's disease, are subject to the generalized motor inhibition of NREM and REM sleep. They are most suppressed in stages 3 and 4 NREM sleep, less prominent in REM sleep and most marked in stages 1 and 2 NREM sleep and particularly at times of arousals from sleep. This indicates that they are selectively suppressed by NREM sleep since muscle activity is normally at its least in REM rather than NREM sleep.

LOWER MOTOR NEURONE MOVEMENT DISORDERS

These conditions, such as palatal myoclonus, hemifacial spasm and fasciculations, usually persist in sleep, probably because the disorder causing the movement at least partially disrupts the supraspinal inhibition of the lower motor neurones.

Effects of movement disorders on sleep

They frequently cause EDS through leading to sleep fragmentation, but it is important to be aware of the indirect effects that they have on sleep, and to treat these appropriately. The ways in which these movement disorders influence sleep are described below.

1 Degenerative disorders disrupt sleep in a similar way to the normal changes in the elderly. Sleep efficiency and total sleep time are reduced with an increase in the number of arousals and sleep-stage transitions. Stages 3 and 4 NREM sleep are shortened. These abnormalities may improve with drug treatment of the movement disorder.

2 There may be associated sleep disorders. Huntington's disease, for instance, is associated with PLMS and RLS, and multiple system atrophy is associated with the REM behaviour disorder. Children with tics are predisposed to sleep walk and talk.

3 Some disorders, particularly the degenerative ones, are associated with respiratory abnormalities such as obstructive or central sleep apnoeas which cause sleep fragmentation.

4 There may be indirect effects on sleep due to, for instance, dementia which alters the regulation of sleep. Changes in environmental stimuli such as a reduction in exposure to light may also affect sleep control, and other factors such as depression and sleep fragmentation due to discomfort and pain are features of many of these conditions, particularly Parkinsonism.

5 Drugs used therapeutically may help to relieve the movement disorder, but may also cause other sleep disorders.

TYPES OF MOVEMENT DISORDER

Chorea

In this disorder there are frequent irregular movements which migrate from one part of the body to another and affect particularly the face and limbs. The movements are worse with activity. In Sydenham's chorea the movements can persist during REM sleep, but little is known about the other types of chorea except for that seen in Huntington's disease. This causes dementia, depression, psychosis and personality changes as well as chorea. It is steadily progressive and is due to widespread cerebral degeneration. The initial complaint is insomnia, but as the disease progresses sleep becomes increasingly fragmented with loss of sleep efficiency, increased sleep latency, increased number of arousals, and a reduction in duration of stages 3 and 4 NREM and of REM sleep. The density and amplitude of sleep spindles is increased, in contrast to Parkinsonism, possibly because of increased dopamine levels within the brain. The chorea is most prominent in stages 1 and 2 NREM sleep and during arousals and least prominent in stages 3 and 4 NREM sleep.

Unilateral chorea (hemiballism) is usually due to contralateral damage to the subthalamic nucleus or its connections, most often because of ischaemia. These movements persist in stages 1 and 2 NREM sleep and REM sleep, although both this and stages 3 and 4 NREM sleep are reduced in duration.

Myoclonus
This diverse group of conditions is characterized by abrupt jerking movements separated by a longer pause than in chorea, but the degree of sleep disruption that they cause and the effect of sleep on the movements depends on where they are generated.

Cerebral cortex. The movements are not detectable during sleep.

Basal ganglia. These movements are partially suppressed in sleep, as in Huntington's disease.

Brain-stem and spinal cord. Movements such as spinal myoclonus and palatal myoclonus persist, although their amplitude and frequency may be reduced during sleep. This suggests that some higher inhibitory control persists over the largely autonomous oscillators which are responsible for these movements, and which in palatal myoclonus probably arises in the region of the dentate nucleus. The myoclonic jerks of Startle disease (hyperekplaxia syndrome) are less intense than during wakefulness, but persist even during stages 3 and 4 NREM sleep in response to minor stimuli. The repetitive twitches of one side of the face in hemifacial spasm, which is due to damage to the facial nerve nucleus, persist, but are reduced in frequency in both stages 3 and 4 NREM sleep and REM sleep.

Torsion dystonias
This is a heterogeneous group of disorders which cause sustained distorting or twisting postures and movements, but do not appear to impair the motor inhibition of sleep. They usually persist in stages 1 and 2 NREM and REM sleep, but with a reduced frequency and amplitude of movement and then become less marked in stages 3 and 4 NREM. As they become more severe they tend to increase the fragmentation of sleep with a low sleep efficiency, long sleep latency, loss of stages 3 and 4 NREM and of REM sleep, and in some patients exaggerated sleep spindles are seen.

Tics
These are rapid, repetitive twitching movements which may be simple or complex. In the Gilles de la Tourette syndrome which arises in childhood and adolescence, multiple tics with vocalizations, including grunting and squealing noises, and often obscenities are associated with obsessive and compulsive thoughts and behaviours. The tics are most pronounced in stages 1 and 2 NREM and less obvious in REM and stages 3 and 4 NREM sleep, but the larger body movements are most frequent in REM sleep. Sleep becomes fragmented with loss of both NREM and REM sleep, and other disorders such as sleep walking are occasionally seen. Insomnia may gradually improve but sleep terrors and sleep walking are common.

Parkinsonism
This is due to degeneration and loss of dopamine in the basal ganglia and causes bradykinesia, tremor and rigidity. There are two main forms which are discussed below.

Idiopathic Parkinsonism. This may have direct effects on sleep and its control since the EEG shows a reduction in amplitude and frequency of sleep spindles which can be reversed by L-dopa therapy. Muscle tone is often increased in REM sleep with a pattern similar to REM sleep behaviour disorder and, interestingly, REM sleep onset blepharospasm is an association. Periodic limb movements in sleep are also more common in Parkinsonism than in normal subjects, and respond to L-dopa. The Parkinsonian tremor is most prominent at the moment of arousal from sleep or at transitions from a deeper to a lighter stage of sleep, and in stages 1 and 2 NREM sleep. Motor function is usually best soon after waking. It often deteriorates during the day, but the mechanism whereby sleep may be beneficial is uncertain. Idiopathic Parkinsonism is associated especially with DMS and EMW insomnia, but may cause an ASPS and even sleep reversal. Several factors contribute to these problems.

Firstly, there are fewer position shifts during sleep than in normal subjects because of difficulty in initiating movements. This may lead to discomfort and pain, and to the complaint of being unable to turn over during sleep and of difficulty in getting out of bed, for instance to urinate. There is difficulty in swallowing saliva and drooling may cause discomfort and sleep fragmentation. Leg cramps are frequent and back pain may disrupt sleep. Depression is also a common complication, especially in the later stages, and leads to insomnia. The effects of L-dopa and dopamine agonists may also cause sleep problems.

Idiopathic Parkinsonism is associated especially with DMS and EMW, but may also cause an ASPS and even sleep reversal. Several factors contribute to these problems.

Polysomnography shows, in addition to spindle abnormalities, a reduced sleep efficiency, an increase in arousals and reduction in REM sleep. These abnormalities are related to abnormal movements due partly to the movement disorder and partly to arousals from PLMS and REM behaviour disorder, and discomfort from being unable to change position. The CNS degenerative changes may also impair the sleep mechanisms and circadian rhythms leading to difficulty in maintaining sleep, which is exacerbated by depression.

The quality of sleep may be improved with good daytime control of Parkinsonism, although L-dopa, dopamine agonists and anticholinergic drugs may increase the frequency and intensity of nightmares. These side-effects are seen particularly with long-acting drugs and those taken late in the evening.

Secondary Parkinsonism. In general, patients with these disorders have the same difficulties with sleep as those with idiopathic Parkinsonism, but they have additional problems as well. The effects on sleep of post-encephalitic Parkinsonism are described in Chapter 6.

In mutliple system atrophy there is widespread CNS degeneration with loss of control of the autonomic nervous system. Insomnia occurs with frequent awakenings, reduction in stages 3 and 4 NREM sleep and especially in the olivo-ponto-cerebellar atrophy variant, loss of REM sleep duration and density, and with prolonged episodes which are difficult to classify either as NREM or REM sleep. Rapid eye movement sleep behaviour disorder may appear early in its natural history and precede other features by as long as 2–3 years. Involvement of the nucleus ambiguous impairs control of the vocal cords and leads to episodes of adduction associated with stridor and choking, often at night, but also occasionally during the day. These cause OSAs and a tracheostomy may be required. An irregular respiratory pattern with prolonged central apnoeas also develops.

In progressive supranuclear palsy (PSP) Parkinsonism is combined with a dystonic gait, a disturbance of axial rigidity and a vertical voluntary gaze palsy. Degeneration develops in the core or tegmentum of the pons and midbrain, particularly in the region of the locus coeruleus. The sleep disturbance is proportional to the degree of motor abnormalities and can be severe. Depression, nocturia and discomfort due to immobility may all contribute to the sleep disruption. The main symptoms are DMS and EMW insomnia. Polysomnography shows a reduction in total sleep time, increased sleep latency, frequent awakenings, reduction of sleep spindles, fewer REM sleep episodes and a shortened total duration of REM sleep [9]. Dream recall is reduced or absent, due to damage to the REM sleep generating mechanisms, and there is little response of the sleep disturbances to L-dopa or dopamine agonists.

References

1 Kavey NB, Whyte J, Resor SR, Gidro-Frank S. Somnambulism in adults. *Neurology* 1990; 40: 749–52.
2 Schenck CH, Mahowald MW. Review of nocturnal sleep-related eating disorders. *Int J Eat Disord* 1994; 15: 343–56.
3 Meierkord H, Fish DR, Smith SJM, Scott CA, Shorvon SD, Marsden CD. Is nocturnal paroxysmal dystonia a form of frontal lobe epilepsy? *Mov Disord* 1992; 7: 38–42.
4 Crespel A, Baldy-Moulinier M, Coubes P. The relationship between sleep and epilepsy in frontal and temporal lobe epilepsies. *Epilepsia* 1998; 39: 150–7.
5 Pollmacher T, Schulz H. Periodic leg movements (PLM): their relationship to sleep stages. *Sleep* 1993; 16: 572–7.
6 Coleman RM, Pollak CP, Weitzman ED. Periodic movements in sleep (nocturnal myoclonus): relation to sleep disorders. *Ann Neurol* 1980; 8: 416–21.
7 Sforza E, Krieger J, Petiau C. REM sleep behavior disorder: clinical and physiopathological findings. *Sleep Med Rev* 1997; 1: 57–69.
8 Mahowald MW, Schenck CH. Status dissociatus—a perspective on states of being. *Sleep* 1991; 14: 69–79.
9 Aldrich MS, Foster NL, White RF, Bluemlein L, Prokopowicz G. Sleep abnormalities in progressive supranuclear palsy. *Ann Neurol* 1989; 25: 577–81.

8 Experiences, Autonomic and Immunological Disorders in Sleep

Introduction

Experiences during sleep include abnormalities of awareness, sensations, thoughts and emotions. These are usually the presenting symptoms, and occur immediately after waking. Autonomic and immunological disorders tend to cause symptoms that are specific to the individual disorder. Nocturnal angina, for instance, usually leads to the complaint of pain, but it may also cause insomnia or excessive daytime sleepiness (EDS) by disrupting the quality and duration of sleep. All these conditions may have an impact on the bed partner and also be a source of anxiety and embarrassment. The conditions described in this chapter do not primarily involve any abnormality of behaviour during sleep or alterations in the control of skeletal muscle. These are described in Chapter 7.

Many of the phenomena observed during sleep are not diseases or disorders, but simply manifestations of the change in balance between the sleep and wake processes. These are not as distinct as is usually thought, and at any moment different parts of the brain may be functioning as if they are asleep, while others are apparently awake. Normal or near-normal events merge into those that are more clearly pathological, but the distinction between them is often hard to make and may be unnecessary.

Sleep is characterized by a decreased awareness of as well as responsiveness to, external and internal stimuli. Problems of awareness, autonomic function and motor activities during the night occur either during sleep or wakefulness, at the transition from a deeper to a lighter stage of sleep or at the moment of arousal from sleep. The threshold for arousal is highest in young children and lowest in old age and higher in stages 3 and 4 non-rapid eye movement (NREM) than in 1 and 2 NREM and rapid eye movement (REM) sleep. Arousal is a non-specific response which can be induced by any nociceptive stimulus such as a distended bladder or pain. Once arousal has taken place the nature of the stimulus and its location can be identified by the waking brain and an appropriate response made. Often, however, the arousal is only partial and an inappropriate response takes place. These events should be distinguished, if possible, from those that occur simply during wakefulness during the night. The inability to recall sensations and thoughts after the event is not a reliable indicator of whether the subject was asleep at the time.

Assessment

A careful history is essential to accurately assess awareness and autonomic and immunological activity (Chapter 4). The issues that should be considered are as follows.

The nature of the symptoms
Details of the awareness of sensations, thoughts and emotions should be sought into. The nature and vividness of dreams and the recall of any movements and other activities are important.

Assessment of the relationship of the event to sleep and wakefulness, or the transition between these
The time during the night, degree of recall, dream activity and the nature of any movements may help to establish when the episodes are occurring.

Physical examination may reveal abnormalities specific to the disorder and investigations relevant to the system involved may be required. Polysomnography is occasionally needed to establish the nature of the nocturnal episodes, for instance to distinguish gastro-oesophageal reflux from obstructive sleep apnoeas (OSA) as a cause of nocturnal choking.

Principles of treatment

The aims of treatment are as follows.
1 To explain the nature of the disorder to the subject and to reassure when appropriate.

2 To provide specific treatment for the disorder. This may be, for instance, drug treatment for asthma or nocturnal angina.

3 Modify sleep wake patterns by:

(a) sleep hygiene—the aim is to reinstate the normal sleep–wake pattern and prevent these episodes;

(b) behavioural therapy, e.g. in nocturnal enuresis;

(c) drug treatment, e.g. tricyclic antidepressants which reduce REM sleep-related episodes, such as nightmares.

Experiences during sleep

Introduction

Experiences during sleep may be recalled but once arousal has taken place the awareness of a sensation, such as pain, is strictly speaking no longer occurring in sleep, although the stimulus causing the sensation may have developed during sleep. The same applies to recall of dreams or nightmares, and sensations of choking or breathlessness with, for instance, OSA, or the feeling of a need to move the legs with periodic limb movements in sleep (PLMS) (Table 8.1).

Disorders of awareness may also have autonomic or motor features, or both. A confusional arousal is characterized by a combination of subalertness and abnormal behaviour, but in this chapter only those conditions which present primarily with abnormal sensations, thoughts and emotions, will be considered.

Wakefulness—non-rapid eye movement sleep-transition disorders

Sensory hypnic jerks

Hypnic jerks are common (page 138), but their sensory equivalents are under-recognized. A sensation of falling or occasionally floating is common, but flashes of light, or even fragments of visual hallucinations may occur, and usually accompany the motor jerk.

Auditory sensations such as snapping noises or loud bangs may be heard and may be associated with a sensation of bursting in the head. These are often frightening and are probably responsible for what has been termed the 'exploding head syndrome'. These sensations occur at the transition from wakefulness to stage 1 or 2 NREM sleep, and are followed by an arousal to wakefulness, often with a tachycardia. They may generate a fear of initiating sleep if they recur frequently.

Investigations are not usually required and reassurance is usually sufficient.

Wakefulness—rapid eye movement sleep transition disorders

Hypnagogic and hypnopompic hallucinations (pre- and post-sleep dreams)

Dreams normally occur during sleep but they may arise before any other features of sleep have developed. This occurs particularly in normal subjects who are extremely sleep deprived and during drowsiness in narcolepsy, in which they are particularly vivid. The images and forms that these presleep dreams, or hypnagogic hallucinations, take may be so realistic that it may be subsequently impossible to be sure whether the events were true or were simply dreamt. Similar dreams can occur at the transition from sleep to wakefulness, particularly at the end of the night (hypnopompic hallucinations), especially in narcolepsy. The content of these experiences is often auditory with repetitive sounds or voices, visual including shadowy outlines or shapes of people, a sense of pressure or of floating or flying, or the awareness of the presence of a person or spirit, such as a demon. The latter is often associated with fear which may be intense. 'Out of body' experiences are probably due to changes in the processing of proprioceptive sensory input and are often associated with lucid dreams and sleep paralysis.

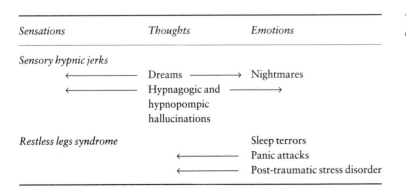

Table 8.1 Sensations, thoughts and emotions in sleep and on arousal.

Sensations	Thoughts	Emotions
Sensory hypnic jerks		
⟵———————	Dreams ⟶	Nightmares
⟵———————	Hypnagogic and hypnopompic hallucinations	⟶
Restless legs syndrome		Sleep terrors
	⟵———————	Panic attacks
	⟵———————	Post-traumatic stress disorder

Table 8.2 Dream recall.

Increased recall	Decreased recall
Pregnancy	Old age
REM rebound after sleep deprivation or drug withdrawal	Drugs
Insomnia	Progressive supra-nuclear palsy
Fever	Multiple system atrophy
Narcolepsy	Obstructive sleep apnoeas

REM, rapid eye movement.

Dream abnormalities

The neurophysiological basis of dreams has been discussed in Chapter 1, but several types of dream abnormality can develop.

ABNORMALITIES OF RECALL

Dream recall usually fades rapidly after the onset of wakefulness, suggesting that dreams are not incorporated into either short- or long-term memory (Table 8.2). Although dreaming occurs around 40 times each week, only two to three of these are usually recalled. The rate of recall falls with age, despite the percentage of REM sleep remaining constant even in the elderly. Dream recall may be absent in conditions such as progressive supranuclear palsy and multiple system atrophy, particularly the olivo-ponto-atrophy cerebellar atrophy type, in which there is pontine degeneration. Loss of dream recall is usually associated with loss of saccadic eye movements, although pursuit movements are retained. Drugs such as benzodiazepines, barbiturates and alcohol also reduce dream recall. This is uncommon in OSA despite the frequent arousals from REM sleep, probably because the extreme fragmentation of REM sleep prevents dreams from becoming fully formed. Drowsiness or even confusion on arousal may also inhibit recall of dreams.

Recall of dreams is increased in narcolepsy (because REM sleep intrudes into partial wakefulness), pregnancy, fever, insomnia (in proportion to the number of awakenings during the night) [1], and sleep deprivation with REM sleep rebound or when REM sleep rebound occurs with withdrawal of tricyclic antidepressants, benzodiazepines, barbiturates and alcohol.

DREAM VIVIDNESS

Vivid dreams are a feature of narcolepsy, the REM behaviour disorder and the post-traumatic stress disorder, as well as with drugs such as such as L-dopa

and lipophilic beta blockers such as propranolol, metoprolol, labetalol and pindolol.

DREAM THEMES

The content of dreams reflects both current preoccupations and activities, and previous experiences. These gradually become attenuated with time in normal subjects, but in the post-traumatic stress disorder, repetitive dreams recapitulating the traumatic event persist. These are associated with anxiety attacks, causing awakening from sleep and often lead to sleep deprivation and EDS.

In the REM sleep behaviour disorder the dreams are vivid and often have a violent content. Schizophrenics are said to dream particularly of strangers, but the dreams of subjects with obsessional compulsive disorders do not contain rituals similar to those that these individuals need to perform during the day.

EMOTIONAL CONTENT

The degree of pleasantness of dreams is influenced by the mood of the subject during the day time as well as recent and previous emotional experiences and concerns. Dreams tend to be sad if the dreamer is sad. During depression dreams are often negative or unpleasant, but revert to normal once the depression is treated. Dreams which cause intense anxiety are termed nightmares and are discussed separately below.

DREAM ENACTMENT

Physical acting out of dreams is uncommon, but is a feature of REM sleep behaviour disorder, and possibly delirium.

Nightmares

OVERVIEW

Nightmares are dreams which are terrifying and lead to intense anxiety on arousal from sleep. They occur in REM sleep but because of the intense motor

Characteristic	Nightmare	Sleep terror
Age of onset	Usually 3–6 years	Usually 2–6 years
Gender	M = F	M > F
Time in night	Last third	First third
Dream content	Long and complex, terrifying	Nil
Recall	Good	Very little
Behaviour	No movement	Very active
Autonomic response	Little	Intense
Post event	Orientated	Confused

Table 8.3 Nightmares and sleep terrors.

inhibition they rarely lead to any detectable movement until arousal occurs.

OCCURRENCE

They are equally common in males and females in childhood, but are more common in females in adult life. Nightmares are rare before the age of three years, but occur in 10–50% of 3–6 year olds. They become less frequent after the age of six, but are present occasionally in 40–50% of adults and less frequently in the elderly. In adults they are most common in the post-traumatic stress disorder, narcolepsy, REM sleep behaviour disorder, schizophrenia and schizoid personalities, in acute or chronic anxiety states associated with stress or during drug treatment such as L-dopa or propranolol or withdrawal of REM suppressant drugs such as tricyclic antidepressants.

PATHOGENESIS

The strong emotional content of nightmares distinguishes them from dreams, and reflects the processing of ideas and associations within the brain during REM sleep.

CLINICAL FEATURES

Nightmares are often long and complex but are only recognizable and recalled if the subject awakens from sleep. There is little autonomic overactivity and no motor enactment during the nightmare, except in REM behaviour disorder where muscle tone is retained. The subject is not confused on awakening, has vivid recall of the nightmare and often has difficulty in returning to sleep. The nightmares of the post-traumatic stress disorder have a recurrent theme which is related to the traumatic event. Nightmares occur most frequently and intensely during the last third of the night when REM sleep is more prolonged, especially after sleep deprivation which leads to REM sleep rebound.

INVESTIGATIONS

Polysomnography is rarely required but may show increased REM density for around 10 min before an abrupt awakening from the nightmare, together with some respiratory and heart rate variability. Nightmares almost invariably arise from REM sleep, but occasionally, for instance in the post-traumatic stress disorder, they may occur in stages 1 or 2 NREM sleep.

DIFFERENTIAL DIAGNOSIS

1 REM sleep behaviour disorder.
2 Nocturnal panic attacks.
3 Epilepsy in which the aura may be mistaken for a nightmare.
4 Sleep terrors, although these have little dream imagery and occur early in the night (Table 8.3).

PROBLEMS

Nightmares are frightening for the patient.

TREATMENT

Treatment is not usually required, but any drugs that predispose to nightmares, such as L-dopa or beta blockers, may need to be discontinued and those with REM sleep suppressant action should be tailed off slowly. Reduction of stresses that have precipitated the nightmares, improvement in sleep hygiene and occasionally psychotherapy may be of help. If nightmares persist, REM sleep suppressant drugs such as tricyclic anti-depressants may be required.

Autonomic disorders

Introduction

During NREM sleep parasympathetic activity predominates over sympathetic activity to an increasing extent through stages 1–4. The metabolic rate falls proportionally, but within each stage autonomic act-

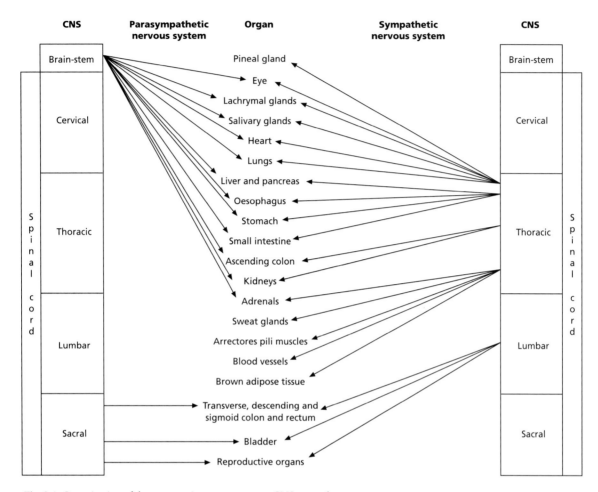

Fig. 8.1 Organization of the autonomic nervous system. CNS, central nervous system.

ivity remains fairly constant. The converse is true of REM sleep, particularly phasic REM sleep. The balance between the parasympathetic and sympathetic activity constantly changes, although overall there is still a tendency towards parasympathetic predominance compared to wakefulness (Fig. 8.1).

The autonomic disorders during sleep reflect these changes. In this section some examples of how modification of autonomic function contributes to symptoms or diseases are given, but there are many other disorders in which this plays an important part.

Neurological conditions

MIGRAINE

Migraines have a complex relationship to sleep. They are often relieved during the day by sleep, but conversely, may develop after waking from sleep, partic-

ularly REM sleep, at night. Migraines are commoner in sleep walkers and narcolepsy than in normal subjects and changes in 5HT neurotransmission may be responsible. The link between migraine and sleep may, however, reflect changes in autonomic function between sleep and wake states.

Migraines occurring on waking need to be distinguished from other causes of early morning headaches. These include those due to OSA, possibly due to raised intracranial pressure, other causes of raised intracranial pressure (see below), sleep bruxism and following alcohol intoxication.

CLUSTER HEADACHES (MIGRAINOUS NEURALGIA)

These are often intense, occur unilaterally around the eye, and are associated with lachrymation, nasal discharge and facial vasodilatation. They are 10 times more common in males than females, occur particularly between the ages of 40–60 years and last for 30–180 min. They are most frequent in spring and autumn when the change in the length of exposure to light is greatest and are also associated with low peak melatonin and cortisol blood concentrations.

Seventy-five per cent of cluster headaches occur during sleep and they often appear at the same time each night for several weeks before going into remission. They are most common in REM sleep, and metabolic activity is increased during these episodes in the cingulate gyrus and hypothalamus close to the suprachiasmatic nuclei (SCN). This probably alters the balance between parasympathetic and sympathetic systems to cause the unilateral vascular and secretory changes which underlie the clinical features. The headaches may worsen during REM sleep rebound when REM sleep suppressant drugs such as tricyclic antidepressants are discontinued.

Chronic paroxysmal hemicrania is probably a variant of cluster headaches and is associated with vasomotor symptoms. The episodes are brief and more frequent with up to 10–20 attacks occurring each 24 h. They occur at a regular time each night and are closely related to REM sleep, which they often cause to become fragmented.

The diagnosis of these conditions is based on the history. Sleep investigations such as polysomnography are rarely needed.

HYPNIC HEADACHE
This unusual condition has been described in the elderly. The headaches are diffuse and may be associated with dreaming. They occur at a consistent time each night for each individual and last for 30–60 min. They are said to be related to REM sleep but no cause has been established. They may respond to lithium.

INTRACRANIAL HYPERTENSION
The intracranial pressure rises during REM sleep, possibly because of an increase in the cerebral blood flow. If the pressure rises sufficiently it may cause a headache which leads to awakening from REM sleep, and which usually clears within 20–60 min after arousal. Distortion of the dura mater or vasodilatation, at least partly related to the action of nitric oxide, stimulates pain receptors in the intracranial vessels.

The headaches are usually bifrontal, may be associated with nausea and vomiting, and tend to occur when these physiological changes are superimposed on the changes in cerebrospinal fluid dynamics associated with space occupying intracranial lesions, severe hypertension, hypercapnia, cerebral oedema following a hypoglycaemic episode and with benign intracranial hypertension.

Cardiovascular conditions
The metabolic rate and cardiac output fall during NREM sleep and the loss of sympathetic vasoconstriction reduces the systemic vascular resistance so that the blood pressure falls. In contrast, in REM sleep autonomic control is unstable. Fluctuations in heart rate and blood pressure are common and the cerebral blood flow increases. These changes protect against some cardiovascular problems during sleep, but predispose to others.

CARDIAC DYSRHYTHMIAS
The increased parasympathetic activity in sleep reduces the heart rate and atrioventricular node conduction, and increases the threshold for ventricular fibrillation. The heart rate accelerates at the moment of an arousal through an increase in sympathetic activity.

Prolonged sinus arrests may be seen in REM sleep, particularly in young males. Asystole for up to 2.5 s is conventionally regarded as normal, but this may be as long as 9 s in otherwise healthy subjects, probably because of an increase in parasympathetic activity. This is probably a normal variant, although it has been termed the 'REM sleep-related sinus arrest' syndrome. Sinus dysrhythmia is also prominent in young males, particularly during phasic REM sleep, and occasionally even Mobitz Type 1 second-degree atrioventricular block may occur.

In general, sleep tends to prevent supraventricular tachycardias, paroxysmal atrial fibrillation and ventricular dysrhythmias, especially in stages 3 and 4 NREM sleep. Ventricular ectopics are frequent on arousal from sleep, presumably due to increased sympathetic activity and can be prevented by beta blockers. Sudden death presumed to be cardiac in origin is most common between 7.00 and 11.00 AM and may be associated with the increase in sympathetic activity and circulating catecholamines after sleep leading to ventricular tachycardia and fibrillation. Hypoxia associated with OSA or chronic lung disease may also cause dysrhythmias.

These dysrhythmias can present with arousals and awareness of palpitations, breathlessness or angina, but they are often asymptomatic. Continuous 24-h electrocardiogram (ECG) recording is required to establish the diagnosis, but polysomnography is rarely needed. Drug treatment depends on the type of dysrhythmia.

HYPERTENSION

The blood pressure normally falls by 5–15% during NREM sleep, but to a lesser extent and in a much more variable fashion during REM sleep, in which both the cardiac output and peripheral vascular resistance fluctuate considerably. The dip in blood pressure during sleep is often absent when hypertension is present during wakefulness, possibly because of persistence of sympathetic vasoconstrictor over-activity.

The blood pressure rises rapidly on waking, either during a brief arousal from sleep or at the end of the sleep episode at night. This and blood pressure fluctuations during sleep may contribute to the increased risk of stroke. The risk is greatest in OSA where the rapidly alternating parasympathetic and sympathetic activity leads to transient rises in blood pressure of up to 50%. Strokes are most frequent between 6.00 and 9.00 AM and the increase in circulating catecholamines and in platelet aggregation on waking may contribute to this.

ANGINA AND MYOCARDIAL INFARCTION

Cardiac ischaemia is common in sleep, particularly during the second half of the night. It is more often silent (asymptomatic) than during exercise. During sleep, cardiac output falls as a result of a slower heart rate rather than any change in stroke volume. In NREM sleep, blood pressure also falls and the drop in perfusing pressure reduces the coronary artery blood flow. An exaggeration of this hypotension (over dipping), especially in stages 3 and 4 NREM sleep, may cause clinically significant cardiac ischaemia, especially in the presence of coronary artery disease. Despite this, NREM sleep is largely cardio-protective because of the low metabolic rate and the low and constant cardiac output.

In REM sleep, however, the major change is that the myocardial oxygen requirements increase. Sympathetic activity is enhanced, although erratically, and there is vasoconstriction within the skeletal muscles. The heart rate, blood pressure and peripheral vascular resistance all rise, but are unstable. Depression of sleep time (ST) segments of the electrocardiogram by more than 1 mm is frequent and angina is also more common in REM than in NREM sleep. Rapid eye movement sleep is also associated with the Prinzmetal variant angina in which coronary

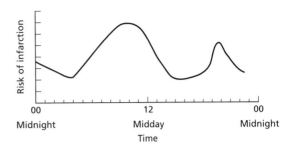

Fig. 8.2 Timing of myocardial infarction.

artery spasm, presumably due to a shift towards sympathetic dominance, leads to ST segment elevation. This is commonest between 4.00 and 8.00 AM.

The process of awakening is probably even more of a risk for cardiac ischaemia than REM sleep. The chance of a myocardial infarction rises between 4.00 and 9.00 AM and is three times more common at this time than in the evening (Fig. 8.2). Unstable angina and sudden cardiac death both show a similar pattern. This is probably due to increased sympathetic activity, increased platelet activation and aggregability and an increase in the fibrinogen level together with the onset of physical exertion which raises the blood pressure and heart rate. The coronary artery vasoconstriction, together with changes in heart rate and blood pressure probably lead to plaque rupture which triggers the thrombotic process.

Obstructive sleep apnoeas can also induce cardiac ischaemia especially in REM sleep. This is partly due to hypoxia, but also to shift of the interventricular septum to the left as the right ventricle dilates. This reduces the volume of the left ventricle during systole, reduces the left ventricular compliance and increases its work. Increase in sympathetic activity also contributes to ischaemia by causing coronary artery vasoconstriction. Angina occurs occasionally, but cardiac dysrhythmias are more common (page 202).

Coronary artery bypass grafting is usually followed by insomnia which gradually improves over several weeks or months and occasionally for up to 2 years. The total ST is reduced together with a reduction in the duration of stages 3 and 4 NREM sleep [2]. These changes may be partly due to postoperative anxiety and pain, and poor sleep hygiene, due, for instance, to noise in the hospital ward, but also to cerebral dysfunction due to the general anaesthetic and extracorporeal circulation.

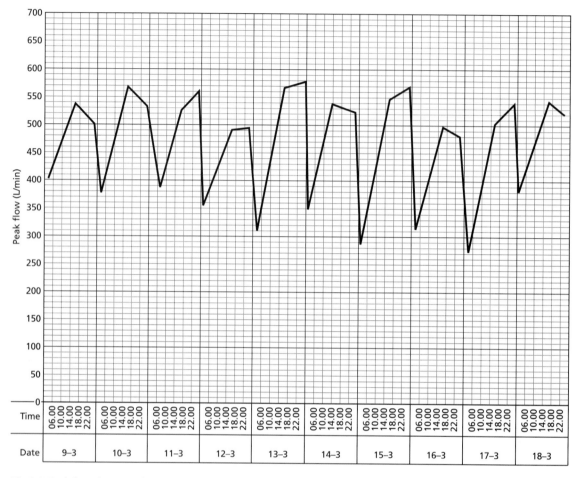

Fig. 8.3 Peak flow chart in asthma showing diurnal pattern with early morning dips.

CARDIAC FAILURE AND CHEYNE–STOKES
RESPIRATION

Left heart failure causing orthopnoea at night has
been recognized for many years. It is related to the
altered hydrostatic forces in the lungs in the supine
position. Reduced ventricular function leads to a slow
circulation time and predisposes to Cheyne–Stokes
respiration (CSR). This may cause arousals from sleep
leading to insomnia and EDS (Chapter 9).

Cheyne–Stokes respiration may also cause cardiac
complications. The oscillations in hypoxia and
increase in sympathetic activity lead to changes in
heart rate and blood pressure which cause fluctuations in the cardiac output and coronary artery blood
flow which may lead to cardiac ischaemia.

Respiratory conditions

The changes in respiration which affect the respirat-

ory pump are described in Chapter 9 and upper airway disorders in Chapter 10. This section covers only
those conditions in which the autonomic control of
lung function is important.

ASTHMA

Asthma is characterized by a widespread but variable
increase in airflow resistance together with hyperinflation of the lungs. It has a circadian rhythm irrespective of the many environmental factors that affect
its severity (Fig. 8.3) [3]. Nocturnal asthma may cause
frequent arousals from sleep, particularly after the
first cycle of NREM and REM sleep and it may lead to
EDS. The arousals are partly due to the increased
work of breathing, but also to frequent coughing and
they improve once the asthma is controlled.

The lowest peak flow rates in asthmatics are recorded at around 4.00 AM. There is a normal circadian

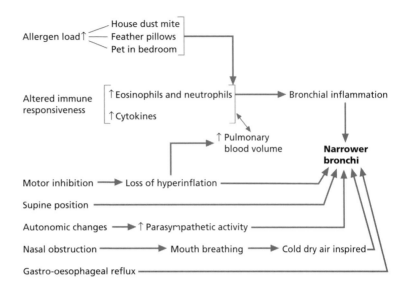

Fig. 8.4 Causes of nocturnal asthma.

fluctuation in peak flow rates of less than 10–15% with the highest values at around 4.00 PM, but this is exaggerated in asthmatics perhaps with a slight shift in the time of the lowest peak flow rates as well.

The cause of the increase in amplitude of the airflow obstruction changes is uncertain (Fig. 8.4). It is probably not primarily related to the onset of sleep itself since the peak flow rates fall even if the subject remains awake at night, although the fall is greater during sleep. The changes are not related to any particular sleep stage, but a major factor appears to be the reduction in lung volume. This is probably due to the generalized inhibition of motor activity during sleep, particularly REM sleep, which leads to relaxation of the chest wall muscles with abolition of any reflex hyperinflation in response to airflow obstruction and failure to respond to any intrapulmonary reflexes during sleep which would increase the lung volume. As the lung volume falls the diameter of the airways decreases and if they are already narrowed, the increase in airflow resistance may be considerable. The reduction in lung volume is greater in the supine position, but posture by itself is not the only factor since there is still a circadian fluctuation even if the subjects lie in bed continuously throughout the 24 h.

During sleep the intrapulmonary blood volume increases. This reduces the volume of air within the lungs slightly, but more importantly increases the number of inflammatory cells and the quantity of mediators within the lung. This increases the potential for any bronchial inflammation. Broncho-alveolar lavage has shown more eosinophils and neutrophils

in the aspirate at 4.00 AM than at 4.00 PM and the quantity of cytokines, for instance IL-1β, is also increased. Transbronchial biopsies have shown an increase in the eosinophilic alveolar infiltrate at night in proportion to the severity of nocturnal asthma. The increase in lung inflammation does not appear to be related to nocturnal changes in cortisol levels, or to serum IgE which peaks at midday, but the antigen load due to house dust mite is increased at night.

There are several other factors which could affect airway function at night in asthma. Firstly, the increase in parasympathetic activity causes bronchoconstriction and the importance of this is indicated by the degree of improvement which can be obtained with atropinic drugs at night. The lower blood levels of adrenaline at night compared to the day time are probably not significant, but the increased nasal resistance associated with the alternating changes in the patency of the right and left nasal airways (nasal cycle) may cause mouth breathing which leads to cool, dry air entering the lungs, which can induce asthma. Gastro-oesophageal reflux is also common during sleep and this can cause reflex bronchoconstriction. Temperature changes in the bedroom and exposure to allergens, such as feathers in pillows and the hair or fur of pets who may have slept in the bedroom, may also exacerbate the nocturnal tendency of asthma to worsen, but are not usually the prime cause.

Respiratory failure due to asthma usually occurs at night partly because asthma is more severe during sleep, but also because of abnormalities of respiratory control. Asthmatics at risk of developing respiratory

Headaches	Cluster headache, raised intracranial pressure, e.g. hypercapnia, hypnic headache
Chest pain	Angina, myocardial infarction, gastro-oesophageal reflux, oesophageal spasm, peptic ulcer
Breathlessness	Asthma, left ventricular failure, bilateral diaphragmatic paralysis, CSR, CSA, OSA
Cough	Asthma, post nasal drip, gastro-oesophageal reflux
Choking	OSA, pharyngeal pooling of saliva, gastro-oesophageal reflux, vocal cord adduction asthma, left ventricular failure
Nocturia	OSA, prostatic hypertrophy, renal disease, diabetes mellitus or insipidus

Table 8.4 Sleep-related causes of some common symptoms.

CSA, central sleep apnoeas; CSR, Cheyne–Stokes respiration; OSA, obstructive sleep apnoeas.

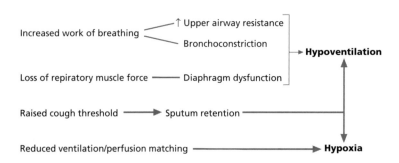

Fig. 8.5 Effects of sleep on chronic obstructive pulmonary disease (COPD).

failure often have a reduced hypoxic and hypercapnic ventilatory response to bronchoconstriction and some also increase their inspiratory time which reduces the time available for expiration and so predisposes to air trapping.

The differential diagnosis of nocturnal asthma includes left ventricular failure, OSA, choking during sleep due to, for instance, gastro-oesophageal reflux, and occasionally nocturnal angina (Table 8.4). Nocturnal cough due to asthma should be distinguished from a postnasal drip and gastro-oesophageal reflux.

It is not only important to avoid any factors that may precipitate nocturnal asthma, but also to use long-acting drug treatments which last throughout the night. Care should be taken with theophyllines and systemic glucocorticoids which, although they are often effective in relieving nocturnal asthma, can also cause insomnia.

CHRONIC BRONCHITIS AND EMPHYSEMA
(CHRONIC OBSTRUCTIVE PULMONARY DISEASE)
In chronic bronchitis and emphysema (chronic obstructive pulmonary disease, COPD) the arterial Po_2

falls during sleep, partly due to hypoventilation which leads to a rise in the arterial Pco_2 and partly to worsening of ventilation and perfusion matching within the lungs. The cardiac output is maintained, but the pulmonary artery pressure rises, because of hypoxic vasoconstriction. Rapid eye movement sleep is initially fragmented and later there is loss of stages 3 and 4 NREM sleep. Chronic hypoxia may lead to polycythaemia, hypercapnia during wakefulness and other physiological changes described in Chapter 9.

The essential physiological feature of chronic bronchitis and emphysema is expiratory air flow limitation (Fig. 8.5). The expiratory phase is prolonged and if it cannot be completed before the onset of the next inspiration, air trapping with intrinsic positive end expiratory pressure (PEEP) develops. The impaired ventilation–perfusion matching requires an increase in the ventilation to normalize gas exchange, but the pattern of respiratory rate and tidal volume adopted by the patient fluctuates continuously. The reduced lung compliance and hyperinflation increase the work of breathing and also reduce the length of the inspiratory muscles, particularly the diaphragm, and thereby impair their effectiveness.

During sleep the upper airway narrows, particularly in REM rather than NREM sleep, increasing the airflow resistance. This prolongs the inspiratory time, thereby reducing the expiratory time, and increasing the risk of air trapping and intrinsic PEEP. The alternative strategies of reducing the tidal volume (hypopnoea) or of slowing the respiratory rate both lead to alveolar hypoventilation.

The combination of upper-airway obstruction with chronic airflow limitation has been termed the 'overlap syndrome', although this term is of little value. The combination of these two conditions predisposes to hypercapnia, both during sleep and wakefulness. This is partly because the airflow obstruction prevents the respiratory muscles from normalizing the blood gases rapidly enough after arousal and before the next apnoea, and because once hypercapnia is established during the night it leads to hypercapnia while awake as well. This sequence of events can be suspected if daytime hypercapnia occurs when the forced expiratory volume in one second (FEV1) is greater than about 1.0–1.5 l.

Diaphragmatic dysfunction during sleep is related to hyperinflation, in which the diaphragm shortens and alters its configuration so that it contracts horizontally and draws the lateral rib cage inwards instead of expanding it. These ineffective contractions are particularly important in REM sleep when the diaphragm is the only active inspiratory chest wall muscle. Prolonged and deep oxygen desaturations associated with hypercapnia may result.

A third factor is the fall in lung volume during REM sleep which increases airflow resistance, reduces ventilation–perfusion matching and leads to an increase in the work of breathing and a fall in the Po_2. The higher cough threshold during REM sleep and the deeper stages of NREM sleep predisposes to retention of secretions in the airways which increases the airflow resistance and the work of breathing.

These changes are superimposed on a fluctuating chemoreceptor drive in response to rapid micro-oscillations in the arterial Pco_2 and Po_2 and changes in the activation of mechanoreceptors according to the tidal volume, respiratory rate and airflow during each breath. The Po_2 is often located near the inflection point of the oxyhaemoglobin dissociation curve so that any slight fall causes a disproportionately large oxygen desaturation compared to normal.

The central sleep apnoea (CSA) and OSA that result from these abnormalities cause repeated arousals and fragmentation of sleep. Rapid eye movement sleep is particularly shortened and fragmented, and later in the natural history stages 3 and 4 NREM sleep are similarly affected. Hypercapnia occurs, particularly in REM, and later in NREM sleep as well. Arousals may be associated with a sensation of breathlessness on waking, and lead to EDS. Early morning headaches due to carbon dioxide retention may appear. Most patients prefer to sit upright rather than lie flat, in order to optimize diaphragmatic function.

The approach to treatment is similar to that described in Chapter 9 for nocturnal respiratory complications due to neuromuscular and skeletal disorders. Long-term oxygen treatment is advisable if the Po_2 remains persistently below around 7.3 kPa during the day and night, but if this is associated with significant daytime hypercapnia (Pco_2 greater than about 8 kPa) ventilatory support with or without supplemental oxygen is preferable. Improvement in survival, symptoms and in the physiological abnormalities has been demonstrated. The ventilator should be set with a slow respiratory rate, short inspiratory time, high inspiratory flow-rate, small tidal volume, long expiratory time and PEEP, together with a sensitive triggering system in order to coordinate the patient's respiratory activity with the ventilator and to minimize the risk of air trapping.

PARENCHYMAL DISORDERS

The effects of these on sleep has been very little studied, but interstitial lung diseases can cause frequent arousals from sleep. The respiratory frequency, which is rapid during wakefulness, hardly changes during NREM sleep. In REM sleep an unstable respiratory pattern appears and leads to oxygen desaturations which are often considerable because of the low initial Po_2 which is often close to the inflection point of the oxyhaemoglobin dissociation curve. These desaturations are, however, usually less marked than during exercise. They may be relieved either by treatment of the lung disease itself or by supplemental oxygen at night. This is often needed during the day as well. Ventilatory support is rarely required.

Gastro-intestinal conditions

SWALLOWING DISORDERS

The flow of saliva almost ceases during sleep, and the frequency of swallowing falls, particularly in stages 3 and 4 NREM sleep. Each swallow is associated with a brief arousal.

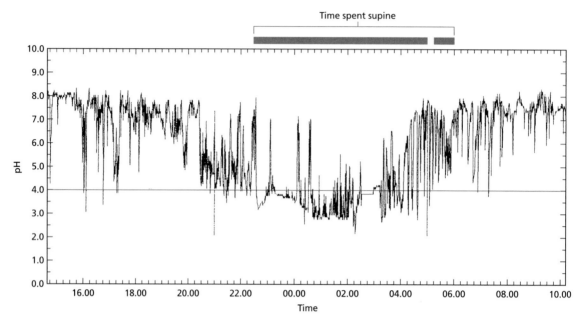

Fig. 8.6 Oesophageal pH recording showing acid reflux in sleep. The oesophageal pH frequently falls below 4 at night, whereas it rarely does so during the day.

Waking with a sensation of choking due to pooling of saliva in the pharynx occasionally occurs in elderly subjects. It appears to be unrelated to gastro-oesophageal reflux, but is precipitated by hypnotic and other central nervous system (CNS) depressant drugs. It probably reflects a deterioration in the swallowing mechanism with age and which is amplified by sleep. This condition has been termed the 'sleep-related abnormal swallowing syndrome'.

Choking during sleep has several other causes. The most common is vocal cord adduction triggered by gastro-oesophageal reflux (see below). Waking feeling unable to breathe in or out or to speak is often terrifying. The sensation of choking is located in the throat and may last for a few seconds or up to half a minute. There is often a need to get out of bed and occasionally consciousness may be lost. The attacks may recur several times over a few weeks, before going into remission. They can be relieved by anti-acid secretion preparations, e.g. proton pump inhibitors. These episodes may be similar to the sensation of choking with OSA (although these are usually briefer), nocturnal asthma (which can occasionally affect the larynx as well as the trachea and bronchi), and vocal cord adduction, due to, for instance, motor neurone disease. The 'sleep choking syndrome' probably does not exist as a discrete entity.

GASTRO-OESOPHAGEAL REFLUX

This is more common during sleep than wakefulness. The lower oesophageal sphincter tone is reduced during sleep, and gastric fluid can reflux into the oesophagus, particularly in the supine position. The tone of the upper oesophageal sphincter (cricopharyngeus) may also fall during sleep, allowing oesophago-pharyngeal reflux.

The refluxed gastric acid may stay in contact with the oesophageal and pharyngeal mucosa for prolonged periods because of the infrequency of swallowing and this slow clearance of acid contributes to oesophagitis. If swallowing does occur more readily it may lead to sufficiently frequent arousals to cause EDS. Reflux can be diagnosed by continuous oesophageal pH recordings which show the duration as well as the extent of the fall in pH (Fig. 8.6). The frequency of episodes of reflux is usually taken as the number in which the pH remains less than 4 for at least 12 s.

Nocturnal gastro-oesophageal reflux may cause sudden awakening due to retrosternal pain due to oesophagitis, or occasionally choking caused by vocal cord adduation, coughing or wheezing. These latter symptoms are due to reflex induced asthma due to reflux of acid into the distal oesophagus and, less commonly, to a direct effect of the refluxed fluid on the airways. The negative intra thoracic pressures during each OSA facilitate acid reflux. Diffuse oesophageal spasm is also most common during sleep and causes arousal with chest pain.

PEPTIC ULCERATION

Gastric acid secretion is partly under parasympathetic control. Basal secretion reaches a peak between 9.00 PM and 2.00 AM is not closely related to NREM or REM sleep. In patients with duodenal ulcers the secretion of gastric acid increases both during the day and at night compared to normals. This can be abolished by a vagotomy indicating that autonomic changes both during awake and asleep contribute to these abnormalities.

Epigastric pain may cause awakening which usually occurs 1–4 h after the onset of sleep, and may be relieved by food. The differential diagnosis includes nocturnal angina. Upper gastro-intestinal endoscopy may be required to establish the diagnosis.

INTESTINAL MOTILITY DISORDERS

The contractions of the stomach are less frequent in sleep and gastric emptying is slower than during wakefulness. This probably also applies to the small and large intestines. The changes in motility may underlie the worsening of abdominal pain at night in the irritable bowel syndrome. Colonic motility is particularly reduced in stages 3 and 4 NREM sleep and its reduction during sleep is associated with the infrequent need to defaecate and the common requirement for this soon after wakening, particularly after food. Nocturnal diarrhoea is a feature of extensive inflammation in, for instance, ulcerative colitis, and of diabetes when this causes an autonomic neuropathy. This may modify the control of bowel motility or secretion of bile salts during sleep.

Genito-urinary tract disorders

NOCTURNAL ENURESIS (BED WETTING, ENURESIS NOCTURNA)

Overview

Nocturnal enuresis is the persistent involuntary incontinence of urine during sleep after the age of 5 years. It usually represents a transient phase of inadequate neurological control over the detrusor muscle of the bladder.

Occurrence

It is slightly more frequent in males than females. It is more common in monozygotic twins and is often familial. It affects 15% of children at the age of 5 years, 10% at 6 years and 5% at 10 years, but is rare in adults unless there is an organic cause.

Pathogenesis

Nocturnal enuresis is probably due to an immaturity of the CNS which fails to inhibit contraction of the detrusor muscle. Once this generates a sufficiently high pressure within the bladder, involuntary relaxation of the bladder neck occurs and this is followed by micturition. The failure to inhibit the detrusor may be provoked by stress or other psychological problems. Some subjects may also have a small or non-compliant bladder which contributes to nocturnal urinary frequency. Failure to arouse from stages 3 and 4 NREM sleep, which is more prolonged and consolidated in children than in adults, may also predispose to enuresis.

Clinical features

Nocturnal enuresis is normal up to the age of around 5 years, but not after this age if it is persistent and frequent or if control of micturition has been acquired during wakefulness. It is often exacerbated by family stresses or over attentiveness to the problem of bed wetting. Sedative drugs may exacerbate it by impairing neurological control of the bladder during sleep. The child may awaken unaware of having wet the bed and dreams relating to bed wetting may follow rather than cause the event. In children enuresis tends to occur during the first third of the night and may be associated with other conditions such as OSA and respond to treatment of these.

Investigations

Polysomnography is not required to make the diagnosis, but often reveals partial or complete arousals, usually from stages 3 and 4 NREM, occasionally from 1 and 2 NREM, and least commonly from REM sleep. Sleep cystometry shows an increase in bladder reactivity to external stimuli and an increase in detrusor muscle contraction prior to micturition. The pressure within the bladder rises to a level which is sufficient to trigger involuntary micturition during wakefulness and therefore probably during sleep as well.

Differential diagnosis

1 Anatomical abnormalities, e.g. bladder neck obstruction, ureteric stenosis. These often cause daytime enuresis or sleep enuresis after a period of continence has been established (secondary enuresis).

2 Vesico-ureteric reflux. This is often associated with detrusor instability and detrusor-sphincter incoordination which leads to enuresis.

3 Central nervous system abnormalities, e.g. lumbar spinal cord disorders.

4 Acquired disorders, e.g. recurrent urinary tract infections.

5 Disorders causing increased volume of urine, e.g. diabetes mellitus, diabetes insipidus, OSA.

6 Nocturnal epilepsy causing urinary incontinence.

Problems

1 Embarrassment, particularly for older children.

2 Secondary psychological reactions.

Treatment

1 Treat any contributory factor, e.g. OSA.

2 Discontinue hypnotic drugs.

3 Reduce oral fluid intake in the evenings and avoid any diuretics, such as caffeine, in drinks.

4 Family support.

5 Training methods:

  (a) bladder training exercise during wakefulness, such as attempting to hold increasing volumes of urine before micturition;

  (b) sphincter training exercises involving repeatedly interrupting the urinary stream while micturating;

  (c) conditioning methods involving, for instance, alarms which are triggered by urination which wake the child. This leads to an increase in the awareness of incontinence and earlier sensing of detrusor muscle activity; and

  (d) arousal techniques involving setting an alarm at regular intervals during the night before bedwetting occurs so that the child can urinate before the bladder fills.

6 Drug treatment. This may be used to stabilize the detrusor muscle, e.g. oxybutynin, tricyclic antidepressants and nasal desmopressin, a synthetic analogue of vasopressin (antidiuretic hormone, ADH) may reduce the volume of urine even in the absence of diabetes insipidus. These drugs should only be used in children over the age of 7 years, for courses of less than 3 months and after other therapies have been tried.

IMPAIRED SLEEP-RELATED PENILE ERECTIONS

Penile erections occur predominately during REM sleep, although they may persist into NREM sleep and after awakening. They become less frequent and briefer from childhood onwards but in adults their absence indicates either an alteration in sleep architecture with reduction or fragmentation of REM sleep, as in OSA and PLMS, or an organic cause for impotence. This may be diabetes mellitus or drugs including selective serotonin re-uptake inhibitors (SSRI) and tricyclic antidepressants, beta blockers and REM-suppressant drugs, including amphetamines and related drugs. Erections during sleep and on waking are retained with most psychogenic causes of impotence.

PAINFUL PENILE ERECTIONS

In this rare condition erections during sleep cause a deep penile pain, whereas those during wakefulness, such as during intercourse, are painless [4]. The pain is most intense and prolonged during the second half of the night when REM sleep is most prominent, although the erections are often more prolonged than normal and less closely linked to REM sleep so that they extend into NREM sleep. They may cause frequent nocturnal awakenings with fragmentation, particularly of REM sleep. They appear to be triggered by anxiety, particularly regarding sexual relationships, and fluctuate in severity, often remitting spontaneously.

They are not associated with Peyronie's disease, which causes penile pain during erections in wakefulness as well as sleep, and in which the pain is related to local anatomical abnormalities. Benzodiazepines and beta blockers may be of help, possibly through relieving anxiety, but there is usually only a temporary response to antidepressants.

Renal disorders

There is considerable diurnal variation in renal function. Water and sodium are, for instance, retained at night and of the 1–2 l of urine that is normally excreted in the 24 h, around 80% is produced during the day. This diurnal rhythm is, however, abolished or even reversed in chronic renal disease, adrenal gland insufficiency and in the presence of oedema. This leads to the symptom of nocturia which may also occur if there is bladder outflow obstruction, due, for instance, to prostatic hypertrophy.

The diurnal fluctuation in renal function may also be related to the tendency for episodes of gout to arise during sleep. Most of the uric acid which is produced by purine metabolism is excreted through the kidneys and a reduction in urate clearance at night may be responsible for hyperuricaemia.

Cutaneous disorders

NIGHT SWEATS (SLEEP HYPERHIDROSIS)

There are two to four million cutaneous eccrine sweat glands which are innervated by the sympathetic nervous system with acetylcholine as the neurotransmitter. The volume and tonicity of the sweat is controlled largely by the preoptic nucleus in the hypothalamus in order to regulate the body temperature.

Night sweats may be a physiological response to a rise in temperature, but many normal subjects complain of excess sweating at night without any demonstrable fever. This is probably due to an increased sympathetic stimulation of sweat glands and is often related to anxiety or stress, or is a response to sleep disorders such as OSA. Menopausal night sweats are related to fluctuations in blood oestrogen levels.

Sweating at night can lead to frequent awakenings from sleep. Treatment is unsatisfactory, except for the sweats related to the menopause which respond to oestrogen replacement treatment. If night sweats are drenching and require frequent changes of night clothes either extensive tuberculosis or a lymphoma, such as Hodgkin's disease, should be suspected.

NOCTURNAL PRURITUS (ITCH)

Pruritus during sleep may be due to an identifiable skin disorder, but often occurs in the absence of this. It is most common in stages 1 and 2 NREM sleep and is probably secondary to cutaneous vasodilatation. It may also occur during REM sleep, but is least frequent in stages 3 and 4 NREM sleep. Sedating antihistamines, such as chlorpheniramine, are usually effective.

Immunological disorders and infections

The changes in immune function in sleep are less well documented than the autonomic changes, but the blood eosinophil and cortisol levels, and natural killer (NK) cell activity fluctuate with a circadian pattern. There is a relationship between melatonin, cytokines and interferon, all of which have immunological actions and influence sleep. The T-lymphocyte level rises in sleep, but the peripheral blood monocyte concentration falls, largely because the cells are sequestered in the spleen. In additon, changes in autonomic activity regulate the local immune responses through, for instance, alterations in regional blood flow. Peripheral release of cytokines may also affect sleep through stimulation of vagal afferents which reach the brain-stem as well as through direct transfer across the blood–brain barrier.

Immune responses are also affected by acute sleep deprivation. This increases the white blood cell count and the number of killer lymphocytes, reduces antibody production and may increase the frequency of infections. Alterations in melatonin secretion or autonomic activity may be responsible for these changes.

Fever and infections

The immune responses to fever and infections and the changes in sleep that these cause are described on page 134.

Systemic mastocytosis

This rare disorder is associated with profound lethargy, possibly due to liberation of sleep promoting mediators such as PGD2 from mast cells.

Paroxysmal nocturnal haemoglobinuria

In this uncommon condition lysis of red blood cells intravascularly during sleep leads to nocturnal haemoglobinuria. It usually presents with the passing of red or brown urine after waking or with symptoms of anaemia. The condition is equally common in males and females and occurs usually between the ages of 20–40 years. The red cells are deficient in CD59 and HRF proteins which inhibit the C9 fraction of complement from binding to the cell membrane. C5 convertase complexes, produced by the alternative pathway of complement activation, bind to the cells. The lack of CD59 and HRF leaves the cells vulnerable to insertion of terminal complement components, especially C9, into the membrane and this leads to cell lysis. This occurs particularly at night but it is uncertain how sleep influences these events.

Sudden infant death syndrome

Sudden infant death syndrome (SIDS) is a heterogeneous disorder that affects children, usually between the age of 2 and 4 months. It is thought to occur only during sleep and is common in premature infants and in the winter. It usually follows or is associated with an upper-respiratory infection. Similar apparently life-threatening events (ALTE) occur, but the child recovers fully.

The cause of SIDS has never been satisfactorily explained despite intense investigation. It is probably multifactorial and the relative contributions of each component are likely to differ in each child. It has been thought to be due to sleep apnoeas associated with immaturity of the respiratory control system. Apnoeas of prematurity are more common if the birth weight is low, but are less frequent at postconception ages of greater than 40 weeks, which is when SIDS usually occurs. Congenital malformations of the mandible may cause OSA and defects in the medullary respiratory centres could lead to central apnoeas, but the link between these and SIDS has never been firmly demonstrated.

Another possibility is that an abnormal immune response during sleep to aspiration of small quantities of allergens, such as cow's milk protein, into the tracheo-bronchial tree could result in a local anaphylactic reaction in the small airways leading to their obstruction [5]. The altered immune response during sleep could be related to the secretion of melatonin which begins around this age, and immaturity of the CNS may lead to a failure to arouse or to increase ventilation in response to the sudden change in air-flow resistance. There may also be an abnormality of small airway function associated with the increase in smooth muscle which has been demonstrated.

References

1 Schredl M, Schafer G, Weber B, Heuser I. Dreaming and insomnia: dream recall and dream content of patients with insomnia. *J Sleep Res* 1998; 7: 191–8.

2 Edéll-Gustafsson UM, Hetta JE, Arén CB, Hamrin EKF. Measurement of sleep and quality of life before and after coronary artery bypass grafting: a pilot study. *Int J Nurs Prac* 1997; 3: 239–46.

3 Martin RJ, Banks-Schlegel S. Chronobiology of asthma. *Am J Respir Crit Care Med* 1998; 158: 1002–7.

4 Calvet U. Painful nocturnal erection. *Sleep Med Rev* 1999; 3: 47–57.

5 Coombs RRA, Holgate ST. Allergy and cot death: with special focus on allergic sensitivity to cows' milk and anaphylaxis. *Clin Exp Allergy* 1990; 20: 359–66.

9 Respiratory Pump Disorders

Introduction

The respiratory pump comprises the muscles, bones and soft tissues of the chest wall, including both the rib cage and the abdomen, their controlling mechanisms in the brain and spinal cord and the peripheral nerves. It provides the force required to draw air through the upper and lower airways into and out of the gas-exchanging areas of the lungs. The control of the respiratory pump during sleep differs from wakefulness and this has important consequences for oxygen uptake and carbon dioxide elimination.

The origin of the respiratory rhythmicity lies in the medulla. Two main groups of neurones have been identified. The dorsal respiratory group (DRG) is situated in the ventro-lateral nucleus of the solitary tract and receives afferent impulses from the vagus nerve and other sources, and integrates information from the chemoreceptors and lung receptors. The respiratory rhythm generator is probably located in the DRG which projects to the ventral respiratory group (VRG) which is located close to the nucleus ambiguus and extends throughout the length of the medulla. It innervates all the main respiratory muscles through bulbo-spinal fibres. These reach the phrenic nerve nucleus in C3 to C5 segments and other motor nuclei.

The medullary respiratory centres are influenced by impulses from several types of receptors. Chemoreceptors sensitive to hypoxia are located in the carotid bodies and their impulses travel along the carotid sinus nerve, a branch of the glossopharyngeal nerve, to the DRG. Chemoreceptors sensitive to changes in pH, and thereby indirectly to PCO_2, are located both in the carotid bodies and near to the ventro-lateral surface of the medulla. These respond to changes in the pH of the cerebrospinal fluid. Hypoxia or hypercapnia increase respiration either through increasing the tidal volume or raising the respiratory frequency. A similar effect results from stimulation of mechanoreceptors in the upper and lower airways, muscles, joints and tendons of the chest wall and in the lung parenchyma. Respiration may also be modified by impulses from cough receptors, which are mainly in the large airways, and from other receptors, particularly those leading to the sensation of pain.

The medullary respiratory centres are influenced by descending impulses from the cerebral cortex and by a variety of brain-stem centres. Inactivity of the cerebral cortex during NREM sleep leaves the medullary centres predominantly under reflex control, but in REM sleep the cortex is irregularly active.

The limitations imposed on the respiratory pump by neuromuscular, thoracic cage and pulmonary disorders are often exposed in sleep before they appear in wakefulness, despite a reduction in the metabolic rate of up to 10–25% during sleep. This fall is due both to a reduction in body temperature at the onset of sleep and to inhibition of motor activity, particularly during rapid eye movement (REM) sleep. In normal subjects alveolar ventilation is reduced slightly more than the metabolic rate since the arterial PCO_2 rises by about 0.5 kPa. The greater fall in PO_2 of 0.5–2.5 kPa reflects worsening of ventilation and perfusion matching in the lungs.

The blood gas changes differ in non-rapid eye movement (NREM) and REM sleep according to the modifications in respiratory control and pattern of activation of the respiratory muscles that occur in each of these sleep states (Fig. 9.1). In this chapter the effects of sleep on the respiratory pump and its disorders are examined. Respiration during sleep in lung disorders, in which changes in the autonomic nervous system are prominent, are discussed in Chapter 8 and the disorders of the upper airway are detailed in Chapter 10.

Respiration in rapid eye movement sleep

Arousal in response to stimulation from mechanoreceptors in the lungs, airways and chest wall, cough receptors and chemoreceptors occurs at a higher

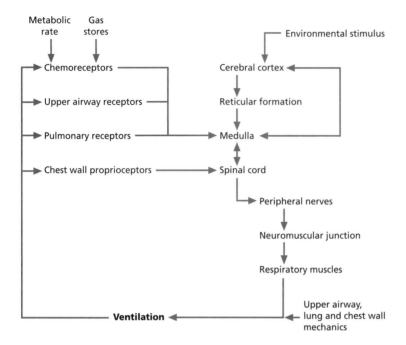

Fig. 9.1 Control of ventilation.

threshold in REM sleep than in NREM sleep. The ventilatory responses to hypercapnia and hypoxia are also reduced to a greater extent in REM than in NREM sleep and the combination of a reduction in reflex responsiveness and irregular cerebral cortical activity leads to an erratic and unpredictable pattern of respiratory activity [1]. This is especially marked in phasic rather than tonic REM sleep. The intervals between respirations may be sufficiently prolonged to be classified as central sleep apnoeas (CSAs) according to the conventional criterion of a lack of airflow for 10 s or more associated with a lack of respiratory effort. Central apnoeas are more frequent and prolonged during REM sleep if other factors such as sleep deprivation, chronic hypercapnia, alkalosis, sedative drugs or alcohol are present.

The intense supraspinal inhibition of motor activity in REM sleep contributes to the reduction in reflex responsiveness and is manifested by a reduction in tone in the postural muscles, including all the respiratory muscles except the posterior crico-arytenoid muscles which abduct the vocal cords and maintain glottic patency, the diaphragm and to a lesser extent the parasternal intercostal muscles. Loss of activity in the upper airway dilator muscles increases the upper airway resistance in REM sleep and predisposes to closure of the airway with obstructive sleep apnoeas (OSA) [2].

Selective sparing of diaphragm activity in REM sleep leads to abdominal expansion increasing relative to the rib cage expansion. Loss of activity in the other chest wall muscles alters the compliance of the chest wall so that the functional residual capacity falls. This not only reflexly reduces the upper airway dimensions, but worsens ventilation and perfusion matching, reduces lung compliance and reduces the volume of the stores of oxygen in the lungs.

Respiration in non-rapid eye movement sleep

The threshold for arousal from NREM sleep rises progressively from stage 1 to stage 4, but remains lower than in REM sleep (Table 9.1). The reflex mechanisms that control respiration during wakefulness remain intact but the responses are quantitatively different to wakefulness. Within each sleep stage they remain constant and a regular respiratory pattern is seen until the sleep stage changes, when a new stable pattern develops. The threshold for the ventilatory response to $P\text{co}_2$ increases from wakefulness to stage 1 NREM sleep and progressively into the deeper levels of NREM sleep with the effect that a $P\text{co}_2$ which stimulates respiration during wakefulness may lead to apnoeas during sleep.

The stage of NREM sleep oscillates frequently at

Table 9.1 Effects of REM and NREM sleep on respiration.

	REM sleep	REM and NREM sleep	NREM sleep
Physiological changes from wakefulness	↓↓ Drive ↓↓ Upper airway dimensions ↓↓ Chest wall muscles ↓ Functional residual capacity		↓ Drive ↓ Upper airway dimensions ↓ Chest wall muscles
Reversible pathological changes		Alkalosis Sedatives and alcohol Obesity Hypokalaemia Malnutrition Hyperinflation	
Irreversible pathological changes	Diaphragm weakness	Upper airway abnormalities Reduced chest wall muscle strength Impaired chest wall mechanics	Reduced reflex drive

NREM, non-rapid eye movement; REM, rapid eye movement.

sleep onset and the threshold for carbon dioxide to act as a respiratory stimulus fluctuates correspondingly. This may lead either to frequent CSA or to a Cheyne–Stokes respiration (CSR) pattern of breathing. During the apnoeic phases the P_{CO_2} rises progressively at a rate determined by the metabolic rate and when it exceeds the apnoeic threshold respiration restarts, often with a phase of hyperventilation until the P_{CO_2} again falls below the threshold and the next apnoea begins.

The upper airway resistance increases in NREM sleep compared to wakefulness, but to a lesser degree than during REM sleep. It increases the work of breathing and predisposes to OSA. The activity of the chest wall muscles is globally reduced, unlike REM sleep in which the diaphragm is selectively spared. The reduction in respiratory activity parallels the reduced ventilatory requirements needed to cope with the lower metabolic rate during NREM sleep. The ratio of rib cage to abdominal movement is greater in NREM than REM sleep.

Respiratory-related arousals from sleep

Causes

Any stimulus to respiration can lead to arousal from NREM or REM sleep to wakefulness. These include hypoxia, hypercapnia, an increased work of breathing and other stimuli which activate the mechanoreceptors. Each cough during sleep is associated with a brief arousal, either to a lighter stage of sleep or to wakefulness, and the same is probably true of each act of swallowing.

Whether arousal occurs or not depends both on the intensity of the stimulus and the stage of sleep. The threshold for arousal for all these receptors is higher in REM than NREM sleep, and rises progressively from the lighter to the deeper stages of NREM sleep.

Effects on sleep

These respiratory stimuli characteristically cause brief, or micro, arousals which can be frequent and contrast with the longer awakenings seen, for instance, in narcolepsy. They have the protective effect of enabling the respiratory system to come temporarily under the control mechanisms of wakefulness which tend to improve the blood gases, but have the disadvantage that they lead to sleep fragmentation. Arousals are almost invariably seen initially in REM sleep and the first abnormality of sleep architecture is fragmentation of REM sleep with REM deprivation. If effective treatment is applied REM sleep rebound appears. Loss of stages 3 and 4 NREM sleep occurs later when the respiratory abnormalities encroach into NREM sleep.

Respiratory-induced arousals minimize the duration and extent of apnoeas and hypoxia in the short term, but the sleep fragmentation reduces ventilatory drive and probably both the strength and the endurance of the respiratory muscles in the upper airway and

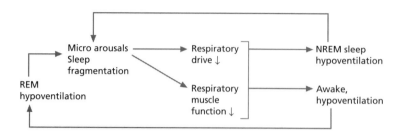

Fig. 9.2 Cycle of effects of hypoventilation on sleep and respiration. EDS, excessive daytime sleepiness; NREM, non-rapid eye movement; REM, rapid eye movement.

chest wall. As a result, hypoventilation worsens and hypoxia, which is initially a respiratory stimulus, can depress respiration if it becomes more severe. Hypercapnia causes progressively less respiratory stimulation as the cerebrospinal fluid bicarbonate concentration rises and buffers the chemoreceptor response to $P\text{CO}_2$ changes. Hypoventilation tends to persist and once it appears in NREM as well as REM sleep it soon appears during wakefulness. Loss of NREM sleep then leads to progressively worsening EDS (Fig. 9.2). The effects on respiratory drive are reversible and improve once sleep fragmentation is relieved, but are exacerbated by, for instance, sedative drugs and alcohol.

Effects on wakefulness

Sleep fragmentation and sleep deprivation affect particularly the function of the prefrontal cortex. Initially the ability to maintain attention and alertness during prolonged monotonous tasks is impaired and this is followed by mood changes, loss of memory, poor concentration and impairment of motor performance. As sleep fragmentation becomes more severe, excessive daytime sleepiness (EDS) worsens and automatic behaviour and even hallucinations, which are probably due to intrusion of REM sleep into wakefulness, with vivid imagery develop.

Assessment

History

A careful history is essential to accurately assess respiratory disorders during sleep (Chapter 4). The issues that should be considered are as follows.

1 How severe is the sleep disruption? How frequent are the arousals from sleep and what is their cause? Is the patient aware of any breathlessness or choking? Are there early morning headaches on awakening, suggesting carbon dioxide retention?

2 How severe is the EDS? This can be assessed by the techniques described in Chapter 4. Respiratory disorders and EDS may be due to sleep fragmentation caused by central or obstructive apnoeas or to the sedative effect of hypercapnia (carbon dioxide narcosis).

3 Are there any features to indicate worsening of pulmonary or cardiovascular function, such as deteriorating breathlessness, ankle swelling or orthopnoea? This may be caused either by pulmonary oedema or bilateral diaphragm weakness.

4 What is the cause? Is there a history of a previous relevant illness such as poliomyelitis or of a muscular dystrophy or other chronic neurological disorder? Is there a scoliosis or kyphosis or has the subject undergone a thoracoplasty? Are there features of chronic bronchitis or emphysema (chronic obstructive pulmonary disease, COPD) or asthma? Is there any inappropriate drug treatment which may be acting as a respiratory sedative, e.g. opiate analgesics or benzodiazepines?

Physical examination

Physical examination may reveal central cyanosis indicating hypoxia, or signs of hypercapnia such as a tachycardia with a large-volume pulse, warm hands and feet, a flapping tremor of the hands, reduction of tendon reflexes, small pupils and occasionally, confusion and papilloedema. Neurological examination may show features of a neurological disorder including respiratory muscle weakness. There may be physical signs of a chest wall deformity and of airflow obstruction with hyperinflation as well as right heart failure and pulmonary hypertension.

Investigations

Most patients with significant symptoms of a respiratory disorder during sleep, or abnormal physical signs, require referral to a specialist centre unless there is a treatable cause such as significantly reversible airflow obstruction. A sleep study with analysis of oxygen saturation, transcutaneous $P\text{CO}_2$, and ideally, airflow, rib cage and abdominal movement and sound is of value. Polysomnography is only needed if other causes of sleep disturbances, such as PLMS, are considered.

If CSR is diagnosed cardiac, and occasionally neurological, function requires investigation. In hypercapnic respiratory failure investigation of the status of the respiratory pump with lung function tests, including lung volumes, maximal inspiratory and expiratory mouth pressures, vital capacity in the lying and sitting position, and occasionally ventilatory responses to oxygen and carbon dioxide are needed. A chest X-ray, electrocardiogram (ECG) and echocardiogram are also usually indicated.

Principles of treatment

The aims of treatment are as follows.
1 Explain and, where appropriate, reassure. This may be sufficient if the respiratory disorder is mild.
2 Treat the cause. This is rarely possible although airflow obstruction and cardiac failure may be amenable to treatment.
3 Optimize respiratory mechanics. Subjects with diaphragmatic weakness prefer to sit up and those with an asymmetrical thorax due to, for instance, scoliosis or following a thoracoplasty may prefer to sleep on one side or the other. Treatment of airflow obstruction and hyperinflation of the lungs may improve respiratory mechanics, but there are no effective inotropic drugs to improve respiratory muscle contractility.

Specific approaches are applicable to the following situations.

Central sleep apnoeas and Cheyne–Stokes respiration

When the subject demonstrates central sleep apnoeas and CSR with a normal or low arterial $P\text{CO}_2$ during sleep, the treatment is as follows.
1 *Stabilize respiratory drive.* This can be achieved by administering oxygen which reduces the hypoxic drive; giving acetazolamide which lowers the apnoea threshold for carbon dioxide, or providing nasal continuous positive airway pressure (CPAP) which has several reflex effects.
2 *Modify sleep pattern.* This can be achieved either by stabilizing the sleep stage, e.g. with benzodiazepines which consolidate stage 2 NREM sleep, or by reducing the duration of REM sleep if this is the state of sleep in which the respiratory abnormalities are most frequent. Protriptyline, a non-respiratory sedative tricyclic antidepressant is usually used.

Central sleep apnoeas with a raised arterial $P\text{CO}_2$ during sleep

Where the subject demonstrates central sleep apnoeas with a raised arterial $P\text{CO}_2$ during sleep, the treatment should be as outlined below.
1 *Increase respiratory drive.* This can be achieved by lowering the arterial $P\text{CO}_2$, relieving sleep deprivation and any metabolic alkalosis, and discontinuing any respiratory sedative medication. Ventilatory stimulants are of little value except theophyllines which may have some benefit in the long term.
2 *Modifying sleep patterns.* The respiratory abnormalities are usually worse in REM sleep and this can be reduced in duration by tricyclic antidepressants such as protriptyline.
3 *Oxygen treatment.* This relieves hypoxia but there is a significant risk of worsening hypercapnia. In practice, nocturnal oxygen therapy is only safe and effective when the disorder is moderately severe. Respiratory support is usually safer and more effective.
4 *Respiratory support.* This may take the form of either positive or negative pressure ventilation or a phrenic nerve pacemaker. These are indicated when respiratory failure is sufficiently severe to cause troublesome symptoms, potentially serious complications such as polycythaemia or pulmonary hypertension, or is likely to lead to these problems or to premature death.

Central sleep apnoeas associated with eucapnia or hypocapnia

Pathogenesis

These apnoeas may appear during sleep through physiological mechanisms such as, for instance, variations in respiratory rate in REM sleep with intervals of greater than 10 s between breaths, or as a result of upper airway reflexes or changes in the apnoeic threshold for carbon dioxide with NREM sleep stage transitions. During the apnoea the $P\text{CO}_2$ gradually rises and when it exceeds the apnoeic threshold a period of hyperventilation occurs which lowers the $P\text{CO}_2$ again. If the hyperventilation causes the $P\text{CO}_2$ to fall below the apnoeic threshold or if there is a sleep stage shift so that the threshold itself rises, a CSA will occur (Fig. 9.3). An increased ventilatory response to changes in $P\text{CO}_2$ has been found in patients with this type of CSA and is probably responsible for the slightly low $P\text{CO}_2$ seen during wakefulness as well as sleep.

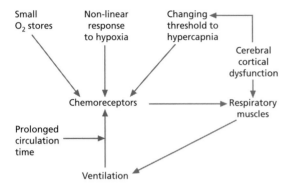

Fig. 9.3 Mechanisms of Cheyne–Stokes respiration.

Clinical features

Central sleep apnoeas associated with a normal or low P_{CO_2} may be asymptomatic, but can lead to arousals from sleep with or without a sensation of breathlessness. If the arousals are frequent EDS may develop, but the arousals tend to be less frequent than in OSA because of the absence of increased inspiratory muscle effort as a stimulus for arousal. Observation during sleep reveals an absence of respiratory movements and muscle activity which differentiates these apnoeas from OSA. These findings can be confirmed by sleep studies. The arousals from sleep may be perceived as sudden awakenings for no reason.

Treatment

Treatment is not usually required for central apnoeas with a normal or low P_{CO_2} unless they cause significant insomnia or EDS. One or more of the following may be helpful.
1 Consolidation of NREM sleep with benzodiazepines in order to minimize the number of sleep stage shifts.
2 Relief of hypoxia with supplemental oxygen usually given by nasal cannulae to stabilize the respiratory drive.
3 Alteration of respiratory reflexes with nasal CPAP. This modifies upper airway reflexes, increases the lung volume and the quantity of oxygen stored in the lungs.

Cheyne–Stokes respiration (periodic breathing)

Cheyne–Stokes respiration is closely related to CSA. It is characterized by a regular waxing and waning of tidal volume with little change in respiratory frequency during the phases when breathing is taking

place. Between these cycles there may be a short or prolonged period of apnoea which if it exceeds 10 s is classified as a CSA using conventional criteria. Occasionally, however, the waxing and waning of tidal volume occurs without any cessation of breathing (Cheyne–Stokes variant).

Pathogenesis

The cyclical changes in respiration are due to an instability in the respiratory control system (Fig. 9.3). Within each stage of NREM sleep the respiratory drive remains constant, but it differs between stages. The frequent changes, at the onset of sleep and with arousal, lead to an unstable respiratory pattern. As the stage of sleep deepens, the arterial P_{CO_2} which is required to act as a respiratory stimulus (the apnoeic threshold) rises. This leads to a central apnoea until the carbon dioxide reaches the apnoeic threshold at which time it stimulates the chemoreceptors, particularly in the carotid bodies, which initiate an episode of hyperventilation to reduce the P_{CO_2} below the apnoeic threshold again [3].

The ventilatory response to carbon dioxide is greater than normal in CSR. This magnifies the hyperventilation response to the rise in P_{CO_2} and also causes the arterial P_{CO_2} to be slightly low during wakefulness and the mean P_{CO_2} to be low during sleep [4]. The exaggerated hyperventilation causes a rapid and deep fall in the arterial P_{CO_2} and in CSR there is usually a prolongation of the time for the arterial blood to reach the peripheral chemoreceptors in the carotid body and thereby to influence respiration. The degree of this delay determines the length of the hyperpnoeic phase of CSR and the crescendo–decrescendo pattern of the tidal volume. The length of the apnoeic phase is largely determined by the extent to which the P_{CO_2} falls below the apnoeic threshold and its rate of rise, which is related to the metabolic production of carbon dioxide.

In CSR, but not in CSA, there are usually other factors which increase the ventilatory response. These include the presence of hypoxaemia. The ventilatory response to hypoxia increases hyperbolically as the P_{O_2} falls and this gain in ventilatory response accentuates the episodes of hyperventilation. The cycle of CSR is shortest in individuals with the greatest hypoxic ventilatory drive. Pulmonary vagal afferent stimulation, which in heart failure, for instance, is associated with pulmonary venous distention and stimulation of pulmonary C-fibres, also increases the respiratory drive.

Causes

Cheyne–Stokes respiration is associated with several conditions; these are described below.

HYPOXIA

This may be due to a low arterial Po_2, including situations when this is the result of breathing gas with a low inspired oxygen concentration or air at low pressure. The low Po_2 at altitude increases the hypoxic ventilatory response which destabilizes respiratory control and causes 'high-altitude periodic breathing'. This type of CSR occurs in NREM sleep which becomes fragmented because of frequent arousals. The duration of stages 3 and 4 NREM sleep is reduced.

REDUCTION IN LUNG VOLUMES

This reduces the body stores of oxygen and makes hypoxia more marked during any transient apnoea.

CARDIAC DYSFUNCTION

This is associated with CSR for several reasons. Firstly, the hypoxia and pulmonary venous distention increase respiratory drive. Secondly, the prolonged circulation time, which is often a feature of cardiac failure or low cardiac output states, leads to the CSR pattern. Lastly, cardiac disease is often associated with changes in the cerebral circulation so that its reactivity to changes in Pco_2 is lost and this alters the ventilatory response to Pco_2 [5].

Cheyne–Stokes respiration is associated with a poor prognosis if cardiac dysfunction is present. The 3-year survival is only around 50%. The high mortality may reflect the increased sympathetic activity during sleep which causes vasoconstriction leading to hypertension with a reduced cardiac output, dysrhythmias, a tachycardia with reduced stroke volume and an increase in the myocardial oxygen consumption.

CEREBRAL CORTICAL DYSFUNCTION

Cheyne–Stokes respiration is common in disorders of the cerebral hemispheres which reduce the inhibition of the medullary respiratory centres so that reflex responses become accentuated. This probably contributes to the increased prevalence of CSR in the elderly.

Clinical features

Cheyne–Stokes respiration causes frequent arousals from sleep, especially in stages 1 and 2 NREM sleep. These may be detected as awakenings and insomnia, and if they are sufficiently frequent may result in EDS. The total sleep time and duration of stages of 3 and 4 NREM and REM sleep are reduced if the CSR frequency is greater than around 20 episodes per hour. Occasionally the airway closes during the central apnoea and this combination of a CSA and OSA is termed a mixed apnoea. The CSR cycles are associated with an increase in sympathetic activity during the hyperpnoeic phase. At this time a tachycardia, an increase in cardiac output, a rise in blood pressure and an increase in the cerebral blood flow occur [6]. These effects are reversed during the apnoea. Cardiac dysrhythmias, such as atrial fibrillation, ventricular ectopics and atrioventricular block may appear transiently during each CSR cycle.

Observation of the respiratory pattern is diagnostic and there may be snoring, usually because the upper airway closes towards the end of the apnoeic phase. During the apnoea neurological changes including eye closure, upward rotation of the eyes, conjugate gaze deviation, hyporeflexia, up-going plantar reflexes, pupillary constriction and a reduction in tone of the limb muscles may be seen. These are all reversed during the hyperpnoeic phase.

Treatment

Treatment is often not required, but if CSR is symptomatic the following should be considered.

1 *Treatment of the underlying cause*, e.g. heart failure.

2 *Oxygen*. This stabilizes the respiratory control and is usually effective. Inspired 3% carbon dioxide also stabilizes the respiratory control, but leads to sympathetic hyperactivity and is impractical for long-term use.

3 *Respiratory stimulants*. These lower the threshold of the ventilatory response to Pco_2. These include theophylline, but this also increases the gain of the respiratory control system by increasing the slope of the ventilatory response to carbon dioxide. Acetazolamide is effective through inducing a metabolic acidosis and has been used especially in high-altitude periodic breathing [7].

4 *Sedative drugs*. Benzodiazepines consolidate sleep and reduce the number of sleep-stage changes.

5 *Nasal CPAP and nasal ventilation* (Fig. 9.4). These increase the mean intrathoracic pressure which reduces pulmonary oedema and pulmonary venous congestion due to cardiac failure. The venous return to the right heart lessens, the left ventricular end-diastolic volume, left ventricular transmural pressure-gradient and the left ventricular after-load are all

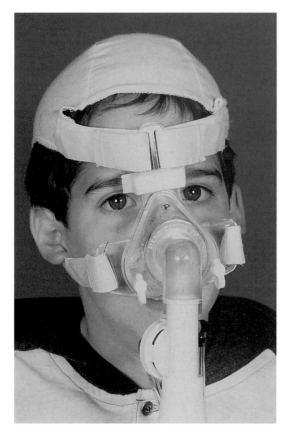

Fig. 9.4 Mask and headgear for nasal ventilation.

Table 9.2 When to suspect ventilatory failure.

High risk disorder, e.g. previous poliomyelitis, muscular dystrophy, thoracoplasty, scoliosis

Plus relevant symptoms, e.g.	Worsening breathlessness
	Awakenings from sleep
	Excessive daytime
	sleepiness
	Early morning headaches
	Swollen ankles

Plus vital capacity < 1.0–1.5 l

reduced. Functional residual capacity rises which enlarges the oxygen stores and may reduce the work of breathing, thereby reducing oxygen consumption and carbon dioxide production. Upper-airway reflexes may also be altered but occasionally the additional expiratory resistance due to the applied expiratory pressure causes the $P\text{CO}_2$ to rise and if it remains persistently above the apnoeic threshold the respiratory pattern stabilizes. Nasal ventilation in particular reduces the respiratory muscle work and the oxygen consumption, and these various effects of CPAP and ventilation often reduce the sympathetic drive and plasma noradrenaline levels [8].

Central sleep apnoeas associated with hypercapnia

It is essential to distinguish 'central' apnoeas due to a loss of respiratory drive from those that are due to impaired respiratory mechanics or to widespread respiratory muscle weakness so that even a normal respiratory drive cannot be translated into detectable respiratory movements (see Fig. 9.5). This latter group are better considered as 'pseudocentral' or 'peripheral' apnoeas than due to any central abnormality [9]. They are characteristic of neuromuscular disorders that cause diaphragmatic weakness so that in REM sleep no functioning inspiratory chest wall muscles are left (Table 9.2). Impaired respiratory mechanics in, for instance, emphysema, may also cause even a normal drive only to be able to develop a small tidal volume (hypopnoea) or even no detectable airflow. These lung disorders have been described in Chapter 8.

Respiratory drive disorders

True central apnoeas due to a defect in reflex respiratory control are, unlike most respiratory disorders during sleep, most common in NREM sleep when respiration is predominantly controlled by reflex mechanisms. The causes of these apnoeas can be either reversible or irreversible.

REVERSIBLE

Sleep deprivation and fragmentation reduce the respiratory drive and predispose to CSA. Drugs such as benzodiazepines and opiates, and a metabolic alkalosis have a similar effect. Chronic hypercapnia increases the cerebrospinal fluid bicarbonate concentration, which increases its buffering capacity and thereby reduces the responsiveness to changes in $P\text{CO}_2$.

IRREVERSIBLE

Certain disease processes are associated with permanent or at least only partially reversible defects of reflex respiratory control. These include the following.

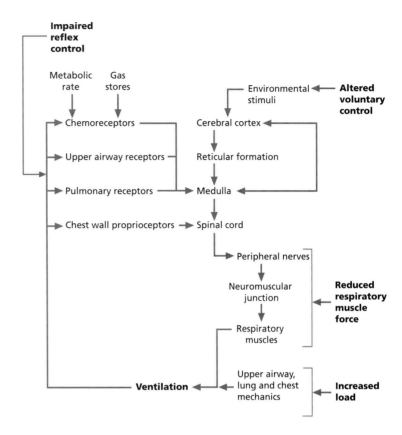

Fig. 9.5 Causes of ventilatory failure.

Carotid body disorders
The carotid bodies increase ventilation in response to hypoxia during sleep and cause arousal if hypoxia becomes severe. Carotid body dysfunction may lead to failure to terminate either central or obstructive sleep apnoeas, and can lead to respiratory failure.

Central alveolar hypoventilation
This disorder occasionally occurs neonatally, in which case it may be associated with other conditions such as Hirschsprung's disease, or more usually in early adult life. In this group it is usually idiopathic and presumably due to a functional defect in the medullary respiratory centres or their connections, but occasionally it is due to organic brain-stem disease such as previous encephalitis, a stroke or tumour. The ventilatory response to hypoxia or hypercapnia or both is reduced. Central sleep apnoeas are seen initially most frequently in NREM sleep and are associated with hypercapnia which, when it becomes more severe, is present during wakefulness as well. It is more marked during intercurrent illnesses such as chest infections in which the work of breathing

is increased beyond the capacity of the respiratory drive. Polycythaemia and pulmonary hypertension may develop. Treatment with non-invasive ventilatory support or phrenic nerve stimulation is effective.

Other medullary lesions
Any lesions in the medulla may disrupt respiratory control and lead to ventilatory failure during sleep. Tumours, haemorrhage, infarction, encephalitis, trauma, neurosurgery, irradiation, multiple sclerosis, syringobulbia and multiple system atrophy may all be responsible. These conditions usually cause a complex clinical picture because of the site of the lesion and this may make it difficult to assess the respiratory complications.

Arnold–Chiari malformation
This is a combination of syringomyelia and herniation of the cerebellar tonsils through the foramen magnum and caudal displacement of part of the medulla. It can cause stretching or compression of the ninth cranial nerve and thereby leads to denervation of the carotid body, causing central apnoeas.

Cervical cordotomy

The main indication for this procedure is the relief of chronic pain, but if it is performed bilaterally the efferent pathways from the medullary respiratory centres can be severed so that the chest wall muscles are disconnected from their control. Central sleep apnoeas during NREM sleep arise and may be prolonged and cause fatal cardiac dysrhythmias, particularly during the first few nights after surgery. The degree of recovery varies.

Respiratory muscle and chest wall disorders

RESPIRATORY FAILURE

The limitations of the respiratory pump in neuromuscular and skeletal disorders that affect the thoracic cage are apparent in sleep before they develop in wakefulness (Table 9.3). The ability to respond to the altered physiological environment during sleep is limited by the capacity of the respiratory drive, respiratory muscle function and the mechanical properties of the respiratory system. In general, if the respiratory drive increases the respiratory frequency rises, but the maximal tidal volume is less than in normal subjects. As a result, the physiological dead space is increased and alveolar ventilation falls with a reduction in Po_2 and a rise in Pco_2. As the respiratory frequency increases, the ratio of inspiratory to expiratory time rises so that the inspiratory muscles contract for longer with a risk of incipient respiratory muscle fatigue. This is usually avoided by the central respiratory control mechanisms adopting a strategy of either recruiting additional respiratory muscles such as the accessory muscles, alternating, for instance, diaphragmatic and intercostal muscle activity during each breath, or by inducing CSAs. Each of these strategies reduces the work of the inspiratory muscles, but the alternative response is to cause an arousal from sleep (see above).

If alveolar ventilation cannot be maintained, the respiratory control system sets the ventilation at a level which avoids muscle fatigue even though it leads to hypercapnia. This is a respiratory stimulant acutely, but becomes progressively less so when it is prolonged (see above). It also increases the cardiac output, leads to a tachycardia, an increase in systolic blood pressure, and to cerebral and cutaneous vasodilatation but visceral vasoconstriction. Its neurological effects include reduction in tendon reflexes, a flapping tremor of the hands and frontal headaches which characteristically occur on awakening from sleep in

Table 9.3 Neuromuscular and thoracic cage disorders causing respiratory failure during sleep.

Neurological
Carotid body disorders
Brain-stem lesions
Central alveolar hyperventilation
Arnold–Chiari malformation
Cervical cordotomy
Spinal cord lesions
Motor neurone disease
Multiple system atrophy
Poliomyelitis
Spinal muscular atrophy

Disorders of peripheral nerves
Acute idiopathic polyneuropathy (Guillain–Barré syndrome)
Charcot–Marie–Tooth disease

Disorders of neuromuscular junction
Myasthenia gravis
Lambert–Eaton syndrome
Botulism

Disorders of respiratory muscles
Duchenne's muscular dystrophy
Myotonic dystrophy
Congenital myopathies
Acid maltase deficiency

Skeletal disorders
Scoliosis
Kyphosis
Thoracoplasty
Asphyxiating thoracic dystrophy (Jeune's disease)

the morning. It may also lead to confusion and even coma (carbon dioxide narcosis), but hypercapnia does enable more carbon dioxide to be excreted in a given volume of expired gas than with eucapnia for any level of respiratory muscle work. This adaptive mechanism tends to stabilize the arterial Pco_2.

As the Pco_2 rises the arterial Po_2 falls and this may be accentuated, particularly in REM sleep, by a reduction in lung volume and a worsening of ventilation–perfusion matching and often to a disproportionate fall in oxygen saturation according to its position on the oxyhaemoglobin dissociation curve. If hypoxia persists it may lead to polycythaemia in response to increased erythropoietin secretion by the kidneys. This increases the oxygen carrying capacity of the blood to maintain oxygen delivery to the tissues despite the low arterial Po_2. It also increases the blood viscosity, predisposing to venous and arterial thrombosis, and increases both the pulmonary and systemic vascular resistance, thereby contributing to the risk of right and left ventricular hypertrophy and failure. Hypoxia also has a direct vasoconstrictor effect on the pulmonary arterioles and raises the pulmonary artery pressure.

The respiratory drive is intrinsically normal in most patients with neuromuscular and thoracic cage disorders, although it can be transiently impaired by, for instance hypercapnia. Disorders which also affect the cerebral cortex, such as myotonic dystrophy, modify respiratory control but through loss of the normal cortical inhibition of brain-stem reflexes.

RAPID EYE MOVEMENT SLEEP
The respiratory abnormalities are seen in REM before NREM sleep in all these disorders other than those in which the medullary respiratory reflex control is directly affected [10]. Rapid eye movement sleep becomes fragmented and reduced in duration with frequent arousals, and only at a later stage is there loss of stages 3 and 4 NREM sleep. The main effects of REM sleep are as follows.

Increase in upper airway resistance
Weakness of the upper airway dilator muscles combines with the intense loss of muscle tone in REM sleep to predispose to upper airway obstruction. The risk of this is greater if the chest wall muscles are selectively spared and remain able to generate a sufficiently negative intra-airway pressure. Conversely, if the chest wall muscles, particularly the diaphragm, are involved then OSAs are less likely. The upper airway diameter is reduced through a reflex mechanism related to the loss of lung volume in REM sleep. The obstruction may occur at any level from the base of the tongue to the larynx, in which case stridor-like noises are often heard at night. If, however, the chest wall muscles are too weak to generate rapid airflow rates there may be little noise despite the upper airway obstruction (Table 9.4).

The high threshold for arousal during REM sleep prolongs the OSAs and, together with the small oxygen stores in the lungs, tends to accentuate the oxygen desaturations. Resaturation after each apnoea is also slow because of the inability of the chest wall muscles to increase alveolar ventilation rapidly once arousal has occurred, either because of their weakness or, in thoracic cage deformities, because of the reduced chest wall compliance. With these neuromechanical defects hypercapnia between apnoeas is partly related

Table 9.4 Neuromuscular causes of obstructive sleep apnoeas.

Multiple system atrophy
Syringobulbia
Posterior inferior cerebellar artery syndrome
Motor neurone disease
Arnold–Chiari malformation
Poliomyelitis
Muscular dystrophies, e.g. myotonic dystrophy, Duchenne's muscular dystrophy
Congenital myopathies

to the inability to normalize the blood gases before the next apnoea begins. Secondary adaptive changes which maintain hypercapnia, as described above, develop and even between apnoeas the weak muscles may be unable to compensate for the increase in the work of breathing through the narrowed upper airway. These effects are accentuated if the subject is obese, takes sedative drugs or alcohol or has any specific dysmorphic features which narrow the upper airway as in, for instance, nemaline myopathy.

Diaphragmatic dysfunction
The diaphragm is the only active inspiratory chest wall muscle in REM sleep, and hypoventilation may result if its function is impaired either due to intrinsic weakness, or to derangement of chest wall mechanics which may put the diaphragm at a mechanical disadvantage, alter its length or reduce the chest wall compliance [11]. The most common causes are congenital myopathies such as acid maltase deficiency, muscular dystrophies such as Duchenne's muscular dystrophy or myotonic dystrophy, previous poliomyelitis and motor neurone disease, and chest wall disorders such as scoliosis, kyphosis or after a thoracoplasty.

Reduction in functional residual capacity
This reduces the upper airway diameter, oxygen stores in the lungs, impairs ventilation–perfusion matching and reduces lung compliance, all of which may contribute to hypoxia, CSA or CSR and hypoventilation.

Reduction in respiratory drive
This, as mentioned above, is rarely due to any intrinsic disorder related to the neurological condition but may be a consequence of sleep fragmentation or hypercapnia.

NON-RAPID EYE MOVEMENT SLEEP

Reflex control of respiration is retained during NREM sleep with little modification by cerebral cortical activity. Central alveolar hypoventilation and cervical cordotomy can impair this control and lead to CSA and respiratory control can also be transiently altered as described on page 187. In general, however, the main effects of NREM sleep in neuromuscular and skeletal disorders are as follows.

Increase in upper airway resistance

This increases to a lesser extent than in REM sleep and OSAs are less common. They may, however, occur in degenerative disorders such as multiple system atrophy and motor neurone disease in which vocal cord adduction develops due to lesions in the nucleus ambiguus.

Cheyne–Stokes respiration

This arises with changes in sleep stage within NREM sleep and may lead to frequent arousals. The slow circulation time due to a cardiomyopathy in disorders such as Duchenne's muscular dystrophy and Friedreich's ataxia contribute to the CSR. Disorders affecting the cerebral cortex with loss of its inhibitory effect on the medullary reflexes also predispose to CSR together with any hypoxia that may be present.

Inactivation of chest wall muscles

There is a global reduction in chest wall muscle activity in NREM sleep in contrast to REM sleep. Neuromuscular disorders affecting these muscles accentuate this and predispose to hypoventilation. Disorders of the thoracic cage such as scoliosis which reduce its compliance may increase the work of breathing sufficiently for hypoventilation to occur even if the chest wall inspiratory muscles are intrinsically normal.

CLINICAL FEATURES

Respiratory disturbances during sleep may be asymptomatic but as they worsen they cause arousals from sleep which may become sufficiently frequent to cause EDS and insomnia of the difficulty in maintaining sleep (DMS) type. Early morning headaches due to carbon dioxide retention may develop but are a late feature of OSA. The partner may be aware of snoring or stridor-like noises as well as an irregular respiratory pattern. Worsening breathlessness on exertion and ankle swelling are common and diaphragm weakness may cause orthopnoea so that sleep takes place in a chair instead of in bed.

Physical examination may reveal cyanosis, signs of weakness or atrophy of the respiratory muscles, thoracic cage abnormalities such as a scoliosis, kyphosis or the appearances following a thoracoplasty in which case there may also be paradoxical movement of the region of the chest where the ribs have been excised. Abdominal paradoxical inward movement during inspiration in the supine position is a sign of diaphragm weakness.

Age has an important influence on the clinical features. Below the age of around 3 years respiration is more dependent on the diaphragm than in later life and the rib cage is very compliant. Any weakness of the diaphragm predisposes to its fatigue and to respiratory failure, particularly since there is a greater proportion of REM sleep than in adults, and this is when respiration is particularly dependent on the diaphragm.

The rate at which the clinical features develop depends on how the balance between the capacity of the respiratory pump and its load changes. A transient intercurrent and often treatable illness such as a chest infection or asthma may precipitate nocturnal (and waking) respiratory failure. Age-related changes in respiratory drive, respiratory muscle strength and endurance, and in the compliance of the chest wall may switch the balance in favour of hypoventilation. The rate of progression of the underlying disorder is another important factor. Stable conditions such as childhood proximal spinal muscular atrophy hardly alter for many years, whereas some conditions are rapidly progressive such as motor neurone disease and multiple system atrophy, and in others, such as multiple sclerosis, the course fluctuates unpredictably. The sequence of progression of abnormalities is fairly predictable in some disorders such as Duchenne's muscular dystrophy and knowledge of this is important in managing the respiratory complications that appear during sleep. In other conditions, such as motor neurone disease, there may be any combination or sequence of weakness of upper airway and chest wall muscles together with bulbar weakness which can cause aspiration of saliva, food and drink into the tracheobronchial tree.

The respiratory effects of these conditions during sleep can also be influenced by unrelated disorders. These include obesity which not only increases upper airway resistance but also mass loads the chest wall muscles, impairs ventilation–perfusion matching and, if it is gross, can impair muscle contractility. Tobacco smoking can increase upper airway resistance as well as intrapulmonary airflow resistance and if it causes emphysema the lung compliance increases leading to hyperinflation.

INVESTIGATIONS

Chest X-ray, ECG and lung function tests including maximal mouth pressures help to establish the severity of the underlying disorder. Arterial blood gases while awake and a sleep study including continuous oxygen saturation and transcutaneous P_{CO_2} recordings will document the severity of any respiratory failure. Recording of airflow and chest and abdominal movements will indicate whether there are any CSA or OSA. Polysomnography may occasionally be required to assess the sleep architecture or the contribution of other sleep disorders. Ventilatory responses to hypercapnia and hypoxia and tests of respiratory muscle endurance may be of help.

TREATMENT

A range of treatments are available and in general the simpler measures should be tried first. Assisted ventilation and phrenic nerve pacing should only be employed in subjects once these have been optimized.

Treat the underlying disorder

Very few of the neuromuscular and thoracic cage disorders are amenable to curative treatment but measures such as physiotherapy may be of help and prompt, energetic treatment of infective exacerbations is essential. Treatment of unrelated conditions which adversely affect respiratory function, such as obesity or tobacco smoking, may also be of value.

Oxygen

Supplemental oxygen can relieve hypoxia during sleep, but by removing the hypoxic ventilatory drive it may prolong both CSA and OSA, worsen hypoventilation and lead to a rise in P_{CO_2}. If oxygen is administered then the oxygen saturation and transcutaneous P_{CO_2} should be carefully monitored during sleep and the flow rate kept to the minimum that is required to raise the oxygen saturation to an acceptable level, such as 90%.

Respiratory stimulants

A variety of drugs such as almitrine and progesterone have been tried, but none of these is effective in improving ventilation during sleep. Methylxanthines can improve CSR partly through an effect on cerebral blood flow and also by lowering the threshold for the ventilatory response to hypercapnia. Acetazolamide, which is a carbonic anhydrase inhibitor and causes a metabolic acidosis, may relieve CSR particularly at altitude and reduces the arterial P_{CO_2} slightly in other disorders.

Inotropic drugs

These have been used to try to improve respiratory muscle contractility, but the results have been disappointing.

Rapid eye movement sleep suppressants

Tricyclic antidepressants and selective serotonin reuptake inhibitors (SSRIs) reduce the duration of REM sleep-related abnormalities including upper airway obstruction. Protriptyline 5–20 mg nocte has been most widely used and is non-respiratory sedating.

Nasal continuous positive airway pressure

This is effective in relieving OSA and may also improve CSA and CSR, possibly by reducing the hypoxic drive through increasing the functional residual capacity and improving ventilation–perfusion matching and also through raising the P_{CO_2} above the threshold for a ventilatory response.

Phrenic nerve pacemaker (diaphragmatic stimulation, electrophrenic respiration)

This treatment is effective if the phrenic nerve, its nucleus in C3–C5 and the diaphragm are intact. Its indication is in respiratory failure due to brain-stem disorders that have disturbed medullary respiratory control and high cervical tetraplegics, but not in patients with, for instance, phrenic nerve damage or muscular dystrophies in whom the contractility of the diaphragm is impaired.

Ventilatory support

Mechanical ventilatory support is in effect an external source of energy which reduces the work of breathing and compensates for apnoeas, hypopnoeas and hypoventilation. It can be provided during wakefulness as well as during sleep.

Indications and effects. Long-term ventilatory support is indicated if respiratory failure is causing troublesome symptoms, potentially serious complications such as polycythaemia or pulmonary hypertension, or is likely to lead to these problems or to premature death. It appears to improve survival in neuromuscular and skeletal disorders, although in rapidly progressing conditions the prognosis is mainly determined by the appearance of other complications such as bulbar dysfunction. The quality of life can be improved, symptoms due to respiratory sleep disturbances abolished and the arterial blood gases both during the day and night normalized within a few days.

Mechanisms of action. The benefits of ventilatory support are due to a variety of actions. The respiratory drive increases, probably both through a reduction in cerebrospinal fluid bicarbonate concentration which resets the ventilatory response to carbon dioxide and through relief of sleep fragmentation and an improvement in sleep quality. Respiratory muscle strength and endurance may improve and the work of breathing may be reduced due to the ventilator taking this over and to an increase in the chest wall and lung compliance through the increase in the tidal range of respiratory movements. Prevention of distal airway closure within the lungs may improve lung compliance as well.

The relief of upper airway obstruction by ventilatory support, particularly if a positive expiratory as well as inspiratory pressure is applied to the airway, may be of benefit and changes in lung volume may improve the function of the chest wall muscles, alter the configuration of the rib cage and improve ventilation–perfusion matching. The frequency of arousals from sleep and of apnoeas is reduced. Rebound REM sleep is seen once the REM sleep respiratory abnormality has been corrected and sleep architecture may return almost to normal.

Techniques. Non-invasive techniques are preferred to tracheostomy ventilation unless there is upper airway obstruction which prevents them from being effective, if the airway has to be protected because of a risk of aspiration, or if ventilatory support is needed almost continuously.

The methods of ventilatory support are as follows.
1 Positive pressure ventilation. This can be achieved during sleep by the following methods.
(a) Tracheostomy ventilation. This invasive method of ventilation is surprisingly well tolerated but requires a higher level of care in the home than the non-invasive methods. Complications such as tube displacement, obstruction, impairment of swallowing and occasionally a tracheo-oesophageal fistula or tracheo-innominate artery fistula may develop.
(b) Mask and mouth-piece ventilation (page 215). Ventilation using a nasal mask, or occasionally a face mask which includes the mouth as well, is usually well tolerated although several difficulties are recognized (see Fig. 9.4). Ulceration of the skin of the bridge of the nose is a common problem. The mask may become displaced during sleep, air-leaks around the mask or through the mouth may develop and upper airway symptoms such as a dry or blocked nose may develop. Functional upper airway obstruction may be seen and if air enters the oesophagus rather than the trachea, abdominal distention with frequent belching, nausea and the passing of flatus may arise. These complications can usually be overcome by careful attention to the mask and ventilator settings, but occasionally ventilation through a mouth-piece is required. This may lead to dental complications, and air-leaks through the nose.
2 Negative pressure ventilation. With these techniques the chest and abdomen are enclosed in an air-tight rigid chamber from which air is evacuated by a venti-

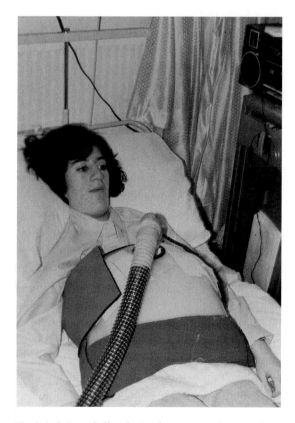

Fig. 9.6 Cuirass shell enclosing the patient's rib cage and abdomen with tubing connecting it to a negative pressure ventilator.

lator connected to it through wide-bore tubing. Air is drawn in through the mouth and nose. Three types of negative pressure ventilation are available.

(a) Tank ventilation (iron lung). The patient lies supine on a mattress within the chamber which encloses the whole body up to the neck. Access to the subject is limited and this equipment is large, heavy and expensive, but effective. It is rarely used for long-term nocturnal respiratory support, for which a cuirass or jacket are usually preferable.

(b) Jacket ventilation. A framework of metal or plastic provides the rigidity and this is covered by an airtight garment from which air is evacuated by a negative pressure ventilator.

(c) Cuirass ventilation. The properties of rigidity and impermeability to air are combined in a single structure, the Cuirass shell, which is usually individually constructed to fit the patient so that it encloses the antero-lateral aspects of the rib cage and abdomen (Fig. 9.6). A cuirass is light and durable and, unlike a mask, does not lead to claustrophobia, but it can induce upper airway obstruction due to loss of the normal sequence of activation of the upper airway muscles during inspiration.

References

1 Douglas NJ, White DP, Pickett CK, Weil JV, Zwillich CW. Respiration during sleep in normal man. *Thorax* 1982; 37: 840–4.
2 Wiegand L, Zwillich CW, Wiegand D, White DP. Changes in upper airway muscle activation and ventilation during phasic REM sleep in normal men. *J Appl Physiol* 1991; 71: 488–97.
3 Khoo MCK, Gottschalk A, Pack AI. Sleep-induced periodic breathing and apnea: a theoretical study. *J Appl Physiol* 1991; 70: 2014–24.
4 Fanfulla F, Mortara A, Maestri R *et al.* The development of hyperventilation in patients with chronic heart failure and Cheyne–Stokes respiration. A possible role of chronic hypoxia. *Chest* 1998; 114: 1083–90.
5 Naughton MT. Heart failure and central apnoea. *Sleep Med Rev* 1998; 2: 105–16.
6 Lorenzi-Filho G, Dajani HR, Leung RST, Floras JS, Bradley TD. Entrainment of blood pressure and heart rate oscillations by periodic breathing. *Am J Respir Crit Care Med* 1999; 159: 1147–54.
7 Swenson ER. Carbonic anhydrase inhibitors and ventilation: a complex interplay of stimulation and suppression. *Eur Respir J* 1998; 12: 1242–7.
8 Philip-Joet FF, Paganelli FF, Dutau HL, Saadjian AY. Hemodynamic effects of bilevel nasal positive airway pressure ventilation in patients with heart failure. *Respiration* 1999; 66: 136–43.
9 Shneerson J. Sleep in neuromuscular and thoracic cage disorders. *Eur Resp Mono* 1998; 3: 324–44.
10 Bye PTP, Ellis ER, Issa FG, Donnelly PM, Sullivan CE. Respiratory failure and sleep in neuromuscular disease. *Thorax* 1990; 45: 241–7.
11 White JES, Drinnan MJ, Smithson AJ, Griffiths CJ, Gibson GJ. Respiratory muscle activity and oxygenation during sleep in patients with muscle weakness. *Eur Respir J* 1995; 8: 807–14.

10 Obstructive Sleep Apnoeas and Snoring

Obstructive sleep apnoeas (OSA) are due to transient closure of the upper airway during sleep. They prevent air from entering the lungs and thereby interrupt the continuous exchange of gas in the lungs (Fig. 4.8). They merge into the upper airway resistance syndrome (UARS) and simple snoring in which the airway only partially or momentarily obstructs. In this chapter OSA will be discussed separately from snoring, although their aetiology, pathogenesis and treatments have much in common.

Obstructive sleep apnoeas

Obstructive sleep apnoea is common but forms a spectrum ranging between normality with a few obstructions to a life-threatening condition which may present with respiratory, cardiovascular or sleep-related symptoms.

Introduction

The prevalence of OSA is uncertain, at least in part because of difficulties in defining the condition. Its name suggests that the demonstration of airflow obstruction, sufficient to prevent airflow during sleep, should be sufficient to confirm the diagnosis, but in practice there are several difficulties. Firstly, all the surrogate markers of airway obstruction, lack of airflow and the presence of sleep have uncertain degrees of sensitivity and specificity. Obstruction may be inferred from, for instance, clinical observation of paradoxical chest and abdominal movement, but this sign can also indicate diaphragmatic weakness. Most physiological measurements of airflow and respirtory movements during sleep are semiquantitative at best and realistic sleep staging is difficult when there are frequent micro arousals from sleep due to the apnoeas.

Cessation of airflow for 10 s has been widely but arbitrarily used as a definition of an apnoea. There is no physiological basis for this. Hypopnoeas, which often accompany apnoeas, are defined in various ways, although the most common is a reduction for 10 s or more in the tidal volume to less than 50% of the previous values. The appropriate initial value to base this on is difficult to ascertain since flow monitors are only semiquantitative [1]. The true frequency of hypopnoeas is therefore always slightly uncertain. A frequency index of apnoeas and hypopnoeas (AHI) has been developed and greater than five per hour has been considered abnormal. There is no physiological basis for this cut-off point and, in practice, clinical features usually appear when there are more than around 15–20 of these events per hour. The presence of symptoms in addition to the physiological abnormalities has been described by the term obstructive sleep apnoea syndrome (OSAS) or sleep apnoea hypopnoea syndrome (SAHS).

Apnoeas and hypopnoeas are more frequent in the elderly and normal values should take this into account. A related index based on the numbers of oxygen desaturations of 4% or greater has been used, but a 4% desaturation represents a different degree of fall in Po_2 according to the initial Po_2 because of the sigmoid shape of the oxyhaemoglobin dissociation curve. Large desaturations occur more readily, for instance if the initial Po_2 is around 8 kPa than if it is around 12 kPa. This renders the desaturation index insensitive at indicating apnoeas when the initial Po_2 is nearly normal.

The situation is further confused by the observation that similar physiological and sleep effects can arise even if airflow does not cease and, in some patients, even if it remains almost normal. This condition, known as the upper airway resistance syndrome (UARS), causes flow limitation with increased inspiratory chest wall muscle effort and negative intrathoracic pressure, especially at the times of arousal from sleep. Daytime sleepiness due to sleep fragmentation occurs in a similar way to OSA but without nocturnal hypoxia. UARS is relatively more frequent in the non-obese than OSA and while it may be a phase which occurs between simple snoring and the appearance of OSA, it is more commonly a 'variant' of OSA.

There is a spectrum of severity of both UARS and OSA from the occasional events seen in normal subjects without any significant adverse clinical or physiological consequences to the state where they occur several hundred times each night with life-threatening effects [2]. It may be more helpful to assess where each patient is on this spectrum of UARS and OSA and to assess their risks and consequences, rather than to arbitrarily delineate a normal and abnormal range. The term OSAS has been used to describe the combination of symptoms and the presence of apnoeas, but it is probably best to separately assess whether the physiological changes of OSA and any clinically important features are present or absent, and also to grade the frequency and severity of the events. There is only a loose correlation between the presence of symptoms and the demonstration of an elevated AHI or desaturation index because of factors such as shift work and personality differences between individuals which affect the threshold for developing symptoms.

Prevalence

Obstructive sleep apnoeas which are sufficiently frequent or severe to cause symptoms occur around four times more commonly in males than females, although milder degrees of OSA may be more nearly equally distributed between the sexes. They are less common in premenopausal women than postmenopausal women and in men, possibly because of the effects of sex hormones. The prevalence increases during adult life, reaching a peak at around 40–60 years but OSA then becomes less common, probably because of the reduction in chest wall muscle activity during sleep which lessens the negative intrapharyngeal pressure [3]. In the UK approximately 3–4% of middle-aged males have more than 5 OSA per hour, 1% more than 10 per hour and 0.3% more than 20 per hour. The prevalence varies in different countries, mainly according to the prevalence of obesity. Symptomatic OSA is probably at least twice as common in the USA as in the UK.

There is a familial tendency to develop sleep apnoeas. This is partly genetic and probably due to an inherited tendency towards a particular shape or size of the upper airway as a result of the formation of both bones and soft tissues. There may also be a genetically controlled pattern of respiratory control which predisposes to apnoeas. The familial tendency to obesity, which is a risk factor for OSA, may be partly inherited and partly acquired through common eating habits within a family, and other behavioural factors such as taking exercise or the probability of smoking or drinking excess alcohol may also be linked within a family, either genetically or through common behavioural patterns.

Pathogenesis

The patency of the upper airway depends on the balance of forces across it and on its compliance (Fig. 10.1). The airway between the oropharynx and the larynx is a single muscular tube which conducts air in and out of the lungs and food, drink and upper airway secretions into the oesophagus. Above the oropharynx two airways (the nasal and oral) are in parallel so that obstruction of either does not cause airflow to cease. Below the larynx the airway is supported by cartilaginous rings which prevent its collapse.

Any factor which narrows the upper airway, increases the pressure around it, reduces the pressure within it, or increases its compliance, will predispose towards OSA. The more negative the pressure in the upper airway the more likely it is that the walls will be sucked together and that the airway will narrow. Any increase in inspiratory effort above a certain level causes an increase in upper airway resistance so that air flow remains constant, or falls or even ceases if the airway closes.

The site of obstruction varies between individuals (Fig. 10.2). The soft palate may be drawn like a wedge between the posterior aspect of the tongue and the posterior pharyngeal wall. Posterior displacement of the tongue, particularly due to loss of genioglossus activity and the effect of gravity, will close the airway at pharyngeal level. This is more common in adults than children. Laryngeal abnormalities, which may be organic lesions or due to disorders of their innervation, may cause OSA and localized anatomical variations or pathological lesions within the airway may cause obstruction at other levels.

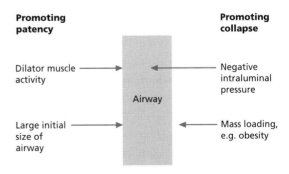

Fig. 10.1 Control of upper airway patency.

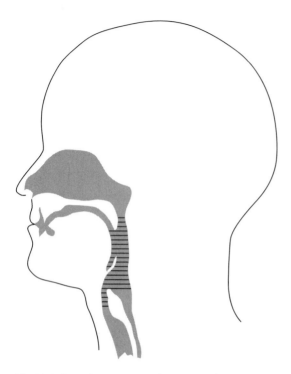

Fig. 10.2 Sites of upper airway obstruction. The hatched area shows the usual area of occlusion of the airway during obstructive sleep apnoeas.

The most important factors which determine whether or not OSA develop are as follows.

SMALL SIZE OF UPPER AIRWAY

The size, and probably the shape, of the upper airway influence whether it is likely to close during sleep. The pharyngeal airway is narrowed laterally in OSA compared to normal subjects but the causes and significance of this are uncertain. The smaller airway is more vulnerable because of the following.

1 By Laplace's law, the narrower the airway the greater the expanding force that is required to generate sufficient wall tension to maintain its patency.

2 If the airway is smaller it takes less change for it to close.

3 A narrow airway increases the resistance to flow and a more negative pressure is required proximally to compensate for this. This tends to cause the airway walls to be sucked together at that point.

UPPER AIRWAY COMPLIANCE

The upper airway is more collapsible in individuals with OSA than in normal subjects because of a combination of neurological and mechanical factors. Its

compliance is influenced by factors such as tissue damage and oedema which can be due to the trauma of OSA or snoring, but the most important factor, which can vary from moment to moment, is the activity in the dilator and constrictor muscles. At the onset of sleep the tonic and phasic activity in both these groups of muscles is reduced. Obstruction of the airway is not due to an increase in constrictor muscle activity, but to a failure of the dilator muscles to counteract the physical forces tending to close the airway.

The changes in dilator muscle contraction vary between the individual muscles. The genioglossus, which protrudes the tongue, and the geniohyoid, which pulls the hyoid forwards, are both upper airway dilators with mainly phasic inspiratory activity which is largely retained at the onset of NREM sleep. In contrast, the tensor palatini, which retracts the soft palate, has mainly tonic activity and this is lost in NREM sleep. The loss of this tonic muscle activity is largely responsible for the increase in upper airway resistance which is seen during normal sleep. Relaxation of the medial and lateral pterygoid muscles lessens the degree of mandibular protrusion, so that the base of the tongue becomes more posterior. The mouth falls open and the pharyngeal airway becomes smaller.

Tonic activity is even further reduced during REM sleep when inspiratory activity is less regular than in NREM. These changes in activity may be mediated through 5HT release by fibres from the dorsal raphe nuclei (DRN) which influence the respiratory centres and lower cranial nerve nuclei in the medulla.

The main neurological factors which determine whether or not the airway is likely to close (Table 10.1) are as follows.

1 The upper airway diameter falls through a reflex mechanism as the lung volume, and in particular the functional residual capacity (FRC), decreases.

2 A negative pressure within the upper airway normally generates activity in the upper airway muscles which prevents airway closure. This reflex may be reduced or absent in individuals with OSA.

3 The normal sequence of activation of respiratory muscles during each inspiration, beginning with the alae nasi, followed by other upper airway muscles and ending with activation of the diaphragm, may be lost. This failure to stabilize the upper airway before the chest wall muscles contract and reduce the pressure within it promotes airway obstruction. It is also seen in certain types of ventilatory support during sleep, particularly in negative pressure ventilation used in the control mode and in phrenic nerve stimulation.

Table 10.1 Factors predisposing to obstructive sleep apnoea.

Small upper airway	Obesity	
	Tobacco smoking	
	Hormonal factors	Menopause
		Acromegaly
		Hypothyroidism
	Supine position	
	Upper airway lesions	Nose: polyps, rhinitis
		Pharynx: tonsils and adenoids, cysts and tumours
		Larynx: congenital webs and cysts
		Crico-arytenoid arthritis
	Skeletal abnormality	Congenital and traumatic abnormalities
		Retrognathia
Loss of upper airway	Sleep deprivation and fragmentation	
dilator muscle activity	Benzodiazepines	
	Alcohol	
	Neurological disorders	Diffuse e.g. poliomyelitis, Duchenne's muscular dystrophy
		Focal, e.g. Arnold–Chiari malformation, strokes
	General anaesthetic	
	Ventilatory support	Nasal and negative pressure ventilation, phrenic nerve pacemakers
Increased chest wall		
muscle force		

4 The upper airway obstruction could be due to an increase in the force of the chest wall muscles relative to what is preserved in the upper airway dilators so that the negative pressure in the airway overcomes the stabilizing effect of dilator muscle activity.

5 The proportion of Type II fast twitch fatiguable muscle fibres in the genioglossus is increased in OSA. This may predispose to a loss of dilator muscle force during sleep, but these appearances may be the result of trauma due to the OSA rather than its cause.

These changes in the sequence or relative force of contraction in the upper airway and chest wall muscles may vary according to, for instance, the $P\text{CO}_2$, stage of sleep, and the individual response to factors such as sleep deprivation and changes in position. There is also breath-to-breath variability within REM sleep which may predispose to apnoeas developing intermittently.

CHEST WALL MUSCLE ACTIVITY

The pressure within the upper airway is determined by the activity of the chest wall muscles and the extent to which this is transmitted to the upper airway. During NREM sleep, the diaphragm, intercostal and accessory respiratory muscles are all active, but in REM sleep the diaphragm alone is responsible for inspiration. The pressure that these muscles generate in the upper airway depends on their contractility, mass, length, rate of shortening and mechanical advantage as well as the compliance and resistance of the lungs and chest wall.

Maintenance and termination of apnoeas

The end expiratory dimensions of the pharyngeal airway lessen progressively during the breaths leading up to airway closure and during an OSA the airway remains closed or almost closed, preventing airflow from occurring. The airway may, however, open temporarily during expiration and allow some gas to leave the lungs. In other situations the airway may only be narrowed and may never completely close. The narrower the airway, however, the greater the pressure required within the lumen to open it by Laplace's law. Surface forces may also be important in holding the mucosa of the airway walls together. The increasingly negative pressure within the airway towards the end of each inspiration tends to maintain closure of the airway during each breath. The respiratory drive and the inspiratory force increase progressively with successive breaths, and this tends

Table 10.2 Maintenance and termination of an obstructive sleep apnoea.

	Onset of apnoea	Maintenance of apnoea	Apnoea termination point	Post apnoea
Upper airway dilator muscle activity	–	–	++	+
Surface forces	–	+	–	–
Respiratory drive	+	++	+++	++
Inspiratory chest wall muscle force	+	++	+++	++
Arousal	–	–	+	+
Airflow	–	–	–	++

to maintain the apnoea until the break point when the airway opens.

The termination of the apnoea occurs at the moment of arousal from a deeper to a lighter stage of sleep, or to wakefulness (Table 10.2). This is determined by the intensity of the inspiratory muscle effort, which rises with the increasing respiratory drive during the apnoea and the tendency to collapse the upper airway which this induces. Intrapleural pressures of -80 cmH$_2$O are often reached, but arousal only occurs when the muscle force reaches a certain percentage of the maximum that can be generated, irrespective of whether the airway is completely occluded or only severely narrowed. The threshold for arousal is higher in stages 3 and 4 NREM sleep than stages 1 and 2, but even higher in REM sleep which explains the longer apnoeas in REM than in NREM sleep. Respiratory stimulation due to hypoxia and to a greater extent hypercapnia contributes to the break point being reached, although these responses are less during sleep than wakefulness. These chemoreceptor influences probably cause arousal both by generating more inspiratory muscle force, and by impulses from the respiratory centres stimulating the reticular activating system.

At the moment of arousal the activity of the upper airway dilator muscles returns and the upper airway resistance falls. The airway often opens suddenly with a loud snorting noise and following this there is compensatory hyperventilation with a reduction in $P\text{CO}_2$ and return of the $P\text{O}_2$ to normal. The respiratory effort wanes and the subject returns to sleep at which time the upper airway dilator muscles become less active again and the OSA may recur. This process may be repeated up to 500 times per night.

Causes of obstructive sleep apnoea
The most important causes of OSA are as follows.

SMALL SIZE OF UPPER AIRWAY
No anatomical abnormality is usually found in the upper airway in OSA, but imaging techniques have shown that the pharyngeal airway is smaller than in individuals without apnoeas. This is probably mainly due to genetic influences which cause variations in skeletal dimensions, such as a slightly shorter mandible, or a more inferior hyoid bone, but soft tissue changes may also be important.

There may also be more readily identifiable causes of a small or abnormally shaped upper airway.

Widespread narrowing
This may be due to one or more of the following factors.

Obesity. Obesity is one of the major risk factors for OSA. The adipose tissue that is most relevant is that which is deposited within the neck rather than elsewhere in the body. The fat is located not within the wall of the airway but around it, and when the muscle tone is reduced during sleep the fatty tissue in effect mass-loads the airway and tends to collapse it. Obesity may also predispose to OSA by reducing the FRC and thereby reflexly reducing the upper airway dimensions. Obesity may be secondary to other sleep disorders, particularly the Prader–Willi and Kleine–Levin syndromes, sleep eating or narcolepsy, all of which can therefore be complicated by OSA. It may also be partly due to loss of the lipolytic action of growth hormone, whose secretion is reduced by fragmentation or loss of NREM sleep.

Neck muscle hypertrophy. Occasionally, hypertrophy of the muscles within the neck can act in a similar way to obesity and compress the upper airway. This is usually seen in those engaged in competitive sports which require strong neck muscles, and following regular physical training.

Diffuse infiltrations. This occurs in mucopolysaccharidoses such as Hunter, Hurler and Scheie diseases.

Tobacco. Tobacco smoking is associated with an increased risk of OSA, probably because it causes a diffuse mucositis affecting the oral and pharyngeal airway, including the soft palate. Nicotine in tobacco may also alter respiratory control. Its pharmacological effects are discussed in Chapter 3.

Hormonal factors. Sleep apnoeas are less common in premenopausal women than postmenopausal women or men. This may be due to a protective effect of oestrogen or progesterone or both, or to an apnoea-inducing action of androgens such as testosterone. These effects may be mediated either through an alteration of the respiratory drive, changes in the dimensions of the upper airway structures or by a reduction in fat deposition in the neck relative to elsewhere in the body [4].

In acromegaly changes in craniofacial skeletal dimensions, overgrowth of the tongue, and diffuse thickening of the upper airway including the larynx, narrow the airway and predispose to its closure. Hypothyroidism leads to OSA because of a myopathy of the upper airway muscles and infiltration with 'oedema' as well as obesity. Abnormality of the control of respiration may lead to central apnoeas as well. In Cushing's syndrome there is no abnormal infiltrate into the upper airway, but a myopathy of the vocal cords and obesity both predispose to OSA.

Sleep position. In the supine position, the weight of the tongue and mandible is unopposed by tonic muscle activity in the upper airway and it tends to fall back into the pharynx and contribute to its narrowing and obstruction. This is more marked in REM than NREM sleep when muscle relaxation is greater. The FRC also falls in the supine position and this reduces the upper airway dimensions. The effect of position on OSA is most apparent in younger adults with mild or moderately severe OSA and in the absence of obesity, presumably because the excess fatty tissue surrounds the airway and causes apnoeas in any position. Neck flexion and opening of the mouth also increase the upper airway resistance and contribute to apnoeas and snoring.

Nasal obstruction
Complete nasal obstruction leads to mouth breathing which may predispose to OSA, and the lack of stimula-tion of nasal pressure and flow receptors may reduce the stability of the upper airway. Partial nasal obstruction leads to a more negative pharyngeal pressure during inspiration to overcome it and this predisposes to OSA. The most important causes are nasal polyps, rhinitis and a deviated nasal septum.

Pharyngeal narrowing
This may be due to enlargement of the tonsils, adenoids, or both. This may be temporary during infections, but chronic enlargement is the most important cause of OSA in children.

Variations in skeletal and soft tissue morphology probably play an important role in contributing to OSA as described above, and may be determined genetically and vary with age. A long soft palate with a margin which falls below the level of the tongue may wedge between this and the posterior pharyngeal wall. The enlargement may be partly due to oedema and other results of the trauma that it is exposed to during the apnoeas, in which case it may improve after treatment of the OSA. Other focal lesions in the pharynx such as tumours or cysts can also cause OSA. Enlargement of the tongue is a feature particularly of acromegaly and amyloidosis and may contribute to pharyngeal obstruction.

Craniofacial abnormalities
Craniofacial trauma and congenital disorders such as Crouzon's, Apert's and Down's syndromes cause mid-face hypoplasia. Down's syndrome is also associated with a narrow nasal airway, large tongue, large tonsils and adenoids, obesity, muscle hypotonia and autonomic dysfunction, all of which may contribute to OSA. Marfan's syndrome causes a high arched hard palate which is associated with a small pharyngeal airway, as well as increased laxity of the pharyngeal airway, which predispose to OSA.

Mandibular abnormalities
Hypoplasia (micrognathia) or a posteriorly positioned (retrognathia) mandible lead to a dental overbite (overjex) and may induce OSA, particularly in the supine position when the tongue tends to fall back into the pharyngeal airway. These abnormalities may be present from birth, as in, for instance, the Pierre–Robin, Hallermann–Streiff and Treacher–Collins syndromes, but OSA may not develop until adult life. Micrognathia may be associated with other skeletal abnormalities of the upper airway, as in Apert's syndrome.

Laryngeal obstruction
Organic disorders of the larynx may cause OSA. These may be congenital webs or cysts, thickening of the laryngeal tissues as in acromegaly and hypothroidism, or crico-arytenoid arthritis due to rheumatoid arthritis in which abduction of the vocal cords is limited.

LOSS OF UPPER AIRWAY MUSCLE ACTIVITY
Loss of the dilator function of the upper airway muscles during sleep may be caused by one or more of the following.

Sleep deprivation and sleep fragmentation
These reduce the respiratory drive and in particular the response of the chest wall muscles to upper airway obstruction, thereby delaying arousal from the apnoeas. This increase in the arousal threshold worsens the degree of oxygen desaturation and of hypercapnia during the apnoeas, and may also reduce the rate of resaturation after the apnoea and even prevent normal blood gases from being attained before the next apnoea begins. The ventilatory response to hypercapnia is reduced.

Benzodiazepines
These increase the level of inspiratory effort which is required to cause arousal at the end of an OSA through their central nervous system (CNS) depressant action. They may also increase the degree of muscle relaxation in the upper airway.

Alcohol
This has similar effects to benzodiazepines. The decrease in arousability prolongs the apnoeas and the reduction in upper airway dilator muscle activity impairs the post apnoea hyperventilation so that the rate of oxygen resaturation is slower. Alcohol also increases the nasal airflow resistance by causing hyperaemia of the nasal mucosa.

Diffuse neuromuscular conditions
Disorders such as poliomyelitis, Duchenne's muscular dystrophy and myotonic dystrophy may diffusely weaken the upper airway dilator muscles and lead to OSA.

Focal neurological disorders
These usually affect the larynx causing either unilateral or bilateral vocal cord adduction, as in achondroplasia, syringobulbia, Arnold–Chiari malformation, multiple system atrophy, and following neurosurgery and neck surgery. Unilateral weakness of the pharynx and larynx occurs in strokes affecting the posterior inferior cerebellar artery territory (lateral medullary syndrome).

General anaesthetic
Central control of the upper airway is altered so that the muscles lose their activity. Obstructive 'anaesthetic' apnoeas occur both during the anaesthetic and in the recovery phase.

Ventilatory support
Loss of the normal sequence of muscle contraction in which the upper airway muscles are activated before the chest wall muscles in negative pressure ventilation using the control mode, and with phrenic nerve stimulation can induce OSA. This can also be provoked by nasal positive pressure ventilation, possibly through a similar mechanism or through changes in airway pressure and flow causing passive closure of the airway.

CHEST WALL MUSCLE ACTIVITY
Obstructive sleep apnoeas are less likely if the chest wall muscles are unable to reduce the intrapharyngeal airway pressure sufficiently to suck the walls of the airway together. This arises in neuromuscular disorders such as Duchenne's muscular dystrophy and to a lesser extent with ageing. Conversely, OSA could theoretically be accentuated by any factor which markedly reduces the intrapharyngeal airway pressure.

Respiratory effects

OXYGEN DESATURATION

Acute effects
Oxygen desaturation is a characteristic feature of OSA, but is not seen in the upper airway resistance syndrome in which the airway narrows but does not completely close. Air flow continues with maintenance of a normal oxygen saturation, but the increased inspiratory muscle work causes arousals from sleep. The depth of oxygen desaturation during an apnoea depends on the prior oxygen saturation, the rate of desaturation and the duration and completeness of the apnoea.

The rate of desaturation is determined by the volume of oxygen stored in the body and the rate of oxygen consumption (Fig. 10.3). Oxygen stores are less in REM sleep than in NREM sleep because of the smaller lung volumes and in REM sleep the impaired ventilation–perfusion matching also reduces

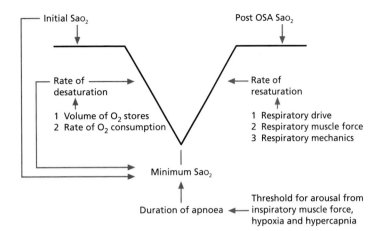

Fig. 10.3 Factors affecting oxygen desaturation in an obstructive sleep apnoea.

the baseline oxygen saturation before the apnoea. This can lead to considerably deeper desaturations because of the sigmoid shape of the oxyhaemoglobin dissociation curve. The rate of oxygen consumption is slower when chest wall muscle activity is reduced as in REM sleep and in the elderly.

Apnoea duration is related to the threshold for arousal from the increased inspiratory muscle force, although hypercapnia, and to a lesser extent hypoxia, also contribute to the break-point. Muscle relaxation is greater in REM than NREM sleep and in general the arousal occurs later in the former.

The rate of resaturation after the apnoea is determined by the respiratory drive and the ability of the chest wall muscles to increase ventilation. This is impaired in neuromuscular disorders and in gross obesity and chronic airflow obstruction where the work of breathing is increased. Sleep fragmentation reduces the arousability in response to increased inspiratory muscle force and thereby prolongs apnoeas. The reduced arousability underlies the longer apnoeas seen later in the night. Sleep fragmentation also reduces the ventilatory response to hypercapnia, facilitating a rise in the $P\text{CO}_2$ both during sleep and wakefulness. In addition, it probably contributes to central apnoeas which develop after the hyperventilation at the end of an OSA. This lowers the $P\text{CO}_2$ below the threshold for the ventilatory response, which is raised with sleep fragmentation.

Chronic effects
Chronic hypoxia may lead to polycythaemia and to metabolic changes, particularly an increase in cyclic adenosine monophosphate (AMP) with a reduction in adenosine triphosphate (ATP). This increases the

production of purine nucleotides such as adenosine and xanthine, which are metabolized to uric acid. The urinary excretion of uric acid is increased in severe OSA and returns to normal with effective treatment.

INTRAPLEURAL PRESSURE SWINGS
The increasingly strong respiratory efforts against the closed airway during an OSA and in the UARS generate large swings in intrapleural pressure. This may fall to as low as −80 cmH$_2$O. This has cardiovascular effects and also leads to changes in the atrial dimensions as their transmural pressure alters. The repetitive stretching of the atria leads to increased secretion of atrial natriuretic peptide (ANP) which increases renal sodium and water loss which lead to nocturia and occasionally urinary incontinence.

HYPERCAPNIC RESPIRATORY FAILURE
Chronic hypercapnia during wakefulness is an infrequent, but well recognized complication of OSA [5]. It may present with early morning headaches in addition to excessive daytime sleepiness (EDS) and other features of OSA. It is often associated with right heart failure and this combination represents the clinical picture of what was in the past known as the 'Pickwickian syndrome' or obesity, hypoventilation syndrome (OHS). This comprised obesity, which is a risk factor for OSA, with EDS and respiratory and right heart failure, which is due to pulmonary hypertension.

Hypercapnia in OSA is usually associated with the presence of one or more of the following.

Gross obesity
This causes narrowing and intermittent obstruction of the upper airway which increases the work of

breathing, but other effects such as the mass loading of the chest wall muscles by the fat around the rib cage and abdomen which reduces the compliance of the chest wall, and the fall in contractility of the chest wall muscles, overstretching of the diaphragm and impairment of ventilation–perfusion matching may all contribute to respiratory failure.

Chronic lung disease
Chronic lung disease, such as chronic bronchitis and emphysema (chronic obstructive pulmonary disease, COPD).

Hypercapnia develops at a greater FEV1 than if apnoeas were absent, in which case the FEV1 is usually < 1.0 l.

Neuromuscular disorders
The weak chest wall muscles may be unable to compensate for the increased work of breathing through a narrow upper airway, so that hypoventilation and hypercapnia develop, particularly if the patient is also obese, takes sedative drugs or alcohol. The most common neuromuscular disorders causing hypercapnia with OSA are congenital myopathies, muscular dystrophies, and previous poliomyelitis.

Cardiovascular effects

During normal sleep the balance of parasympathetic and sympathetic activity shifts towards the former, but this fluctuates during an OSA. Initially parasympathetic activity increases, but with the increasing physiological stress towards the end of the OSA sympathetic activity rapidly rises and continues briefly after the moment of arousal.

This recurring pattern affects the following.

HEART RATE AND DYSRHYTHMIAS
The heart rate initially slows during an OSA and then rises towards the end of it and early in the postapnoea phase. This alternating bradycardia and tachycardia may be mistaken for the brady–tachy syndrome and pacemakers have been implanted unnecessarily on the basis of this erroneous diagnosis. Bradycardias can be profound with heart rates of less than 30 per minute with asystole lasting for greater than 2.5 s. First and second degree atrioventricular heart block may appear in otherwise normal subjects, especially in REM sleep. Inspiratory efforts against a closed airway increase the parasympathetic activity and contribute to the bradycardias. The degree of the subsequent tachycardia is proportional to the fall in Po_2.

Other dysrhythmias are uncommon unless there is pre-existing cardiac disease, usually ischaemic heart disease. They include atrial and ventricular ectopics, atrial fibrillation and ventricular tachycardia. These dysrhythmias are most common if the oxygen saturation falls below around 75% and during REM sleep.

SYSTEMIC BLOOD PRESSURE, MYOCARDIAL INFARCTION AND STROKES

Acute effects
The swings in parasympathetic and sympathetic activity during and after each apnoea lead to a fall in blood pressure early in the apnoea followed by a rise to around 50% above the level seen between the apnoeas [6]. The rise of sympathetic activity is due mainly to the arousal, but also to hypoxia if the apnoeas are frequent and severe. The mean blood pressure may become higher than in wakefulness, especially in REM sleep. The swings in intrapleural pressure also affect the blood pressure. A fall in intrapleural pressure reduces the pressure in the aorta and left ventricular emptying and increases the left ventricular end systolic volume. The lower intrapleural and intrathoracic pressure increases the venous return to the right atrium and the right ventricular end diastolic volume. This shifts the interventricular septum to the left, reducing the compliance of the left ventricle and predisposing to left ventricular failure and a reduced cardiac output.

Chronic effects
The blood pressure may remain elevated during the day as well as intermittently at night. This is probably due to vasoconstriction due to sustained sympathetic hyperactivity, probably related to the degree of sleep fragmentation and may lead to left ventricular hypertrophy.

Epidemiological studies have shown an association between OSA, hypertension, strokes and myocardial infarction. OSA is commonly seen after strokes, possibly because it was present beforehand, but equally the stroke may affect the control of the upper airway muscles. Some of these associations between these conditions and OSA may be due to the presence of common risk factors, such as obesity, alcohol and age, but the link between OSA and strokes is probably a direct one. Strokes appear to be three times more common in patients with severe OSA than in normal subjects and they occur most frequently at 6.00–8.00 AM, suggesting that they are associated with the process of awakening. The causes may be similar to those for myocardial infarction (page 169), but the repetitive hypertensive surges during each apnoea may also contribute. Sustained daytime vasoconstriction, which reduces the ability of the cerebral circulation to respond to haemodynamic changes, may also be a factor. The relevance of cerebral vasodilatation due to hypercapnia in severe OSA is uncertain.

PULMONARY ARTERY PRESSURE

Acute effects
Hypoxia during each apnoea causes pulmonary vasoconstriction with the result that the pulmonary artery pressure rises towards the end of the apnoea and immediately afterwards. This reduces the stroke volume of the right ventricle. This reduction in stroke volume contrasts with the situation towards the start of the apnoea when the right ventricular output is reduced because of the bradycardia although the stroke volume is normal.

The greatly negative intrathoracic pressure increases the venous return to the right atrium and ventricle which then increases the pulmonary artery pressure. The left ventricular compliance, filling and ejection fraction all fall and the left ventricular end-diastolic pressure increases during the apnoea. At the end of the apnoea these haemodynamic changes are reversed and the sympathetic activity increases so that the systemic blood pressure increases rapidly, particularly with the sympathetic induced vasoconstriction. Occasionally, the fall in left ventricular compliance and stroke volume is sufficient to cause pulmonary oedema, especially if there is pre-existing left ventricular dysfunction.

Chronic effects
These changes in pulmonary artery pressure are reversible after the apnoeas, but in certain situations chronic pulmonary hypertension develops. This requires the presence of hypoxia during the daytime in addition to during the OSA at night. The most common situations are when there is coexisting chronic airflow obstruction, severe ventilation–perfusion mismatching due to gross obesity, or hypoventilation usually due to neuromuscular disorders. Right ventricular hypertrophy develops and the pulmonary hypertension together with endocrine and metabolic responses to hypoxia and hypercapnia may lead to right heart failure usually at about the time that daytime hypercapnia develops.

Clinical features in adults
Obstructive sleep apnoeas are often asymptomatic but if they become frequent or severe a variety of clinical manifestations may be seen. The most prominent features are discussed below.

NOISY BREATHING AND AWAKENINGS AT NIGHT
Sleep apnoeas usually follow many years of loud snoring and are associated with a change in the pattern of the noise. At the end of the apnoea the airway snaps open with a loud snorting or similar noise. The variety of irregular and loud snoring noises indicates how many different patterns of hypopnoea, apnoea and arousal take place. Frequency analysis of the noises shows them to be distinct from simple snoring and a stridor-like character suggests that the obstruction is arising at laryngeal level. Noisy breathing during sleep can be confused with asthma or stridor, and in children with grunting.

The noises are usually complained of by the partner rather than the patient, although waking may occur with an awareness of the noise. If the arousal is delayed slightly the subject usually feels that he or she has woken suddenly for no obvious reason, but if it happens earlier there is a sensation of choking since the airway is still closed. These episodes of choking should be distinguished from vocal cord adduction which is often due to gastro-oesophageal reflux, nocturnal asthma and left ventricular failure.

RESTLESSNESS DURING SLEEP
At the end of each apnoea the moment of arousal is associated with movements which may be described as jerking, jumping, or jolting of either the limbs or the whole body. It is the partner who complains of these movements and who can occasionally be injured by them, but the patient is rarely aware of them. These movements should be distinguished from nocturnal epilepsy, periodic limb movements in sleep (PLMS) or other behavioural disorders in sleep.

OTHER SYMPTOMS DURING SLEEP
These include nocturia due to excessive secretion of ANP with reduction in renin and aldosterone secretion. The stimulus to ANP production is right atrial distension due to the increased venous return in response to the increased negative inspiratory intrathoracic pressure and to transient pulmonary hypertension during each apnoea. Nocturia only occurs if OSA is severe, but can be confused with nocturia due

to other causes such as benign prostatic hypertrophy, and it may occasionally lead to incontinence.

Gastro-oesophageal reflux may result from the repetitive Mueller manoeuvres during OSAs and excessive sweating is related to sympathetic overactivity. Confusional arousals are occasionally seen following an arousal from OSA, particularly from stages 3 and 4 NREM sleep. Coronary artery bloodflow falls during apnoeas because of vasoconstriction and changes in left ventricular stroke volume and nocturnal angina may develop. Ischaemic electrocardiogram (ECG) changes appear if there is pre-existing coronary artery disease, but are more common in REM sleep, and during long apnoeas with deep oxygen desaturations.

EXCESSIVE DAYTIME SLEEPINESS AND OTHER NEUROPSYCHOLOGICAL EFFECTS

The most important neuropsychological effect of OSA is EDS [7]. Its severity is largely related to the number of arousals and micro arousals from sleep which fragment the sleep pattern and reduce NREM sleep, but other factors may influence it. These include the motivation to stay awake, the sleep–wake patterns including the total sleep time, the individual's sleep requirements, whether shift work is being carried out, and the presence of other sleep disorders such as PLMS which might impair the quality of sleep. Fragmentation and loss of NREM is probably more important than REM sleep. There may also be a minimum duration of an arousal which contributes to EDS or of sleep between arousals which protects against this.

A common complaint is of waking feeling unrefreshed in the morning and while alertness improves during the morning, sleepiness usually returns during the afternoons, particularly during monotonous activities and in passive situations. The ability to maintain attention and to concentrate falls and short-term memory, verbal fluency and motor skills deteriorate. Alterations in mood, particularly irritability and occasionally depression, may develop. Episodes of automatic behaviour with little recall of the events may occur if the OSA is severe and the risk of road traffic accidents while driving is increased. The risk is related to the degree of EDS, and in severe OSA is around six times greater than normal subjects (page 112).

These neuropsychological changes have important implications for the quality of life. Marital and occupational difficulties, with a loss of productivity, may arise and sickness and inability to develop interpersonal relationships may lead to loss of social contacts and recreational activities with the risk of secondary anxiety and depression. All these changes are reversible with effective treatment of the OSA.

OTHER DAYTIME SYMPTOMS

These include frontal headaches on waking, possibly related to the increased intracranial pressure during OSA particularly in REM sleep and occasionally to hypercapnia. A dry and sore throat on waking is usually due to mouth breathing due to nasal obstruction. A decrease in libido and impotence is partly due to EDS resulting from sleep fragmentation and partly to reduced testosterone levels due to a reduction in gonadotrophin secretion during sleep. There are also fewer penile erections during sleep because of REM sleep fragmentation.

Natural history of obstructive sleep apnoeas and age-related features

The clinical features and significance of OSA vary according to both age and the stage in the natural history of the disorder.

CHILDREN

The most common features are snoring-like noises during sleep, associated with observation by the parents or carers that the child stops breathing and appears to be a physically restless sleeper [8]. Unusual sleeping positions may be seen which probably optimize airway patency. The OSA may be associated with frequent arousals from sleep and enuresis. Excessive daytime sleepiness is unusual. Behavioural disturbances during the day are common and include irritability, hyperactivity, aggression, poor school performance with learning problems and rapid mood changes. There may be developmental delay with short stature which is probably due to reduction in secretion of growth hormone through loss and fragmentation of stages 3 and 4 NREM sleep.

Physical examination commonly reveals enlarged tonsils and adenoids, and occasionally retrognathia and other craniofacial abnormalities. Obesity is less common than in adults, although it may be present in certain syndromes such as the Prader–Willi syndrome. Occasionally OSA is due to a chronic neurological or muscular disorder.

YOUNG AND MIDDLE-AGED ADULTS

The onset of snoring usually precedes the appearance of OSA by many years in adults. There is often a long period of stable snoring which then worsens gradually or sometimes quite rapidly before the symptoms of OSA become prominent. At the time that OSA is evolving from simple snoring, factors such as weight gain (often related to the reduction in physical activity that accompanies this and worsening EDS), may accelerate the deterioration. Snoring which can be reliably dated to childhood and which is still a problem in adult life is often due to enlarged tonsils or to a skeletal abnormality of the face or mandible. Occasionally, OSA arises suddenly in adult life in which case it is usually due to an identifiable event such as a stroke, facial injury or to the development of a contributory disorder such as hypothyroidism. Symptoms such as nocturia, early morning headaches due to hypercapnia and features of right heart failure develop late in the natural history of OSA.

The severity of OSA is related to the increased risk of death. This may be as high as 20% at 5 years and 35% at 8 years in middle-aged males when the apnoea–hypopnoea index exceeds 20 per hour. Death may be due either to accidents, for instance while driving or at work, especially while handling moving machinery, and as a result of strokes, myocardial infarction, cardiac dysrhythmias and consequences of hypertension.

OLD AGE

Obstructive sleep apnoea is probably more frequent in the elderly, but less severe and has less impact on the quality of life. Other respiratory disorders such as central sleep apnoea (CSA) and Cheyne–Stokes respiration (CSR) are more common than in younger adults and may lead to arousals from sleep. The increased frequency of OSA may be related to a deterioration in the coordination or force developed by the upper airway dilator muscles, but as the chest wall muscles become weaker the intrapharyngeal pressure becomes less negative and this tends to reduce the frequency of OSA. These considerations are complic-

ated by the increased need for drug therapy in the elderly, including benzodiazepines, changes in the sleep architecture, increased number of arousals from sleep and the increased prevalence of other sleep disorders such as PLMS.

As a result, there is a less direct link between the presence of OSA and its symptoms or increased mortality, as well as with the relief of these following effective treatment with, for instance, nasal continuous positive airway pressure (CPAP). Obstructive sleep apnoea is in effect a cofactor with other conditions which contribute to morbidity and mortality. It is often only one risk factor, with for instance ischaemic heart disease, in the development of dysrhythmias, and with cerebrovascular disease in the causation of strokes in this age group.

Assessment

HISTORY

A careful history is essential to accurately assess disorders of the upper airway (Chapter 4, Table 10.3). The issues that should be considered are as follows.

1 What noise is generated? Enquiries regarding the duration, severity and type of noise, and whether it is becoming louder or more frequent should be made.

2 What is the respiratory pattern while the noise is being generated? Comments are usually available from the partner who may be aware of how breathing starts and stops, and what noises are associated with this. The patient is occasionally aware of either waking suddenly for no apparent reason, with the noise or with a sensation of choking.

3 Are there any other associated symptoms, e.g. physical restlessness during sleep, nocturia?

4 How severe is the EDS? Is the patient unrefreshed on waking in the morning and does he or she fall asleep only in situations requiring a passive role or in

Table 10.3 When to suspect obstructive sleep apnoeas from the symptoms.	Cardinal symptoms	Snoring and snorting at night, usually with observation of stopping breathing or struggling to breathe *plus* waking unrefreshed and falling asleep readily during the day
	Supportive symptoms	Nocturnal choking or breathlessness Nocturia (if OSA severe) Nocturnal restlessness Poor memory and concentration Irritability

OSA, obstructive sleep apnoea.

those with an active role during the day as well? What is the impact of EDS on the subject's lifestyle, particularly with regard to school or work performance and family, social and recreational activity? Are an excessive quantity of caffeinated drinks taken in order to cope with EDS?

5 What is the cause of any upper airway obstruction? Has the subject gained weight or increased the collar size? Are there symptoms of nasal obstruction? Does the subject smoke, drink alcohol, take any medication and are there any problems with sleep hygiene leading to sleep deprivation? Is there any significant medical history, for instance, of facial or nasal injury, congenital defects, or of neuromuscular disorders such as motor neurone disease which might induce laryngeal obstruction? Has previous surgery for snoring been carried out on the upper airway, particularly the soft palate?

PHYSICAL EXAMINATION

These questions should be supplemented by physical examination, particularly with regard to weight, presence of obesity, any upper airway abnormalities, retrognathia and any abnormalities of the neck. A neurological or thoracic examination is only indicated if neuromuscular or lung diseases may be contributing to the symptoms of upper airway obstruction, but the blood pressure should be noted and signs of pulmonary hypertension and right heart failure sought if OSA is severe.

Observation of the patient during sleep reveals either noisy breathing or intermittent silences during the apnoeas followed by a snort or similar noise at their termination. During the apnoea the rib cage and abdomen move paradoxically, so that, for instance, while the rib cage expands the abdomen is drawn in.

INVESTIGATIONS

Initial investigations include, for instance, thyroid function tests hypothyroidism is suspected, but further investigation is only required if the symptoms are sufficiently severe or if they fail to respond to initial management of the contributory factors (Table 10.4). Investigations are usually carried out in specialist centres and include the following.

Sleep study

There is a wide choice of sleep study techniques for identifying the primary features of OSA, cessation of air flow, obstruction of the airway and arousal from sleep, as well as secondary changes such as oxygen desaturation (Chapter 4). In practice, most of the techniques either give incomplete information or use indirect markers of these three essential features of OSA.

Cortical arousals can be detected by EEG recordings although the conventional scoring system is insensitive for this. It does, however, show frequent sleep stage shifts and a short sleep latency, reduction or even loss of stages 3 and 4 NREM sleep (Fig. 4.5), sleep onset REM, and a reduction in REM sleep duration. Behavioural arousals can be shown by video, electro-myogram (EMG) or actigraphy recordings and autonomic arousals by changes in the heart rate and blood pressure. The beat to beat variation in blood pressure during and after each apnoea has been used to derive the concept of the pulse transit time as a measure of autonomic arousal [9].

The criteria for choosing the most appropriate technique have not been settled and a balance has to be struck between the costs and benefits of the different types of studies. The costs include the price of equipment, the need for the sleep study to be carried out in hospital, the time of the technical and other staff in setting up the study and interpreting the results, and the failure rate of the test. The benefits are usually assessed as the frequency with which the criteria for the diagnosis of OSA are demonstrated or the certainty with which this diagnosis is excluded, but the real value of these tests is more difficult to define. They are useful in confirming or denying the diagnosis of OSA and in assessing the frequency of apnoeas and the events that these cause, but, equally importantly, they should assess the risk to the individual of adverse events if treatment is not provided and be able to predict the effectiveness of any intervention with treatment. None of the available techniques, even polysomnography, has been adequately evaluated from this point of view. An additional complication is that the degree of certainty in the diagnosis that is required before recommending a simple treatment, such as weight loss, is less than what is needed before initiating complex treatments, such as CPAP, and this has implications for the type of sleep study that is required.

Half-night studies have been shown to be less sensitive than overnight studies, although they may be adequate if the OSA is severe. Nap studies during the day have the same problems, but are usually less costly. Occasionally, a second night study is needed, particularly if the patient shows the 'first night effect' and sleeps poorly during the test, or if no REM sleep or sleep in the supine position is obtained during the

Table 10.4 Sleep study techniques for obstructive sleep apnoea.

Technique	Physiological measurement	Abnormality detected
Nasal thermistor End-tidal P_{CO_2} Nasal pressure	Airflow	Apnoea
Plethysmography (inductance, impedance) Magnetometry	Rib cage and abdominal movement	Airflow obstruction
Oximeter	SaO_2	O_2 desaturation
Transcutaneous P_{CO_2}	Transcutaneous CO_2	Hypoventilation
EEG EOG EMG	Awake–asleep Sleep stage	Cortical and behavioural arousals
ECG Pulse transit time Finger plethysmography	Heart rate Blood pressure	Chest wall muscle activity and autonomic arousals
Microphone	Noises due to airflow through upper airway	Snoring and snorting
Oesophageal pressure	Intrapleural pressure	Chest wall muscle activity due to OSA
Actigraphy Video recording	Movements	'Behavioural' arousals and respiratory pattern

ECG, electrocardiogram; EEG, electro-encephalogram; EMG, electro-myogram; EOG, electro-oculogram; OSA, obstructive sleep apnoeas.

first night. In general, studies in the home provide less data than hospital studies, but sleep quality is often better, with more stages 3 and 4 NREM sleep.

These considerations suggest that different types of sleep study should be performed according to the pretest probabilities of each diagnosis and the treatment options. These situations include the following.

Population screening. A cheap, easily applied, sensitive, but not necessarily highly specific test is advisable. Oximetry is the most appropriate.

Low clinical probability for OSA. Excessive daytime sleepiness, but with no known snoring or risk factors such as obesity is an example. A simple screening study such as oximetry, possibly with monitoring of chest wall movements or the pulse transit time may be sufficient to exclude OSA and to raise the probability of a non-respiratory cause of EDS to a sufficient level. An alternative to this approach would be to carry out polysomnography as the initial investiga-

tion, but the use of a simple and cheap screening test avoids the need for polysomnography in those patients in which it does reveal OSA.

Intermediate and high clinical probability for OSA. Snoring with observed apnoeas and EDS is an example. Confirmation of apnoeas or paradoxical rib cage and abdominal movements, or desaturations is required. Oximetry, ideally with a chest wall movement detector and air flow sensor, provides this information and the frequency of arousals can be assessed either from heart rate or pulse transit time variations.

Complex clinical presentation. Excessive daytime sleepiness with snoring and symptoms of the restless legs syndrome is an example. Polysomnography is advisable to evaluate the relative contribution of each of the possible causes.

Failure to respond to CPAP treatment. If compliance with CPAP is satisfactory and an adequate pressure is provided, there is a high probability that an undiagnosed and probably non-respiratory factor is responsible for the persisting symptoms. Polysomnography is the investigation of choice.

Assessment of severity of excessive daytime sleepiness
A measure of daytime sleepiness such as the Epworth Sleepiness Scale is useful and occasionally simple unprepared reaction times, multiple sleep latency tests, maintenance of wakefulness tests and tests of performance such as driving simulators are of value (Chapter 4).

Localization of site of upper airway obstruction

Imaging techniques. Several techniques have been developed to assess the size and shape of the upper airway and the level of its obstruction, but they have a limited application, largely because they are usually carried out while the subject is awake and upright. These methods include X-ray lateral cephalometry, acoustic reflection, computerized tomograph (CT), and magnetic resonance imaging (MRI) scans. Dynamic cine X-ray and CT scans provide information about the changes in the airway during breathing and may be carried out during sleep if EDS is severe.

Endoscopy. Upper airway endoscopy while awake can be useful in selected patients to examine organic lesions of the upper airway and movements of the vocal cords and pharynx. 'Sleep' nasendoscopy has been developed, but is more accurately termed 'sedative' or 'anaesthetic' nasendoscopy since it is carried out under sedation with, for instance, intravenous midazolam or propofol. Nasendoscopy during wakefulness may be combined with a Mueller manoeuvre (a forced inspiration with the mouth and nose occluded) in order to localize the site of obstruction or vibration of the upper airway.

Physiological techniques. Flow-volume loops may indicate the presence of major airway obstruction and show a sawtooth pattern of fluttering, particularly on the expiratory limb.

These localization techniques are of little value, either in mild OSA when simple first-line treatments are envisaged, or if OSA is severe enough to require nasal CPAP treatment, since the effectiveness of these treatments is rarely related to the site of obstruction. There may be value in knowing the level of obstruction before trying a mandibular advancement device,

but this is usually given a therapeutic trial without a localization investigation. The main indication for these techniques is if surgery, particularly on the palate, is being considered, but, as described below, this is usually only indicated for OSA if it is mild. Localization techniques are not often used in assessing whether a tonsillectomy should be performed, but could be of value. They may help in the assessment of major reconstructive surgery for craniofacial abnormalities.

Treatment
The aims of treatment of OSA are:
1 relief of symptoms;
2 prevention of medical complications such as hypertension, myocardial infarction, strokes and premature death;
3 reduction of the risk of accidents; and
4 improvement of the quality of life.

The treatments used to achieve these aims fall into two groups.

FIRST-LINE TREATMENTS
These can be initiated in general practice, often without the need for a sleep study and are aimed at relieving the factors which contribute to upper airway obstruction.

Weight loss
Weight loss should be attempted in patients who are obese, particularly if weight gain has coincided with an increase in neck size indicated by a change in shirt collar requirements and a worsening of symptoms or of sleep study findings. It is of help in around 50% of obese subjects with OSA, but weight is frequently regained.

Alcohol intake
The intake of alcohol should be reduced.

Hypnotics
Benzodiazepines and other hypnotics should be avoided.

Avoidance of sleep deprivation
Sleep deprivation reduces the respiratory drive to both hypoxia and hypercapnia, increases the threshold for arousal, alters sleep architecture and may impair upper airway muscle function.

Sleeping on the side rather than in the supine position
'Postural' or 'positional' treatment is difficult to main-

tain, but sleeping with a pillow wedged under the shoulders to prevent returning to the supine position is preferable to fixing a ball, foam or similar object into the back of the nightclothes since this causes arousal from sleep each time the supine position occurs [10]. This type of treatment is said to lead to a conditioned reflex whereby the lateral position is maintained but there is little evidence for this. Equipment which delivers an electric shock when it detects a snoring sound works on similar principles and has similar disadvantages.

Sleeping with the neck slightly extended may help prevent OSA by increasing the pharyngeal diameter.

Improvement in nasal airway
This may be achieved with treatment for, for instance, rhinitis with inhaled steroids or with external or internal mechanical nasal dilators.

Smoking cessation
Stopping smoking may help, but often leads to weight gain which worsens the OSA.

SECOND-LINE TREATMENTS
These are reserved for subjects who have more frequent and severe OSA (usually greater than 20 per hour), who have daytime hypercapnia, or who are resistant to first-line measures, either because they are ineffective or because of poor compliance. Referral to a specialist centre is usually required for a sleep study and assessment for these treatments (Fig. 10.4). They fall into three groups.

Modification of upper airway muscle control and function
These treatments are usually ineffective and rarely used.

Ventilatory stimulants. A variety of drugs including progesterone, almitrine, doxapram and theophylline have been tried but none is effective.

Oxygen. This may abolish the desaturations detected in sleep studies, but apnoeas may be prolonged because it removes the hypoxic drive to breathe and to arousal. There is also a risk of nocturnal hypercapnia in severe OSA. Little change of sleep quality or daytime symptoms has been reported.

Surface active and muscle activating agents. Application of preparations containing chemicals that alter the surface properties of the upper airway or increase

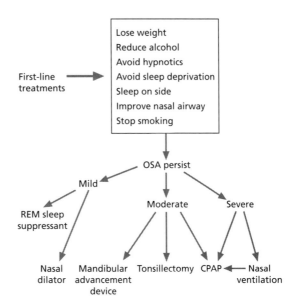

Fig. 10.4 Treatment of obstructive sleep apnoeas (OSA). CPAP, continuous positive airway pressure; REM, rapid eye movement.

the muscle tone have been used, but there is little evidence regarding their effectiveness.

Electrical stimulation of upper airway muscles. Implantation of electrical stimulation devices to 'pace' the pharyngeal dilator muscles in time with inspiration can be triggered by changes in rib cage movements. Direct stimulation of the hypoglossal (12th cranial) nerve with hook electrodes and of the genioglossus muscle have been employed. It is important that the site of obstruction is localized to the base of the tongue before these are attempted [11].

Modification of sleep pattern

REM sleep suppressants. Both tricyclic antidepressants and selective serotonin re-uptake inhibitors (SSRIs) reduce the duration of REM sleep and are effective if OSA are confined or almost confined to REM sleep. Protriptyline 5–20 mg nocte has been most widely used since it is nonsedating, but side-effects such as constipation and urinary retention are common with a dose of more than around 10 mg. Selective serotonin re-uptake inhibitor antidepressants, such as paroxetine, may also reduce the sleep loss of upper airway muscle activity during NREM sleep, possibly through increasing 5HT availability in the DRN. This may reduce the number and frequency of OSA in NREM sleep.

Central nervous system stimulants. Stimulant drugs such as modafinil have been proposed as adjunctive treatment to other measures including nasal CPAP if EDS is not completely relieved. It is important to ensure that the cause of the EDS is OSA rather than an unrelated and undiagnosed disorder such as PLMS and stimulants should only be used after every effort to improve the effectiveness of and compliance with CPAP has been made.

Increase in dimensions of upper airway. This can be achieved by mechanical devices, surgery and pneumatically with nasal continuous positive airway pressure or intermittent positive pressure ventilation.

Mechanical devices
1 *Soft palate supports.* These devices keep the soft palate and uvula elevated but there is little evidence regarding their effectiveness.
2 *Tongue retaining and protrusion devices.* These prevent the tongue from falling back into the pharyngeal airway and in addition may cause mandibular advancement. A suction bulb can be used to anchor the tip of the tongue to the teeth or lips. This is moderately effective in OSA but poorly tolerated.
3 *Mandibular advancement or positioning devices.* These have been quite extensively used and work by holding the mandible in a predetermined relationship to the upper jaw through a gum shield or similar device which is moulded or set to both the upper and lower teeth [12]. Most of these devices are in one piece, but some have two parts which are joined by adjustable hooks and ridges. These allow some lateral and vertical jaw movement so that the patient can talk and yawn, but prevent any antero-posterior movement. The devices can be moulded or set by the patient, or designed individually by a dental surgeon from an impression of the teeth. In general, the position of the mandible should be approximately halfway between the natural resting position and the most protruded position possible as long as this is comfortable. An inability to protrude the mandible less than 0.6 cm is associated with a lack of effectiveness and the devices often fail because of discomfort or increased salivation. The mouth should not be opened excessively since this rotates the mandible and narrows the airway. These devices may work not only by advancing the tongue and mandible, but also by altering upper airway muscle tone.

They are most beneficial if the apnoeas:
(a) originate at the level of the base of the tongue, especially if there is retrognathia;
(b) are worse in the supine position;
(c) are mild or moderate; and
(d) in subjects who cannot tolerate alternative treatments such as CPAP.

These devices may become displaced and compliance is less good with the more bulky devices. They can cause excessive salivation, dental hyper-sensitivity and gagging. They are contraindicated if there is:
(a) temporomandibular joint dysfunction;
(b) insufficient or excessively mobile anterior teeth, dentures which are removed at night, extensive dental crown and bridge work, and periodontal disease;
(c) obesity, which mass loads the airway whatever the body position; and
(d) in nasal obstruction, with some devices, since they can impede oral breathing.
4 *Nasal dilators.* These reduce the nasal resistance to airflow and thereby cause the intrapharyngeal pressure to be less negative and reduce the likelihood that the airway will close. Internal nasal dilators have a spring which stretches the nares. They only dilate the anterior part of the airway, may be difficult to tolerate and often become displaced. External dilators are applied to the nose just anterior to the distal end of the nasal cartilage. They are better tolerated, rarely become displaced and are probably at least as effective as the internal dilators.

Upper airway surgery
Upper airway surgery is more commonly carried out for snoring (p. 217) has been proposed for OSA on the basis that it may widen the airway, cause scar tissue which reduces its compliance and that it may alter upper airway reflexes beneficially [13]. It has the advantage of being a single procedure compared with most of the other treatments for OSA which require regular long-term application. The results of most procedures, except tonsillectomy have, however, been disappointing and, in general, surgery should be avoided in the obese, or if OSA are frequent or severe. In these situations the obstruction occurs at multiple sites or levels in the airway, and a localized surgical approach is unlikely to correct all of these. The operations that have been proposed include the following.

1 *Nasal surgery.* This is rarely effective.
2 *Palatal surgery.* Resection of part of the palate together with a uvulectomy has been practised for many years (uvulopalatopharyngoplasty, UVPPP, UPPP). A similar effect can be obtained with a laser (laser assisted uvulopalatoplasty, LAUP), by refashioning the palate. This can also be used to stiffen it

through applying the laser in various patterns to create burns which heal by fibrosis. Radio-frequency energy applied through a needle also alters the deeper muscular tissues but does not affect the mucosa or alter palatal sensation. It causes necrosis of tissue and submucosal fibrosis with loss of volume of the palate and an increase in its stiffness. It is less painful than the other procedures but often needs to be repeated several times.

Palatal surgery is only effective in around 15% of subjects with significant OSA and even less frequently in those with more severe OSA. If palatal surgery is carried out and is ineffective, application of nasal CPAP may cause mouth leaks since the palate may no longer seal against the back of the tongue. This can be overcome as described on page 214.

3 *Maxillo-facial surgery.* This may be required for complex cranio-facial abnormalities but should be performed only in specialist centres.

4 *Mandibular advancement or osteotomy procedures.* These may occasionally be effective, especially if micrognathia or retrognathia is the cause of the OSA and if the maxilla is also advanced. Mandibular protrusion pulls the tongue base and supra-hyoid muscles forwards, and the soft palate is tightened by maxillary advancement. These procedures may, therefore, be of most value if the airway obstructs at multiple levels.

5 *Tongue volume reduction surgery (linguoplasty).* Resection of the tongue base can be carried out surgically with a laser or radio-frequency technique, but there are little data regarding its value. The technique of suture suspension of the tongue base may be more effective.

6 *Hyoid surgery.* Hyoidoplasty has a limited role. The hyoid is moved forward or rotated and fixed to the anterior margin of the mandible or to the thyroid cartilage. This can be combined with mandibular advancement.

7 *Laryngeal surgery.* This may be of value if there are anatomical or neurological abnormalities affecting the larynx.

8 *Tonsillectomy and adenoidectomy.* These are often effective both in children and in adults if the tonsils and adenoids are markedly enlarged even if OSA are frequent and severe.

9 *Excision of obstructing mass.* Excision of any mass, such as an upper airway benign tumour, which narrows the airway may improve OSA.

10 *Tracheostomy.* This has been recommended in the past because it bypasses the upper airway obstruction, but it is now rarely required. The indications are if

OSA is life threatening and neither nasal CPAP nor intubation are available, and if CPAP is ineffective, as occurs occasionally with laryngeal disorders, or cannot be tolerated. A simple alternative to tracheostomy in these situations is the administration of air at around 5 l/min through a minitrach or trans-tracheal oxygen catheter.

11 *Gastric surgery.* Gastric surgery, including stapling, does not have any direct effect on OSA, but by assisting weight loss may indirectly improve it.

NASAL CONTINUOUS POSITIVE AIRWAY PRESSURE

The principle of CPAP is that it increases the pressure within the upper airway during both inspiration and expiration (Fig. 10.5). It acts as a pneumatic splint, counteracting the forces that tend to close the airway. It may also have effects on upper airway reflexes which tend to activate the upper airway dilator muscles. Continuous positive airway pressure also increases the functional residual capacity slightly. This increases the oxygen stores and therefore reduces the degree of oxygen desaturation during an apnoea, reflexly increases the upper airway diameter, and reduces the left ventricular preload and reduces any pulmonary oedema.

Equipment

A CPAP system comprises the following.

Continuous positive airway pressure pump. This is a pump with a high flow capacity which delivers air at pressures which can be adjusted and then maintained almost constant during both inspiration and expiration (Fig. 10.6). The pressure can be kept at a fixed value throughout the night or varied in two ways. Firstly, the desired pressure level can be gradually reached over 20–30 min at the onset of sleep using a pressure 'ramp'. This may be useful for patients who find it difficult to tolerate the required pressure while they are falling asleep. Secondly, newer variable pressure (intelligent, autocontinuous, auto-CPAP) machines detect when there is inspiratory flow limitation and adjust the CPAP level on a breath by breath basis to prevent this [14]. The aim is to abolish all micro arousals due to airflow limitation, and to minimize the applied pressure. In practice, however, the mean pressure that is achieved is only slightly less than with standard CPAP models, and there is a risk that allowing some airflow limitation will lead to arousals. Leaks due to displacement of the mask or opening of the mouth may be interpreted by the machine as an arousal and

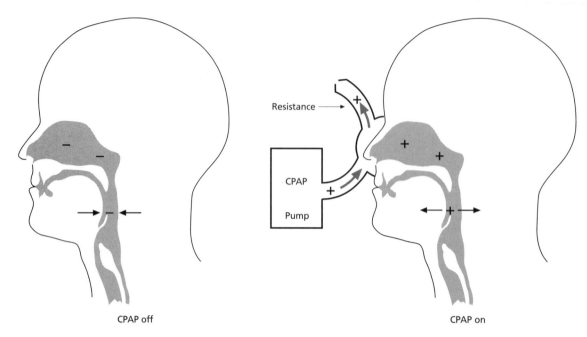

Resistance →

CPAP
Pump

CPAP off

CPAP on

Fig. 10.5 Continuous positive airway pressure (CPAP) principle. The right hand figure shows positive pressure generated by the CPAP pump being conducted to the upper airway and expanding it at pharyngeal level. The left hand figure indicates spontaneous breathing without CPAP with negative pressure in the upper airway drawing the pharyngeal walls together.

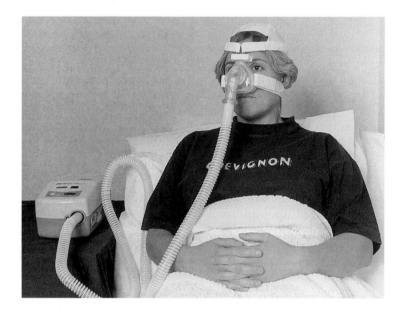

Fig. 10.6 Continuous positive airway pressure (CPAP) mask and pump.

lead to an inappropriate increase in the pressure. These systems are probably only of value in the few patients with variable and high pressure requirements who find CPAP difficult to tolerate.

They have been used as a diagnostic technique, but their accuracy varies according to the methods used to adjust the pressure and they have not been well evaluated. Errors due to, for instance, mouth breathing and displacement of the nasal pressure transducer may be significant.

They have also been employed to assess the level of CPAP that is required when treatment is being initiated. The pressure which relieves 95% of obstructive episodes has been recommended but artefacts and events during arousals often make interpretation of the pressure changes difficult. They have the advantage of reducing the costs associated with the supervision that is needed to 'manually' titrate the CPAP level, but the loss of personal contact may reduce the patient's degree of understanding and acceptance of the equipment. Newer methods, such as the forced oscillation technique, may be of more value in assessing the optimum CPAP level. The use of predictive equations is an unsatisfactory alternative to any of these methods.

Continuous positive airway pressure systems are powered either by mains electricity or an external battery and most have a dual voltage or continually variable voltage facility. Their pressure range is around 4–20 cmH$_2$O, but the degree of pressure stability during each respiratory cycle varies between CPAP systems. The pressure tends to increase during expiration as air is added to the circuit from the patient and to fall in inspiration according to the patient's inspiratory flow rate. The noise of most CPAP systems is around 40 decibels. The air can be humidified with a heated water humidifier if necessary, usually because of nasal symptoms. Most CPAP systems have an electronic clock which either measures the duration for which the machine is switched on or for which a predetermined pressure is applied. The latter is of more value in assessing the patient's compliance since it measures the time for which the CPAP is applied to the face rather than simply the time for which the machine is switched on.

Continuous positive airway pressure circuit. This comprises the connecting tubing between the pump and the mask. An exhalation valve or leak is placed in the circuit close to the patient or in the mask in order to prevent rebreathing and carbon dioxide retention. The efficiency of these leaks or valves varies from system to system.

Mask and headgear. A nasal mask is usually sufficient, but occasionally a full face mask which includes the mouth as well is needed, either because of persistent mouth leaks or if the nasal airway is significantly blocked. The masks are made of silicon or similar inert flexible material and should be fitted individually to provide a comfortable seal around the nose or

Table 10.5 CPAP complications and corrective measures.

Complication	Corrective measure
Air leak	Change mask or headgear Try chin strap or collar Alter head and neck position Consider face mask
Nasal symptoms	Inhaled steroid or ipratropium Minimize mouth leak Heated water humidification
Skin ulceration	Change mask or headgear Protect skin with, e.g., granuflex
Claustrophobia	Use smaller mask or nasal seals
Aerophagy	Reduce level of CPAP
Noise of CPAP	Reassure Earplugs

CPAP, continuous positive airway pressure.

nose and mouth. Nasal plugs or seals which fit into or around the nares are alternatives, particularly in patients who find masks claustrophobic. The mask, plugs or seals are held in place by headgear of a cap or strap design which fits around the skull.

Indications
Continuous positive airway pressure is effective in OSA whether it is mild or severe, but compliance is poor unless there is considerable symptomatic relief. Its use is therefore reserved for patients in whom there are:
1 troublesome symptoms from OSA;
2 frequent and deep oxygen saturation dips (usually more than 30 desaturations per hour) or other indicator of OSA frequency which suggest that complications are likely unless treatment is provided [15]; or
3 hypercapnia during the day time. Treatment for the first few nights with nasal positive pressure ventilation may be needed before transferring to CPAP.

The threshold for initiating CPAP should be lowered in the presence of other cardiovascular risk factors, or a history of angina, myocardial infarction or stroke, or if the patient is particularly at risk from the effects of EDS because of, for instance, the need to drive motor vehicles for long distances.

Side-effects
Several problems may arise while CPAP is being used (Table 10.5). The most important are discussed below.

Air leaks. These may occur around the mask and although the CPAP pump can compensate for considerable leaks these should be minimized, particularly if the air is directed into or close to the eyes when it can cause conjunctivitis. Air leaks through the mouth are common, and can be minimized by the use of a chin strap, collar and attention to the head and neck position, or if necessary the use of a face mask instead of a nasal mask.

Upper airway symptoms. The most common are a sensation of nasal blockage, nasal discharge or occasionally nose bleeds. A blocked nose is often noticed within one or two nights of starting CPAP, and may require inhaled nasal steroids. If the nasal discharge is watery, nasal inhaled ipratropium is of use. These symptoms are worse if there is a large unidirectional airflow through the nose which usually accompanies a significant mouth leak, and correction of this often improves nasal symptoms. If they persist heated water humidification of the inspired air or the use of a face mask which includes the mouth as well as the nose, are usually effective.

Skin problems. Soreness, redness and ulceration of the skin at the contact points with the mask are common. These can be prevented by attention to mask selection and fitting, and to the head gear. Once an ulcer has formed a barrier such as granuflex is usually required to assist healing and this can also be used prophylactically. A *Staphylococcal folliculitis* occasionally occurs and responds to fucidic acid cream.

Claustrophobia. Some patients feel claustrophobic with a nasal or face mask, but may be able to tolerate nasal seals or plugs.

Aerophagy. Air entering the pharynx under pressure may pass through the cricopharyngeal sphincter into the oesophagus instead of entering the trachea. Abdominal distension, belching and the passing of flatus rectally may result. Reduction in the CPAP level usually relieves these symptoms.

Noise. The noise of most CPAP systems is around 40 decibels, but the air leak in the mask or in the circuit close to the patient can also cause a disturbing noise. Ear plugs may be of help to either the patient or the partner.

Failure of continuous positive airway pressure
Continuous positive airway pressure treatment usually causes an improvement in symptoms and in sleep study findings even after a single night at an appropriate level. Failure to improve may, however, be due to one or more of the following.

Incorrect diagnosis. The apnoeas may be central rather than obstructive or the observed desaturations could be due to ventilation–perfusion mismatching rather than to apnoeas. In many patients OSA is not the only diagnosis and symptoms of, for instance, EDS may be mainly due to periodic limb movements in sleep and OSA may be of secondary importance.

Insufficient CPAP level. The usual level of CPAP that is required is 5–15 cm or occasionally up to 20 cm of water. The pressure is usually adjusted so that oxygen desaturations and markers of autonomic arousal, such as heart rate changes, are abolished, but other criteria such as reduction in airflow limitation can be used. If the pressure is too low the apnoeas will only be partially relieved and symptoms may not disappear. A higher pressure is needed in the supine than the lateral posistion and in REM than in NREM sleep. The pressure that is required often falls slightly over the first few weeks after treatment is initiated, possibly because of relief of sleep fragmentation and of oedema of the palate and pharyngeal walls, but if the patient's weight changes the required CPAP level may alter again at a later stage.

Technical problems. Worsening leaks or nasal obstruction may prevent CPAP from being effective.

Poor compliance. Compliance with CPAP is often measured in terms of the number of hours used per night, but a better measure is whether or not the CPAP is used sufficiently to relieve symptoms. This may be only around 4 h per night for many patients. Failure to achieve this may be due to inadequate education and explanation at the time of initiation of treatment, a pressure set too low, pressure-related side-effects, claustrophobia or rejection of the equipment psychologically by the patient or partner. Some patients take the CPAP mask off during their sleep, possibly during a confusional arousal, but use of a low-pressure alarm in the circuit which wakes the subject and alerts him or her to replace the mask is often effective.

Compliance is best if the patient has been well instructed and educated in the need for CPAP when it is initiated, if there is symptomatic improvement and if there are few side-effects. Regular follow-up with attention given to psychological aspects of accepting the

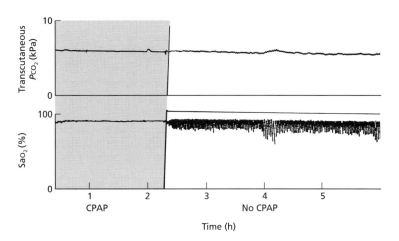

Fig. 10.7 Effects of continuous positive airway pressure (CPAP) on Sao_2 and transcutaneous Pco_2. Oximetry tracing in lower figure shows constant value of 95% using CPAP during the first third of the night, but without this there are frequent desaturations to a minimum of 66%. These are associated with transient rises in transcutaneous Pco_2 shown in the upper tracing indicating episodes of hypoventilation.

equipment, relief of complications and modification of the CPAP level according to its effectiveness are all important in maintaining compliance. The compliance rate varies from 40 to 90% in different centres largely according to the selection of patients for CPAP, and the level of education and supervision that is provided.

Effects of treatment

The effects of CPAP on the pathophysiological responses to OSA are immediate [16]. Symptoms both during the night and day improve within one or two night's treatment and the improvement is virtually complete within around two weeks. Sleep architecture returns to normal, but there is often REM sleep rebound during the first few nights, particularly if sleep onset REM is present before treatment. The ventilatory response to carbon dioxide returns to normal and disturbed circadian rhythms, including changes in the temperature cycle, are normalized. The apnoeas and oxygen desaturations are relieved (Fig. 10.7) and the rapid changes in blood pressure and heart rate disappear. The haemoglobin and erythropoietin level fall and pulmonary hypertension during the apnoeas disappears. Right ventricular function and pulmonary artery pressure during the day also normalize. Mood changes, EDS, difficulty in concentrating and other cognitive problems resolve and as far as is known the risk of cardiovascular complications, particularly stroke, returns to normal, although direct evidence for this is lacking. Fibrinogen levels and platelet activation and aggregation also return to normal with CPAP.

Cessation of treatment

Continuous positive airway pressure does not cure OSA but it is able to control or suppress the tendency to obstruct the upper airway. If CPAP is not used for any reason the OSA returns, although it may be several nights before its full intensity is seen, because of factors such as absence of sleep deprivation on the first night which progress as the time without CPAP increases.

A trial without CPAP is justified if it is possible to treat or relieve the underlying cause of OSA. Loss of weight, treatment of, for instance, hypothyroidism or by tonsillectomy may all enable CPAP to be withdrawn. If some OSA persist, an alternative treatment such as a mandibular advancement device can be tried.

NASAL INTERMITTENT POSITIVE PRESSURE VENTILATION

Nasal intermittent positive pressure ventilation (NIPPV) is occasionally required to treat OSA. The same system is used as for hypercapnic respiratory failure due to other conditions (page 192). A positive inspiratory pressure is combined with an expiratory pressure of approximately one third of the inspiratory level. This combination both provides inspiratory support to increase the alveolar ventilation and prevents the upper airway from closing during expiration. It is indicated in the following circumstances.

1 When daytime hypercapnia is present (Pco_2 greater than about 7 kPa). Hypercapnia indicates that the OSA are severe and it usually occurs either in the grossly obese, in the presence of chronic lung disease, particularly chronic bronchitis and emphysema, with neuromuscular disorders in which respiratory muscle strength is reduced, or occasionally in those who live alone and in whom the lack of social contact delays their presentation until an advanced stage in the natural history has been reached. Nasal positive pressure ventilation may only be required for a few days until sleep deprivation has been relieved and the Pco_2 has

returned to normal. At that stage the transfer to nasal CPAP can be made, although NIPPV is occasionally required in the long term.

2 Poor compliance with CPAP because of a high pressure requirement. The high expiratory pressure may be difficult to tolerate and use of a bilevel pressure system in which the inspiratory pressure is usually around three times the expiratory pressure is often of benefit, and reduces the severity of nasal side-effects.

Snoring

Overview
Simple snoring is a common problem in which noise is generated in the upper airway but is not associated with airflow limitation.

Prevalence
The prevalence of snoring is hard to assess because of the difficulty in quantifying it. It is usually complained of by the patient's partner who is only capable of reporting it if he or she is awake. It is said that around 35% of adults snore occasionally and 10% on most nights, and that it is approximately four times more common in men than women. It becomes less common during the teenage years after involution of the tonsils and adenoids, but becomes more frequent again in early middle age and increases in prevalence up to around age 75 years. Beyond this age it becomes less of a problem, partly because the chest wall muscles are less able to induce a sufficiently negative intra-airway pressure to vibrate the walls of the upper airway and also because of the increase in prevalence of deafness among the partners.

Pathophysiology
Snoring is due to vibration of the tissues of the upper airway, usually during inspiration but occasionally during expiration or alternatively during both. Unlike OSA there is no interruption of airflow into the lungs since the closure of the airway is at most only momentary and is not sustained throughout one or more inspirations. The noise of snoring is generated by turbulent flow in the column of air in the upper airway.

Vibration of the upper airway can occur at any level down to the larynx but usually involves the soft palate, base of the tongue and posterior pharyngeal wall. There is no cortical or autonomic arousal from sleep during simple snoring since the work of the inspiratory muscles does not progressively increase as in OSA and the upper airway resistance syndrome.

Aetiology
The aetiology of simple snoring is similar to OSA.

Clinical features
The complaint of snoring almost invariably comes from a listener, usually the bed partner of the patient (Table 10.6). The complaint usually reflects the degree of sleep disruption or dissatisfaction of the partner and varies according to the partner's arousability from sleep by the noise and the presence of any insomnia. Snoring can lead to significant sleep disruption with EDS and frustration and anger in the partner. This may be expressed by repetitive physical attempts to wake the snorer who may then become secondarily sleep deprived and feel guilty about the sleep disruption that the snoring is causing to the partner. There is no evidence that snoring causes noise induced deafness either in the patient or partner.

The volume of the snoring varies considerably between patients and during any one night. Acoustic analysis has shown that the frequency of sound generated at palatal level is around 200 Hz with frequent harmonics and can be distinguished from tongue base (predominantly around 1000 Hz) and laryngeal snoring. These sound differences can be identified by the experienced observer. A stridor-like sound usually arises from the larynx. Snoring may be continuous or intermittent and can build up to a crescendo in which case the UARS or OSA should be suspected.

Snoring may remain constant or may fluctuate only slightly in severity and frequency over many years, but occasionally it evolves into the UARS or OSA, at which time the character of the snoring changes. Until that point other features of OSA are absent although epidemiological surveys have shown an increased prevalence of EDS and hypertension in snorers. This is probably because these populations included subjects with undiagnosed UARS and OSA.

Physical examination may reveal pathology within the upper airway, obesity or retrognathia as with UARS and OSA. An attempt to simulate snoring may

Table 10.6 Clinical features of snoring.

Noise usually inspiratory
Snoring usually regular, if not suspect UARS or OSA
No EDS unless sleep disrupted by the partner, UARS or OSA
Partner's sleep disrupted

EDS, excessive daytime sleepiness; OSA, obstructive sleep apnoeas; UARS, upper airway resistance syndrome.

be helpful in indicating at which level it is arising, particularly if the noise is recognized by the partner as being identical to snoring during sleep.

Assessment
The assessment of snoring is similar to that of OSA since it is important not only to assess the snoring itself, but also whether the subject has OSA since the management of the two conditions often differs.

The same issues are important in taking the history and on examination. Referral for investigation is required if simple first-line measures are insufficient or if surgery is being considered. Investigation includes the following.

SLEEP STUDIES
These are required to assess whether UARS or OSA are present or whether the problem is simple snoring (page 206).

ASSESSMENT OF THE DEGREE OF EXCESSIVE DAYTIME SLEEPINESS
In contrast to OSA and UARS, EDS is not a consequence of simple snoring unless the partner's response to the snoring causes sleep deprivation.

LOCALIZATION OF THE POINT OF VIBRATION OF THE UPPER AIRWAY
The techniques that are available for localizing where the snoring is originating have been described on page 208. Localization is more important in the management of snoring than OSA since it is important, before undertaking any surgical procedure, to assess whether snoring is arising at the level which is to be operated on. In addition to the techniques described above, an audio tape recording of the snoring, either in the patient's home or in hospital, may help in assessing the level at which the snoring is arising. An alternative is for the patient to generate a snoring sound, for this to be identified as such by the partner and either under direct vision or through nasendoscopy for the site of vibration of the upper airway causing the sound to be visualized.

ASSESSMENT OF THE SEVERITY OF THE SNORING
The primary impact of snoring is on the listener rather than on the snorer. This is subjective and varies not only according to the loudness, frequency and pattern of the snoring, and also with the partner's quality of sleep, sensitization to the snoring noise and the emotional response to the noise and to being woken during the night. A visual analogue score of the severity or frequency of the snoring completed by the partner may be of help in assessing its perceived severity.

Treatment
The aim of treatment of snoring is to render the patient sufficiently quiet for the partner to sleep. Simple snoring does not have any known adverse effects on the snorer. Improvement in the partner's sleep can be achieved by the following.

TREATMENT OF THE PARTNER
It is important that the partner is aware that the snorer is not generating the noise voluntarily and reassurance about the absence of health risks to the snorer may be of help. The partner may be able to sleep better if he or she falls asleep before the snorer and protection in the form of ear plugs or similar equipment may be useful. If these measures are ineffective and the snoring can not be treated, an alternative is for the snorer and partner to sleep in separate bedrooms. Hypnotic drugs are occasionally taken by the partner to minimize the sleep disruption caused by the snoring, but are inadvisable as long-term treatment.

TREATMENT OF THE PATIENT

First-line treatments
These are identical to measures for treating OSA.

Second-line treatments
In general these are similar to the treatments for OSA, but the importance of oral devices and surgery is greater compared with CPAP, both because these treatments are more effective and because compliance with CPAP in simple snoring is poor because of the lack of symptomatic benefit to the patient. Oral devices and upper airway surgery are probably more effective because the upper airway disorder in snoring is more localized than it is in OSA.

Upper airway surgery. Surgery is occasionally indicated for OSA (p. 210) but is more commonly carried out for snoring. It is usually advisable to localize the origin of the snoring before carrying out surgery, and it is essential that a sleep study is performed before surgery is contemplated in order to assess whether OSA are sufficiently frequent to be a contraindication to surgery. Surgery should, in general, not be recommended unless first line treatments, in particular weight loss, have been attempted and failed.

The mechanisms by which surgery may work are similar to those described under OSA. The indication for surgery is that the snoring should be sufficiently troublesome to the listener. The snorer should be aware that he or she will not directly benefit from surgery and that there are risks with all the procedures.

The surgical techniques that have been used include the following.

1 *Nasal surgery.* This is often effective if nasal polyps are present, but usually has little effect in other situations.

2 *Palatal surgery.* This can be carried out with either a surgical, laser or radio frequency technique. It is effective in around 70% of non-obese subjects if snoring has been localized to palatal level, but is less effective in the obese. Snoring recurs in around 20% over the next two years, possibly more frequently with the laser procedures than with a surgical palatoplasty. Side-effects of resection of too much palate include voice change, difficulty in swallowing, and nasal regurgitation of fluids due to palatal incompetence (velo-pharyngeal insufficiency). If too little is resected the chance of snoring being relieved is lessened. These procedures are painful in the immediate postoperative period, and if palatal surgery is carried out when OSA has not been recognized, it may be fatal because of oedema or a haematoma developing postoperatively and obstructing the airway. Complications are less frequent with the laser and radio frequency procedures than with a surgical palatoplasty, and they can be readily repeated if the snoring recurs.

3 *Tonsillectomy and adenoidectomy.* These procedures are usually effective if the tonsils and adenoids are enlarged.

4 *Mandibular advancement or osteotomy procedures.* These are rarely indicated for simple snoring.

Mandibular advancement devices. These are effective, particularly if the snoring is worst in the supine position.

Nasal CPAP. This is effective in treating snoring, although it is rarely recommended because of poor long-term compliance since there is no symptomatic benefit to the patient.

References

1 Tsai WH, Flemons WW, Whitelaw WA, Remmers JE. A comparison of apnea-hypopnea indices derived from different definitions of hypopnea. *Am J Respir Crit Care Med* 1999; 159: 43–8.

2 Exar EN, Collop NA. The upper airway resistance syndrome. *Chest* 1999; 115: 1127–39.

3 Stradling JR. Obstructive sleep apnoea: definitions, epidemiology, and natural history. *Thorax* 1995; 50: 683–9.

4 Whittle AT, Marshall I, Mortimore IL, Wraith PK, Sellar RJ, Douglas NJ. Neck soft tissue and fat distribution: comparison between normal men and women by magnetic resonance imaging. *Thorax* 1999; 54: 323–8.

5 Weitzenblum E, Chaouat A, Kessler R, Oswald M, Apprill M, Krieger J. Daytime hypoventilation in obstructive sleep apnoea syndrome. *Sleep Med Rev* 1999; 3: 79–93.

6 Zwillich CW. Sleep apnoea and autonomic function. *Thorax* 1998; 53(3): S20–4.

7 Engleman H, Joffe D. Neurophysiological function in obstructive sleep apnoea. *Sleep Med Rev* 1999; 3: 59–78.

8 Gaultier C. Obstructive sleep apnoea syndrome in infants and children: established facts and unsettled issues. *Thorax* 1995; 50: 1204–10.

9 Smith RP, Argod J, Pepin J-L, Levy PA. Pulse transit time: an appraisal of potential clinical applications. *Thorax* 1999; 54: 452–8.

10 Jokic R, Klimaszewski A, Crossley M, Sridhar G, Fitzpatrick MF. Postional treatment vs continuous positive airway pressure in patients with positional obstructive sleep apnea syndrome. *Chest* 1999; 115: 771–81.

11 De Backer W. Non-CPAP treatment of obstructive sleep apnoea. *Monaldi Arch Chest Dis* 1998; 53: 625–9.

12 Marklund M, Persson M, Franklin KA. Treatment success with a mandibular advancement device is related to supine-dependent sleep apnea. *Chest* 1998; 114: 1630–5.

13 Sher AE, Schechtman KB, Piccirillo JF. The efficacy of surgical modifications of the upper airway in adults with obstructive sleep apnea syndrome. *Sleep* 1996; 19: 156–77.

14 Braghiroli A, Sacco C, Carli S, Rossi S, Donner CF. Autocontinuous positive airway pressure in the diagnosis and treatment of obstructive sleep apnoea. *Monaldi Arch Chest Dis* 1998; 53: 621–4.

15 Loube DI, Gay PC, Strohl KP, Pack AI, White DP, Collop NA. Indications for positive airway pressure treatment of adult obstructive sleep apnea patients. *Chest* 1999; 115: 863–6.

16 Ballester E, Badia JR, Hernandez L, Carrasco E *et al.* Evidence of the effectiveness of continuous positive airway pressure in the treatment of sleep apnea/hypopnea syndrome. *Am J Respir Crit Care Med* 1999; 159: 495–501.

11 Sleep Disorders and Society

Introduction

Sleep occupies approximately 8 h of each 24 h-cycle, but much less attention has been paid to the medical problems during this phase of life than to those that occur during wakefulness.

There are several reasons for this. Patients are often reticent about events which occur during sleep. They regard this as a personal and private time and are more reluctant to talk about sleep problems than those occuring during wakefulness. They may be unaware of the existence of a sleep disorder, such asa behavioural abnormality or obstructive sleep apnoeas, which may only be reported if the partner becomes alarmed. Sleep-related symptoms are often attributed to problems occurring in everyday life. 'Tiredness', for example, may be thought to be due to age or overwork, rather than to a sleep disorder.

In addition to this under-reporting of sleep problems, medical and other healthcare professionals are generally less aware of sleep disorders and how to assess and manage them than conditions arising during wakefulness. Medical consultations take place while the patient is awake so that direct observation of a sleep disorder by the doctor is unusual. A survey of British medical schools has shown that only a few minutes are spent on the teaching of sleep disorders during the whole of the undergraduate and postgraduate training [1]. An American survey has indicated that the mean number of questions asked in response to the complaint of insomnia is only 2.5. This probably reflects the lack of awareness of the possible causes and effects of this symptom, and how to formulate a management plan for it.

Historical and cultural influences

It is likely that the prevalence and severity of sleep disorders has fluctuated over the centuries, but there is very little quantitative data to support this assertion. As long as artificial light could only be provided by candles and fire, most members of society tended to wake up soon after dawn and go to bed soon after dusk. This pattern maximized the opportunities during day-light hours for farming, hunting and social activities. It not only minimized sleep restriction, except in Polar regions during the summer, but also tended to maintain regular sleep–wake routines. The availability of artificial light, initially with the electric light bulb, and now from a variety of other sources, has, however, extended the time for which waking activities can be performed and has distorted the influence of light on the sleep–wake cycle.

Exposure to light during the natural hours of darkness is often combined with less exposure to light during the day than previously. Modern urbanized indoor life removes many people from sunlight for most of the day, particularly in the mornings. Work, recreation and other activities, including many sports and shopping, often entail remaining indoors for prolonged periods. Atmospheric pollution, particularly in the cities, reduces the amount of sunlight that reaches the eye, and climatic conditions such as rain, cold and early onset of darkness in high latitudes increase indoor rather than outdoor activities. The intensity of light while watching television is often only 1–15 lux (1 lux equals illumination from a candle at one metre from the surface; 1 foot candle equals 10.76 lux), in dim indoor light it is around 100 lux, in most domestic areas 300–500 lux, while outdoors on a cloudy day the light intensity is around 1000 lux and on a bright day 10 000 lux.

The irregularity of the timing of activities using artificial light also disturbs the circadian sleep rhythm by constantly altering the stimuli that regulate sleep and wakefulness. Artificial light has allowed the concept of a '24-hour society' to develop. Shift work, nocturnal entertainment and other activities previously confined to the day time can now be carried out at night. Business activities involving contacts in other continents often require working at night. The increased noise level caused by these and other activities, such as driving, also hinders sleep, especially in urban societies. The development of the 24-hour society has also had an impact on other time givers for sleep, such as meals, exercise and social activities so that the endogenous circadian rhythms increasingly conflict with the often rapidly changing external factors that control them. These effects are magnified by any pre-existing insomnia, excessive daytime sleepiness (EDS) and restriction of sleep duration.

It is not only attitudes to sleep that have changed, but also attitudes to many of the factors that influence this. In westernized societies obesity is becoming increasingly frequent. There may be a direct link between obesity and EDS, but it can also cause this through inducing obstructive sleep apnoeas (OSAs). The lack of exercise during the day removes an alerting stimulus during wakefulness and one which promotes sleep at night. The availability of therapeutic and recreational drugs adds an extra dimension to sleep disorders and, while many of these chemicals have beneficial effects, their influence on sleep may be difficult to cope with.

Cultural influences also affect sleep–wake patterns and the prevalence of sleep disorders to a certain extent, partly through the mechanisms already described. In cold climates it is usual to go to sleep earlier and to wake up later than in hotter areas. In some Mediterranean countries an afternoon siesta is taken which coincides with the normal 2.00–4.00 PM phase of increased drowsiness. In these societies it is usual to stay awake until later at night and it would be expected that the difficulty in initiating sleep (DIS) type of insomnia would be less apparent in hotter climates. The advanced sleep phase syndrome (ASPS) pattern of circadian rhythm disorder would, in contrast, be more apparent in these societies than in colder climates, where an earlier time of sleep onset is normal.

Impact of sleep disorders

Sleep disorders are common. The prevalence rates of some of the major conditions have been given in the earlier chapters, and many of these have important consequences. Chronic insomnia leads to persisting tiredness and frustration due to a lack of energy. Behavioural abnormalities during sleep may cause injury either to the patient or to the partner or carer. Respiratory and other medical conditions in sleep have potentially serious complications which may reduce the life expectancy.

Excessive daytime sleepiness impacts on many areas of life. Social relationships and recreational activities suffer, and it increases the risk of errors at work, loss of productivity and accidents. The efficiency of late committee meetings is often impaired because of irritability and poor concentration of members of the group, and computer errors can be extremely costly. A study of Swedish gas meter readings showed that the greatest number of errors were made when they were read between 2.00 and 4.00 AM, and a second smaller peak was noted between 2.00 and 4.00 PM. Accidents with milling machinery have been documented to increase by 25% during night shifts compared to an early morning shift, and doctors who have been working long hours or shifts tend to operate more slowly and may be prone to errors. The extent to which this occurs depends on the personality of the individual and their ability to develop coping strategies, as well as on the degree of sleep deprivation.

Individual sleep-related accidents can have a major impact on society. In the Chernobyl nuclear plant incident, at 00.28 AM on 26 April 1986 the water circulation around the plant failed because of a stuck valve. This led to over heating of the plant, but the staff were slow to become alert to the problem and to respond appropriately because of the long shifts that they had been working. The nuclear plant was close to meltdown before the fault was corrected. The population of eastern Europe was exposed to considerable radiation and the mean lifespan of men in the Ukraine fell from 74.5 to 63.4 years over the 5 years after this incident. A similar episode occurred at 4.00 AM in the Three Mile Island nuclear plant, Pennsylvania on 28 March 1989 and the failure to act appropriately was again associated with EDS due to shift work.

Sleep-related accidents are particularly important with regard to transport. The combination of shift work, comfortable cabins or similar areas for driving or controlling the mode of transport, and the reduction in the number of staff on each shift have all contributed to the increased risk of accidents. The Exxon Valdez disaster on the 25 March 1989, in which the oil tanker hit a reef off the Alaska coast and liberated 240 000 barrels of oil, was related to the Captain being asleep and a Third Mate being left to navigate difficult waters. His long shift at night caused his tiredness which contributed to the accident in the early hours. Similarly, in the Sante Fe rail accident in 1990, all the crew were asleep at the time of the accident and $4.4 million of damages were paid. Investigation into the crash of flight US2860 at 02.38 AM on the 18 December 1977 near Salt Lake City, Utah, USA revealed that this was due to flight-crew fatigue, coupled with inadequate advice from an air traffic controller who was also sleep deprived.

The reliance on automatic controls, which makes flying more monotonous, and the possibility of jet lag and of sleep deprivation of pilots all contribute to the risk of this type of accident. Frequent brief naps may partially offset the erratic sleep schedules and sleep restriction, but it was sleep deprivation of the managers at National Aeronautics and Space Administration (NASA) that led to the error in the timing of the launch of the Challenger space shuttle that contributed to its explosion.

Legal aspects

The two most common legal problems that arise from sleep disorders are related to road traffic accidents and violence.

Road traffic accidents

The essential question is usually whether or not sleep caused or contributed to the accident. The legal situation is complex, but it is usually considered that it is an offence in law to cause damage or loss of life through falling asleep while driving. This is based on the assumption that falling asleep is under voluntary control. Awareness that this ruling leads to a finding of guilt has probably led to the number of sleep-related accidents being greatly under-reported. They may also be difficult to identify because of a head injury or death of the driver and because the driver may have little recall of the details of why the accident happened. A recollection of feeling sleepy beforehand may persist, but very often alternative possibilities of, for instance, epilepsy, a cardiac dysrhythmia or a 'blackout' are substituted for falling asleep.

It is possible to drive for several miles while partly asleep, or while having repetitive micro sleeps. This is a form of automatic behaviour with reduction of awareness for unusual events happening on the road, restriction of peripheral vision and loss of responsiveness to changes in the driving environment. This combination increases the risk of accidents (Chapter 6). The probability of sleepiness being responsible for the accident is strengthened by the observation by other drivers of changes in lane and speed prior to the accident, an appearance of staring ahead and not responding to signals such as flashing of car lights or sounding the horn, and a lack of any avoiding action when the accident is imminent. The time of day (often

2.00–6.00 AM and 2.00–4.00 PM), the lack of any other medical cause for the error in driving, and the presence of predisposing factors such as a long previous time awake, shift work or hypnotic, antidepressant or antihistamine treatment, all increase the likelihood that sleep is the cause of the accident.

Violence

The essential issue is usually whether the patient was awake and intended to injure or kill, or whether the action took place during sleep, or in a mixed sleep–wake state in which it would be reasonable to assume that the subject was not responsible for his or her actions. This distinction may be difficult to make and requires an understanding of which sleep disorders may lead to violent actions [2]. The most common are as follows.

CONFUSIONAL AROUSALS
These may be caused by, for instance, OSA, periodic limb movements in sleep (PLMS) and idiopathic central nervous system hypersomnia (ICNSH). They occur particularly during the first third of the night. The subject looks confused and disorientated and has no eye contact with the victim.

SLEEP WALKING
Violence is unusual unless the sleepwalker is restrained, which usually causes the sleepwalker to develop a confusional arousal. It is more common in children and young adults and in the first third of the night, especially if there has been sleep deprivation, ingestion of alcohol and if the subject is woken during the first NREM sleep episode. These trigger-factors may initiate a sleep walking episode, even when these do not occur regularly, but a history of childhood sleep walking or a family history of this condition is important. Those with an angry personality during the day may be particularly prone to violence during sleep walking.

NOCTURNAL EPILEPSY
The most common type is frontal lobe epilepsy which causes undeflectable stereotyped movements. Other types of epilepsy may be followed by arousal and then a post-ictal sleep.

RAPID EYE MOVEMENT SLEEP BEHAVIOUR DISORDER
This usually occurs in older males during the second half of the night. The violent actions are explicable in terms of the dream content, which is usually aggressive.

DELIRIUM
The combination of agitation and disorientation can lead to dream-enacting behaviour, including violence.

PSYCHOGENIC DISSOCIATIVE STATES
These imply severe psychopathology and there is usually no recollection of the event.

FUGUE STATES
These are often prolonged and involve complex behaviour including wandering, but there is occasionally compulsive violent behaviour.

DEMENTIA
Alzheimer's disease and other similar conditions can lead to nocturnal confusion during which the patient may attack the partner or carer.

NARCOLEPSY
Violence is rare but can occur when terrifying hallucinations or dreams are enacted due to failure of motor inhibition during REM sleep.

POST-TRAUMATIC STRESS DISORDER
The vividness of the oppressive nightmares and the terror that they are associated with can lead to acts of violence.

It may be difficult to distinguish between many of these conditions in retrospect, but the important features of violence committed during sleep or in a mixed sleep–wake state are that there is no premeditation or planning of the act and no motive. The violence is impulsive and the sleeper usually looks confused and disorientated. There is no attempt to cover up the evidence or leave the scene of the event. There is at most only a vague recall of an unpleasant event. Some memory for the violence is compatible with it occurring during a sleep disorder, such as a confusional arousal due to obstructive sleep apnoeas, rather than during wakefulness. The patient often has a blank, surprised, perplexed or horrified expression once the outcome of the violence is recognized, but is usually uncontactable during the episode.

These conditions may all lead to injury to the patient, including bruises, lacerations, fractures and dislocations due to, for instance, falling out of bed, down stairs or out of a window, or through being forcefully restrained. The actions may be only accidentally directed at the partner or carer, who may be in their way, or they may be targeted at an individual. The actions may be simple, such as punching, or more complex such as strangling and even involve driving a car, as in a confusional arousal.

The case for a sleep disorder being responsible for the violence is strengthened if there is a history of similar episodes such as sleep walking, if the time of the event is characteristic of the stage of sleep during which it is proposed that the actions took place and if specific trigger factors for the behavioural abnormality, such as alcohol consumption, were present. In contrast, it is more likely that the violence took place during wakefulness if there was a motive, any behaviour prior to the violence which suggested planning, if the subject could be communicated with during the event, and if there was eye contact and the actions appeared to be intentional.

Costs of sleep disorders to society

The impact of errors and similar problems at work and while driving, or during social activities has been emphasized [3], but additional costs of sleep-related disorders are the result of the following.

1 Development of other diseases which could have been avoided if the sleep disorder had been recognized and treated earlier. An example is the occurrence of strokes or myocardial infarctions associated with untreated obstructive sleep apnoeas.

2 Reduction in the quality of life. Excessive daytime sleepiness leads to irritability and difficulties in interpersonal relationships, which not only impair social activity, but also reduce productivity at work. Studies of OSA before and after using continuous positive airway pressure (CPAP) have shown a considerable reduction in quality of life which improves with treatment. The same has been demonstrated for those with narcolepsy before and after receiving treatment with modafinil.

3 Financial consequences of sleep related accidents. Excessive daytime sleepiness impairs efficiency at work and leads to accidents which may have considerable financial consequences. The duration of sick leave is increased in those with EDS and insomnia.

These costs could largely be avoided with better awareness of sleep disorders and availability of advice and treatment for them. The cost of providing care for sleep disorders and of education about good sleep hygiene practice has to be offset against these potential savings. Sleep laboratories are expensive, investigations such as polysomnography are costly and require trained staff.

These resources should be used in a cost-effective manner in order to provide the best value for money. The simplest effective test should be used rather than proceeding directly to polysomnography unless the additional information that this provides is required. Most drugs used to treat sleep disorders are cheap, particularly benzodiazepines and other hypnotics and antidepressants, but some drugs and equipment such as CPAP systems and light therapy are more expensive. The cost of ongoing medical or paramedical supervision of the patient also has to be balanced against the benefit that it provides.

The future

The consequences of sleep deprivation and sleep disorders are almost certainly increasing in westernized societies without a corresponding increase in the awareness by the general population of these problems. Greater public education about the needs for sleep and the main components of good sleep hygiene is required. The effects of shift work should be more widely recognized. Awareness of these issues should become an important influence on those who make decisions regarding practices at work, in educational establishments and social activities. If government policy reflected the importance of sleep problems in everyday life, better provision for, for instance, the sleepy driver would be made on motorways, which are the highest risk routes for sleep-related accidents.

It is important that doctors and other health-care workers become aware of the impact of sleep disorders and that these become a regular part of their training programme. Clear check lists or protocols might be helpful for general practitioners to assist identifying significant sleep disorders and providing treatment. The provision of specialist sleep centres should reflect the need for them by society, and within each centre a multidisciplinary approach should be developed.

There is pressure in modern society to carry out an increasing variety of activities during wakefulness and the expectations that these can be achieved tends to push sleep into the background. It can seem a semi-expendable commodity which is to be fitted around apparently more important events. This trend towards sleep deprivation and irregular sleep–wake patterns leads to EDS with impairment in concentration and memory which reduce the quality of life and the ability to fulfil the expectations of enjoying and completing the intended activities. The balance may have to swing back towards an awareness that adequate and regular hours of sleep are required to promote a state of wellbeing during wakefulness. Once aware of this, it becomes the responsibility of each individual to select his or her own combination of sleep and wakefulness by choosing between the opportunities that present themselves every day.

References

1 Stores G, Crawford C. Medical student education in sleep and its disorders. *J R Coll Phys* 1998; 32: 149–53.
2 Schenck CH, Milner DM, Hurwitz TD, Bundlie SR, Mahowald MW. A polysomnographic and clinical report on sleep-related injury in 100 adult patients. *Am J Psychiatry* 1989; 146: 1166–73.
3 Stoller MK. Economic effects of insomnia. *Clin Therapeutics* 1994; 16: 873–97.

Further Reading

1 Aldrich MS. *Sleep Medicine*. New York: Oxford University Press, 1999.

2 Chokroverty S, ed. *Sleep Disorders Medicine,* 2nd edn. Boston: Butterworth, 1999.

3 Cooper R. *Sleep*. London: Chapman and Hall Medical, 1994.

4 Culebras A. *Clinical Handbook of Sleep Disorders*. Boston: Butterworth–Heinemann, 1996.

5 Culebras A. *Sleep Disorders and Neurological Disease*. New York: Marcel Dekker, 2000.

6 Kryger MH *et al. Principles and Practice of Sleep Medicine,* 2nd edn. London: W.B. Saunders, 1994.

7 Parkes JD. *Sleep and Its Disorders*. London: W B Saunders, 1985.

8 Poceta JS, Mitler MM, eds. *Sleep Disorders, Diagnosis and Treatment*. New Jersey: Humana Press, 1998.

9 *Sleep and Breathing*. In: Saunders NA, Sullivan CE, eds. *Lung Biology in Health and Disease,* Vol 71, 2nd edn. New York: Marcel Dekker, 1994.

10 Shapiro CM, ed. *ABC of Sleep Disorder*s. London: BMJ Publishing Group, 1993.

11 Shneerson J. *Disorders of Ventilation*. Oxford: Blackwell Scientific Pubilications, 1988.

12 Stradling JR. *Handbook of Sleep-Related Breathing Disorders*. Oxford: Oxford University Press, 1993.

13 Stevens A. *Private Myths. Dreams and Dreaming*. London: Penguin Books, 1996.

14 Thorpy MJ, Yager J. *The Encyclopedia of Sleep and Sleep Disorders*. New York: Facts on File, 1991.

15 Thorpy MJ. *Handbook of Sleep Disorders*. New York: Marcel Dekker, 2000.

Index

Note: page numbers in *italic* type refer to figures; those in **bold** type refer to tables.